DENTAL BIOMATERIALS

Dental Biomaterials

By

Edward C. Combe, PhD, DSc, FADM

Professor, Minnesota Dental Research Center for Biomaterials and Biomechanics, Department of Oral Science, University of Minnesota
USA

F.J. Trevor Burke, DDS, MSc, MDS, FDS, MGDS RCS (Edin), FDS RCPS (Glas) FADM

Professor of Primary Dental Care
University of Glasgow
Scotland
UK

William H. Douglas, BDS, MSC, PhD, FADM

H.L. Anderson Endowed Professor and Director, Minnesota Dental Research Center for Biomaterials and Biomechanics, Department of Oral Science, University of Minnesota, USA
and
Honorary Professor, School of Clinical Dentistry
The Queen's University of Belfast
Northern Ireland
UK

SPRINGER SCIENCE+BUSINESS MEDIA, LLC

Combe, E. C. (Edward Charles)
Dental biomaterials / by Edward C. Combe, F.J. Trevor Burke, William H. Douglas.
P. Cm.
Includes index
ISBN 978-1-4757-4935-9 ISBN 978-1-4757-4933-5 (eBook)
DOI 10.1007/978-1-4757-4933-5
1. Dental materials. 2. Biomedical materials. I. Burke, F.J. Trevor. II. Douglas, William H., 1937- III. Title.
(DNLM: 1. Dental Materials. 2. Biocompatible Materials. WU 190 C729d 1999)
RK652.5.C65 1999
617.6'95--dc21
DNLM/DLC
for Library of Congress 99-27913
CIP

Originally published by Kluwer Academic Publishers in 1999
Softcover reprint of the hardcover 1st edition 1999

Printed on acid-free paper.

Contents

Foreword

A fundamental knowledge and understanding of dental materials is an absolute requisite to performing optimal dental care. This tenet is true not only for general dentists, but also for specialists alike. It is true not only for the developing dental student, but also for the practicing dentist. It is clearly evident that the authors of *Dental Biomaterials* have both an in-depth knowledge of dental materials and a fundamental appreciation for the importance of this information in contemporary clinical dentistry.

Owing to the broad range of expertise of the authors, this textbook distinguishes itself from most dental materials texts by its remarkable ability to address a myriad of dental materials in the context of actual clinical applications. Emphasizing the clinical significance of dental materials is an obvious and conspicuous goal of this text that pervades the entire content of its pages. In fact, to that end, the authors notably include numerous highlighted sections entitled "Dental Significance" throughout the chapters to underscore the clinical importance of the subject matter. This approach is exceptionally effective at fostering a basic understanding of dental materials for the dental student. It piques the interest without stifling the student with abstract concepts.

This text also is a valuable and reliable resource for the practicing dentist. Dentists today are inundated with new products and associated claims by manufacturers regarding the merits of their materials. Further complicating the area of dental materials are the numerous self-appointed "experts" who disseminate information through publications and lectures based largely on anecdote and opinion rather than sound science and research. Dentists are left with the difficult task of distinguishing between fact and fiction. By contrast, this text is highly objective and evidence-based. The references are all well-selected and current.

This text is amazingly broad in its scope of coverage of dental materials. It provides basic information that is easily understood on topics such as polymers, metals, and ceramics. But beyond its inclusion of fundamental dental materials information, it is very comprehensive and current. It is a text that is very up-to-date including new product categories such as flowable composites, resin-modified glass-ionomers, and compomers. It also provides a very lucid insight into the highly confusing area of dentin bonding systems. It also is very progressive in its approach, including a review of contemporary preventive materials and conservative restorative options. This text also addresses materials used in virtually every discipline including endodontics, periodontics, prosthodontics, orthodontics, and pediatric dentistry. Of particular note is the attention this text affords to esthetic restorative materials and properties. It deals with this topic with particular clarity and aplomb.

In summary, *Dental Biomaterials* is the consummate resource in contemporary dental materials for the dental student as well as the practicing dentist. Its scope of information coupled with its high degree of dental relevance make it an indispensable text for those interested in promoting clinical excellence.

Harald O. Heymann DDS, MEd
Professor and Chair
Department of Operative Dentistry
University of North Carolina at Chapel Hill

Preface

The subject of Dental Biomaterials is dynamic, with the frequent introduction of new products for use during dental treatment. Knowledge of the subject is essential to the dental practitioner, because clinical success depends on, among other things, the wise selection and utilization of materials. Yet information on new materials may be difficult to obtain and the clinician may have to assess information given in advertising material and articles. It is hoped that the information contained in this book may help in this regard.

The book has been written to serve the needs both of dental students and practitioners. To achieve this, there are a number of novel features:

- At the outset, the requirements for materials are systematically discussed, providing criteria for the critique of materials;
- The book contains a blend of scientific background and clinical application;
- The scientific background is based in both the physical and biological sciences;
- The essentials of the materials science background is given, with notes on the clinical relevance of the principles being enunciated;
- There is a discussion of the oral environment into which materials are placed, so that problems in developing materials and achieving longevity of restorations can be appreciated;
- In terms of clinical applications, there is emphasis on the need for prevention of dental disease, and this is discussed *before* materials for the restoration and replacement of teeth;
- The topic of adhesive materials – both theory and practice – is discussed;
- The increasing interest of patients and dentists in esthetic dentistry is reflected by a detailed discussion of tooth colored restorative materials, veneers and bleaching systems;
- In a number of places, particularly in relation to newer types of material, tables are given which describe the technique of use, and give the rationale for the recommended procedures. It is our belief that dental procedures are not a matter of merely following recipes, but of understanding principles;

- In some cases, detailed guidelines are given to material selection – e.g. in relation to restorative materials and luting cements;
- A number of Appendices list and classify some of the more important recent types of dental product.

It is hoped that this structure will benefit the student, who will find the theoretical and practical aspects systematically organized. It will also benefit the practitioner, who may start with the later sections of the book, and turn back to the supporting science, as required.

The authors welcome comments on this text, to facilitate the production of updated versions as required. Comments can be sent by mail or e-mail to the first author, and will be gratefully acknowledged.

E. C. Combe, MDRCBB, Department of Oral Science, University of Minnesota School of Dentistry, 16-212 Moos Tower, 515 Delaware Street S.E., Minneapolis, MN 55455.
[e-mail: combe001@tc.umn.edu]

F. J. T. Burke, University of Glasgow

W. H. Douglas, University of Minnesota

Acknowledgments

The authors are grateful to those who have provided valuable assistance in the production of this book. These include:

- Professor William Saunders and Dr Declan Millett who made comments on sections of the text;
- Dr Daranee Tantbirojn who supplied the SEM pictures in Figures 8.2, 24.1, 26.3, 27.1, 27.2, 28.5, 45.1 and 51.3; she also spent many hours checking the proofs;
- Dr Javier Martinez who supplied Figures 33.7, 47.1 and 47.2.

The advice and assistance of the staff of Kluwer Academic press is greatly appreciated.

Finally the authors acknowledge with gratitude the support and encouragement that they have received in this project from their wives and families.

I

BASIC CONCEPTS

Chapter 1

Introduction

Summary: This chapter considers definitions, applications and classifications of materials for use in dentistry.

Dental significance: Knowledge of dental biomaterials is central to success in the practice of most aspects of dentistry.

1.1 DEFINITIONS

The subject of *biomaterials* is the scientific discipline concerned with synthetic materials for use in the body. *Dental biomaterials* is that aspect of the subject which considers materials for use in the mouth, as well as those employed in dental laboratory procedures. Detailed discussion of materials with pharmacological effects is beyond the scope of the subject.

Biological materials are those which occur in the body. As will be shown, knowledge of the composition and properties of tooth tissues — namely, enamel, dentin and pulp — is relevant to an understanding of the utilization of biomaterials.

1.2 IMPORTANCE OF DENTAL BIOMATERIALS

Knowledge of dental biomaterials is essential because restorative dental treatment involves the selection and utilization of materials, and a substantial proportion of the general dental practitioner's practice is involved in the restoration of teeth. Often there is a considerable choice of materials for any given application. Choice of a dental material with inadequate properties will lead to premature failure of treatment. Likewise, it is important to be able to manipulate a material in such a way that optimum results are obtained.

Furthermore, the design of dental restorations often depends on the material of choice. Examples are:

- The design of tooth cavity preparation is influenced by the properties of the chosen filling material ;
- The design of cast partial dentures and orthodontic appliances depends on the properties of the alloy to be used.

Considerable technical advances are occurring, and new materials may be technique-sensitive. As an example, many currently available materials are capable of adhesion to tooth tissue, and these are often particularly sensitive to mishandling. It is important not only to know how to manipulate such products, but also to understand the scientific principles governing their use.

1.3 APPLICATIONS OF MATERIALS

Materials are used in dentistry for a wide variety of applications. Materials can be employed in certain circumstances to prevent decay (fissure sealants) and to reduce or eliminate the effects of trauma (mouth guards). There are also used in the realignment of teeth (orthodontic treatment) and for the improvement of esthetics (veneers and bleaching systems).

Many products are available for the direct restoration of teeth — that is — they are placed in the unset condition into tooth cavities, where they harden *in situ.* These include well-known materials like amalgam, and a number of different types of tooth colored restoratives. Also to be considered are materials for root canal treatment, as in endodontology.

Indirect restorations — inlays and crowns — are fabricated outside of the mouth from ceramics, cast alloys or resin composites, then cemented in place. Prostheses, for tooth replacement, are also prepared by a laboratory procedure, and may be fixed (e.g. bridges) or removable (e.g. dentures).

Where laboratory fabrication is carried out, a wide range of auxiliary materials is required. An impression material is used to record the form of a patient's tissues. From such an impression, a cast, model or die is prepared, from which the restoration or prosthesis is produced.

1.4 PERSPECTIVE

The order in which the applications of dental biomaterials are introduced in Section 1.3 is based on the fact that synthetic materials are not as durable as healthy tooth tissue. Thus prevention of dental disease and protection from trauma are of paramount importance. Furthermore, treatment must, as far as possible, be carried out to maintain as much healthy tooth tissue as possible. Durability of restorations is important. Each time a tooth filling is replaced, more tooth tissue may be destroyed.

1.5 CLASSIFICATION OF DENTAL BIOMATERIALS

There are three classes of materials - polymers, metals (alloys are mixtures of metals) and ceramics (Table 1.1). Examples of each are used in dentistry. Composite materials, for example polymer-ceramic mixtures, are also used. Dental biomaterials may also be classified according to clinical usage; see Table 1.2.

Table 1.1. Material types

Type of material	General description
Polymers	Large molecules with many repeating chemical groups
Metals	Usually hard and lustrous with good thermal and electrical conductivity
Ceramics	Compounds of metals and non-metals
Composites	Example: mixtures of polymers and ceramics

Table 1.2. Classification according to clinical usage

Clinical application	Examples
Intended to be permanent	Tooth restorations, dentures, implants
Provisional materials	Provisional (temporary) crown and bridge materials and temporary dressings
Short term usage (for example, up to 10 days)	Functional impression materials, tissue conditioners, guided tissue regeneration materials
In the mouth for very short time periods – e.g. up to 3 minutes	Impression materials, fluoride rinses, dentifrices
Not used in the mouth	Laboratory materials – cast, die, pattern and mold materials; abrasives

Chapter 2

Requirements of Materials for Oral Use

Summary: A perspective is given on the stringent requirements of materials for oral use.

Dental significance: Guidelines are given for critiquing any dental material. These principles are used consistently throughout the book.

2.1 INTRODUCTION

There are stringent requirements for materials designed to be placed in the human body, including the mouth. In addition to the usual considerations of strength and other mechanical properties, one has to take into account the biological environment of the material. A number of general questions must be asked:

- What effect will a material have on the oral environment?
- What is the nature of the interface between the biomaterial and human tissue?
- What is the effect of the oral environment on the biomaterial? This is the converse of the first question. Will there be chemical breakdown? Will the material fracture or wear?
- What other physical properties are important - for example, thermal and optical properties?
- Are esthetic considerations important?
- Is the material easy and convenient to use, or is it very technique-sensitive? For example, rheological or flow properties are of importance for materials at all stages of handling - for materials as supplied, as mixed, and during and after setting;
- Is the material cost effective? That is, does a high cost material provide enhanced clinical performance over a low cost material?

2.2 REQUIREMENTS

From the preceding general questions we can formulate a general list of desirable properties, the use of which enables a systematic assessment to be given of any dental biomaterial. This assists in the selection of materials, and also gives an awareness of the limitations and merits of a chosen material.

2.2.1 Biocompatibility

In general terms, a material should have no harmful effects on the mouth or the body. There is a wide range of potential problems that can occur. For example, a material may be irritant, toxic, allergenic, teratogenic, mutagenic or carcinogenic. One example of a material of questionable biocompatibility is the metal nickel, which is allergenic.

In addition it would be useful if materials could confer some benefit to the dental tissues. One example of this is fluoride-containing dental cements; they can leach fluoride into the surrounding tooth tissue, which may inhibit dental caries.

2.2.2 Interfacial properties

The behavior of the interface between a material and the oral tissues is important. Not only does this relate to biocompatibility as above, but also to factors such as adhesion and marginal microleakage of dental restorative materials. Adhesion of restorations (prepared both by direct and indirect techniques) to tooth enamel and dentin is considered to be important. One advantage of achieving this is that there is less likelihood of marginal microleakage of bacteria and toxins at the interface between restoration and tooth tissue. Another benefit is the potential for minimal cavity preparations, as compared to 'traditional' cavity designs for non-adhesive materials which often require substantial preparation of sound tooth tissue to provide retention and resistance form for the restoration.

2.2.3 Chemical properties

One aspect of the effect of the oral environment on materials relates to chemical properties. What effect will saliva and dietary constituents have on a material? Absorption of fluids or dissolution may occur. Metallic materials may be subject to corrosion, leading to loss of mechanical integrity and to the release of corrosion products which may not be biocompatible.

2.2.4 Mechanical and other physical properties

Another effect of the oral environment on a material relates to the possibility of physical breakdown of the material. Mechanical properties relate to matters such as hardness, rigidity and strength. Also, surface properties such as abrasion resistance and wear must be taken into account.

Other physical properties of relevance include thermal and optical properties.

2.2.5 Esthetic considerations

Esthetic properties are important, given the considerable demand for restorations that resemble the appearance of natural teeth, and for treatments such as veneering and tooth bleaching. Dentures should also mimic the appearance of the oral tissues.

2.2.6 Practical questions

Issues of practicability need to be taken into account. Will a material be readily available and easy and economical to use? Will it be stable on storage over a period of time? Will it have the right viscosity when mixed? Will its setting time be sufficient to allow placement of the material? Additionally, environmental considerations must be considered - will disposal of excess material cause environmental difficulties and will production of the material be environmentally friendly?

2.3 SUMMARY

The above six principles: biocompatibility, interfacial properties, chemical properties, mechanical and other physical properties, esthetic properties, and practicability are applied, where relevant, as criteria in the assessment of each type of clinically used material in subsequent chapters of this book.

II

PROPERTIES OF MATERIALS

Chapter 3

Biological Properties

Summary: A review of the methods of assessing biocompatibility is given, followed by some examples of potential hazards of materials.

Dental significance: Biocompatibility is of paramount importance. All materials to be used in the mouth must show an appropriate host response.

3.1 INTRODUCTION

The *biocompatibility* of a material relates to its compatibility with tissues and body fluids. This has often been regarded as complete inertness in the body. According to this principle, the ideal material would be:

- Non-toxic;
- Non-irritant to the oral or other tissues;
- Non-allergenic;
- Non-teratogenic (not causing developmental malformations);
- Non-mutagenic;
- Non-carcinogenic.

In practice, however, no material is totally inert in a biological environment. Thus an appropriate host response, which may be a complex series of events, is important. Furthermore, a material may degrade *in situ*, so biocompatibility of its degradation products also needs to be noted.

The importance of biocompatibility is seen by the fact that there is now legislation covering dental biomaterials. In the USA this is the Medical Device Bill passed by Congress in 1976. Similar legislation has been passed in Europe.

3.2 BIOLOGICAL EVALUATION

A wide range of biocompatibility testing methods is available, and these are detailed in an American (ANSI/ADA Document 41 - 1982) and an International Standard Specification (ISO 7405:1997). A number of questions need to be asked in selecting appropriate methodology. For example, what is the application of the material and with what tissues will it come into contact? For how long will there be contact?

3.3 REQUIREMENTS OF THE AMERICAN STANDARD

3.3.1 Classification of materials

Materials are classified according to usage, into six types, as outlined in Table 3.1.

Table 3.1. Classification of materials (according to ANSI/ADA Document 41 - 1982)

Type	Examples of applications
I	Tooth restorative materials, including: metallic and non-metallic filling materials, cavity liners and bases, cements, pit and fissure sealants, reagents for the treatment of enamel and dentin and coatings for restorations
II	Prosthetic materials, including: impression materials, waxes, baseplates, metallic and polymeric denture materials, artificial teeth, veneer materials
III	Endodontic materials, including: pulp capping, pulpotomy and root filling materials
IV	Periodontal materials
V	Orthodontic materials – both metallic and polymeric
VI	Laboratory materials – not coming into contact with the oral cavity

3.3.2 Biocompatibility tests

Biocompatibility tests are classified into three groups - initial tests, secondary tests and usage tests.

1. Initial tests include:
- Cytotoxicity testing, using HeLa cells to classify materials as non-toxic, slightly toxic, toxic or severely toxic;
- Hemolysis testing, using rabbit blood;
- Mutagenicity testing, using Ames' test or Styles' cell transformation test;

- Acute systemic toxicity measured by the oral and intraperitoneal LD_{50} tests in rats;
- Acute inhalation test in rats.

2. Secondary tests include:

- Mucous membrane irritation test, using hamsters' pouches;
- Dermal toxicity, assessed using rabbits;
- Tissue reaction following subcutaneous implantation in guinea pigs;
- Implantation in bone of guinea pigs;
- Sensitization tests in guinea pigs.

3. Usage tests are carried out in subhuman primates, for dental restorative materials, for pulp capping materials and for endodontic materials.

3.3.3 Selection of tests

Many types of tests in ANSI/ADA Document No. 41 have been listed, but they are not all applied to all materials. A table is supplied in the document, indicating which tests are appropriate for each class of material. The document includes no assessment of carcinogenicity, and a foreword to the document suggests that such testing be only required if positive results are obtained from the mutagenicity testing.

3.4 REQUIREMENTS OF THE INTERNATIONAL STANDARD

3.4.1 Classification of materials

ISO 7405:1997 considers dental biomaterials to be included under the general category of 'medical device.' A classification into four groups may be made, according to the nature of contact with tissue:

- Non-contact devices are excluded from biocompatibility testing – this group includes many materials used in the dental laboratory;
- Surface contacting devices which come into contact with the surface of the oral tissues; examples include fissure sealants and dentures;
- External communicating devices that penetrate and are in contact with the oral tissues and are exposed to the oral environment – for example, tooth restorations;
- Implant devices that are not exposed to the oral environment.

The international standard specification also considers the duration of contact of the device with the oral tissues, namely less than 24 hours, between 24 hours and 30 days and greater than 30 days.

3.4.2 Biocompatibility tests

ISO 7405:1997 classifies biocompatibility tests into three groups. Group I tests relate to the *in vitro* assessment of cytotoxicity. Group II includes a wide range of techniques for acute and subchronic systemic toxicity, skin irritation, sensitization, genotoxicity and local effects after implantation. Group III tests are specific usage tests. These include tests for biocompatibility of materials with dentin and pulp, and pulp capping and endodontic materials.

3.4.3 Selection of tests

As with the American Standard, not all tests are applied to all materials, and it is recognized that alternative methods for evaluation may on occasion be used.

3.5 EXAMPLES OF HAZARDS

In later chapters of this book details are given of many clinically used materials. In presenting an evaluation of each material, its biocompatibility is assessed. Some of the main areas of current concern in this regard are considered to be:

- The potential estrogenic activity of the chemical bisphenol-A, from which resins for pit and fissure sealants (Chapter 19) and resin composites (Chapter 27) are prepared – see Appendix V;
- The toxicity of fluorides (Chapter 20);
- Mercury in dental amalgam (Chapter 24);
- Nickel is allergenic (Chapters 35 and 36);
- Nickel alloys may contain beryllium, which produces toxic dust during finishing and polishing procedures (Chapters 35 and 36);
- Residual monomer in poly(methyl methacrylate) may present problems (Chapter 45);
- Investment materials contain silica, which, if inhaled, can cause silicosis (Chapter 53).

FURTHER READING

Williams D F (1990). Biocompatibility: an overview. *Concise Encyclopedia of Medical & Dental Materials* (editor: Williams D F). Pergamon Press, Oxford, pp 51-59.

Langeland K (1990). Biocompatibility of dental materials. *Concise Encyclopedia of Medical & Dental Materials* (editor: Williams D F). Pergamon Press, Oxford, pp 59-69.

Chapter 4

Mechanical Properties

Summary: A discussion of properties of materials such as strength, rigidity, hardness, etc.

Dental significance: Knowledge of mechanical properties is important in the design of tooth restorations and prostheses. Also, mechanical testing can give some indication of potential clinical indications and contra-indications of materials. It is important however, to realize that *in vitro* testing cannot adequately predict *in vivo* behavior.

4.1 INTRODUCTION

In this chapter we consider *mechanical properties,* which deal with the behavior of materials under applied forces. They are of considerable importance in dentistry since tooth restorations, prostheses and appliances are subjected to forces in the mouth, as detailed in Chapter 9.

Fundamental properties of materials can be obtained by determining the relationship between *stress* and *strain,* as defined in Sections 4.2 and 4.3. These properties are determined by applying a steadily increasing load to a material, and plotting stress *versus* strain. They can give useful information in the selection and application of biomaterials, and are described and defined in Section 4.4.

Other mechanical properties can be determined under conditions that attempt to simulate the service conditions of a material. For example:

- How will a material behave under conditions of sudden loading (Sections 4.5 and 4.6)? For example, will a denture fracture if it is dropped on a hard surface, or if the wearer is in an automobile accident?
- How will a material behave if given repeated small loads (Section 4.7)?

In addition to considering the properties of the bulk of the material, as above, surface characteristics are also of significance:

- What is the surface hardness (Section 4.8)?

– How well will the surface of a biomaterial resist abrasion? Or will it abrade tooth substance with which it comes into contact (Section 4.9)?

Also of relevance is the fact that solids (such as tooth fillings and denture materials) may show undesirable time-dependent deformation (Sections 4.10, 5.6 and 5.7).

It must be emphasized that although mechanical properties are important, the link with clinical behavior is complex and difficult to predict.

Table 4.1 gives a classification of the various properties, distinguishing between properties of the bulk of the material and surface properties. SI units are used, where the standard units are: mass - kilogram (kg); length - meter (m); time - second (s). Appendix I gives some conversion factors for units.

Table 4.1. Classification of mechanical properties

Type of property	Method of testing	Data obtained
Bulk properties	Steadily increasing load	Stress-strain curve 1. Points on the curve - Proportional limit - Elastic limit - Yield point - Proof stress - Compressive strength - Ultimate tensile strength (UTS) 2. Gradient of the straight line portion of the curve - Modulus of elasticity (Young's modulus) 3. Areas under the curve (measures of energy) - Modulus of resilience - Toughness
Bulk properties	Application of a sudden load	Impact strength Fracture toughness
Bulk properties	Repeated low loads	Fatigue Endurance limit
Bulk properties	Time-dependent (viscoelastic) properties	Creep Stress relaxation
Surface properties	Hardness – resistance to indentation	Hardness numbers
Surface properties	Resistance to abrasion	Volume or weight loss of material

4.2 STRAIN

When an external force or load is applied to a material the phenomenon of *strain* occurs. This is a change in dimension of the material, usually measured by its change in length (either an increase or decrease, depending on whether the material is in tension or compression, Figure 4.1) per unit length. Thus strain is equal to e/L, where e is the change in length and L is the original length. Strain may also be expressed as a percentage of the original length, that is 100 e/L. Strain may be either elastic or plastic. If the material returns to its original length after removal of its load, its deformation has been *elastic*. If there is a permanent change in shape this is *plastic deformation*.

It is important to realize that all materials (including tooth substance) exhibit deformational strain under load.

4.3 STRESS

Associated with strain is the phenomenon of *stress* - this is an internal force/unit area in a material, equal and opposite to the applied load or force/unit area. Stress is measured in units of force per unit area. In SI units, the unit of force is the Newton (1 N = the force required to give a body of mass 1 kg an acceleration of 1m/s^2). The stress $S = F/A$, where F is the load or force applied, and A is the cross-sectional area of the material over which the load is applied, and is expressed in N/m^2. 1 N/m^2 is equal to 1 Pascal (Pa).

A material may be stressed in compression, tension, torsion, shear or flexure (Figure 4.1). In practice, the stresses within a material are complex. Thus if a beam is bent as shown in Figure 4.2 (3-point loading, as used in measuring transverse strength), the lower portion of the beam is in tension, and the top is in compression. Shear stresses may also be present in this case, particularly in thick beams.

In materials with cracks, notches, grooves, inclusions, surface scratches, or marked changes in contour due to design, *stress concentration* can occur. This is clearly to be avoided as far as possible in the construction of dental appliances, as it can lead to failure of the material. For example an upper denture with a deep frenal notch is liable to show midline fracture.

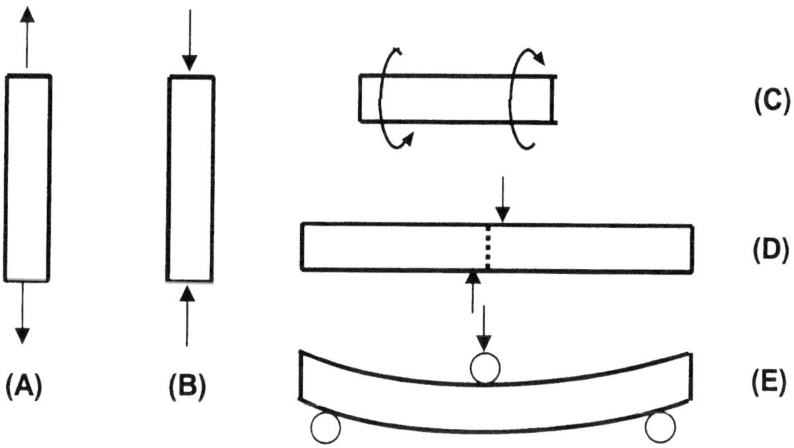

Figure 4.1. Types of stress: (A) tension, (B) compression, (C) torsion, (D) shear, (E) flexure.

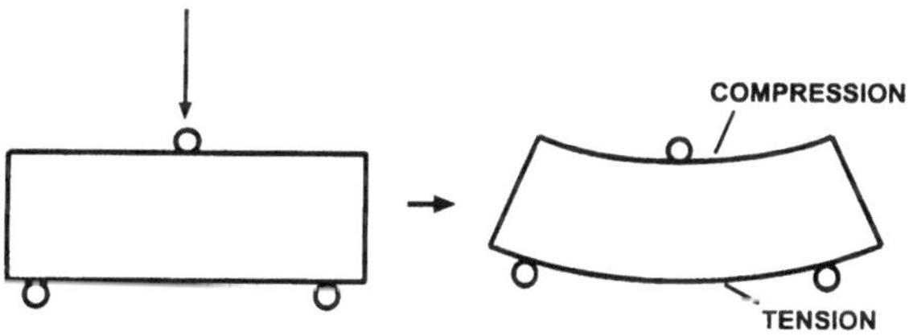

Figure 4.2. Three-point loading of a beam.

4.4 TENSILE AND COMPRESSIVE PROPERTIES

4.4.1 Stress-strain relationship

If stress is plotted against strain for a material in tension or compression, a graph such as Figure 4.3 can result. Figure 4.4 shows typical graphs for a ductile metal, a brittle ceramic and a polymer. From such data many useful properties can be determined, as detailed below.

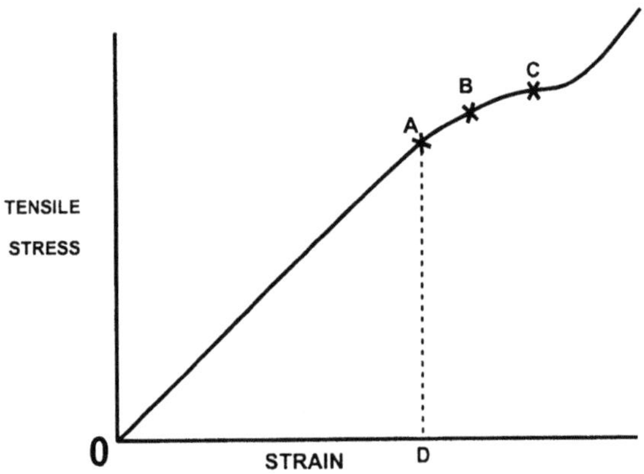

Figure 4.3. Tensile stress-strain diagram. A is the proportional limit, B is the elastic limit, C is the yield point.

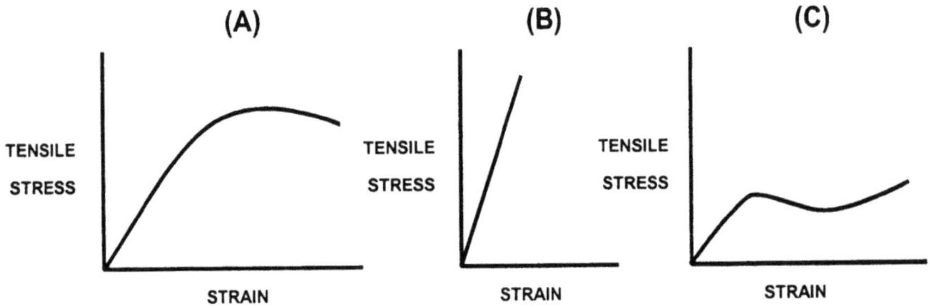

Figure 4.4. Typical tensile stress-strain diagram for (A) a ductile metal, (B) a brittle ceramic and (C) a polymer.

4.4.2 The rigidity of a material; modulus of elasticity

Dental Significance: The modulus of elasticity is a measure of the stiffness or rigidity of a material. This is important in designing partial dentures (Chapter 47) and orthodontic appliances (Chapter 41). Also, in the ideal situation, a filling material should have the degree of rigidity of tooth substance with which it comes in contact.

From Figure 4.3, it can be seen that between points O and A, stress is proportional to strain — this is an example where *Hooke's law* is obeyed. The slope of this linear portion is a measure of the rigidity of the material and is termed the *modulus of elasticity*. For example, portions of the stress-strain graphs of two materials are in Figure 4.5. Material A has a modulus of elasticity of 200 GPa and for material B the modulus is 100 GPa. For a stress of 200 MPa, A is strained by 0.1%, and B by 0.2%. Material A, with a higher modulus is more rigid; material B is more flexible. The tensile modulus is often called *Young's modulus*, and is usually given the symbol *E*. The other corresponding moduli are the shear modulus (*G*) and the bulk modulus (*k*).

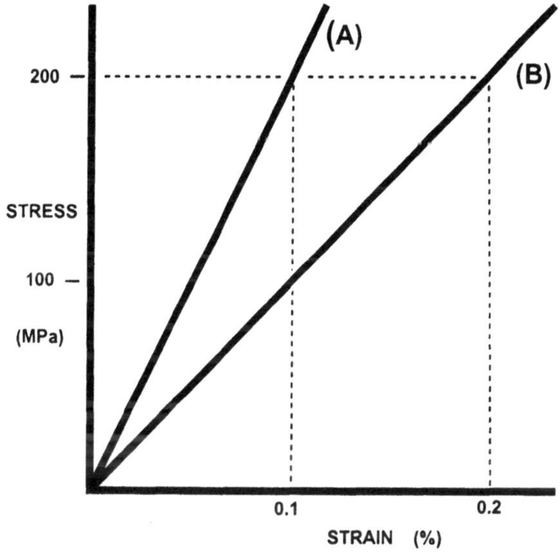

Figure 4.5. Portions of the stress-strain graphs of two materials below the proportional limit.

4.4.3 Proportional limit

Dental significance: It is important to know at what stress level a dental restoration or prosthesis will permanently deform, since this is obviously undesirable.

In Figure 4.3 the proportional limit is represented by point A - the maximum stress at which stress is proportional to strain. Ceramic materials often break in the linear region of the graph (Figure 4.4B).

4.4.4 Elastic limit

Quite commonly, a material may be stressed above its proportional limit, yet behave elastically - that is, on removal of the load, the specimen returns to its original length. The *elastic limit* is the maximum stress that a material can endure without undergoing permanent deformation; it is represented by point B in Figure 4.3.

4.4.5 Yield point

A material reaches a *yield point* (C in Figure 4.3) when there is a rapid increase in strain without a corresponding increase in stress; the deformation is now completely plastic. In some instances there is a drop in stress (e.g. Figure 4.4A). This decrease in stress can be accounted for by the contraction in cross-section (termed *necking*) which accompanies the elongation of the specimen, consequent on the material not changing in volume when it deforms plastically.

For practical purposes there is little significant difference between proportional limit, elastic limit and yield point.

4.4.6 Proof stress

In practice it is very difficult to determine the proportional limit and yield point. Often, the data obtained depend on the accuracy and sensitivity of the testing machine. To overcome this, values of *proof stress* are often quoted, particularly in the tensile testing of metals. For example, the 0.1% proof stress is the stress corresponding to a 0.1% permanent (or plastic) strain (Figure 4.6). A construction line is drawn from the 0.1% strain on the horizontal axis, parallel to the straight-line portion of the stress-strain curve. The 0.1% proof stress is at the point of intersection of this line with the stress-strain graph.

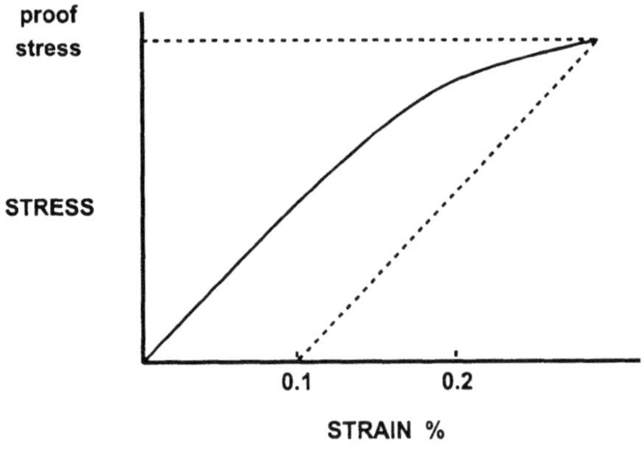

Figure 4.6. 0.1% proof stress.

4.4.7 Ductility and malleability

Dental significance: A cast prosthesis - for example a partial denture clasp - with little ductility (low percentage elongation) may be so brittle that it will fracture easily if an adjustment is made to it – see Chapter 47.

Many metals can be drawn out into the form of a wire - this property is termed *ductility. Malleability* is closely associated with ductility - it is the ability of a metallic material to be deformed to make thin sheets, without breaking or cracking. For example, gold can be rolled and beaten into sheets that are so thin that they can transmit light - it is thus a highly malleable metal.

These properties can be measured by *percentage elongation.* After a metal specimen of known length has been fractured in a tensile test, the broken fragments are pieced together and the new length measured. A high percentage increase in length indicates a very ductile material and a low figure indicates brittleness. Another method is to measure reduction in area of cross-section. The greater the malleability, the bigger is the reduction in cross-sectional area.

4.4.8 Poisson's ratio

Associated with the increase in length of material under tension (axial strain) there is also a decrease in cross sectional area (lateral or transverse strain). *Poisson's ratio* is defined as the ratio of the lateral to the axial strain during elastic deformation. This parameter is important in computer simulations of material behavior using a technique called finite element analysis.

4.4.9 Compressive and tensile strength

Compressive and tensile strength is maximum stress that a material can undergo in compression or tension without fracture. The tensile strength is sometimes written as the UTS, or *ultimate tensile strength.* It is often measured by direct application of a tensile load to a specimen. In order to ensure good gripping of the specimen, its ends are often enlarged in relation to its central portion. Materials with little ductility (brittle materials) are liable to fracture at the gripped ends of the specimen.

An alternative method of measuring the tensile strength of brittle materials is to use the diametral compression test. A cylinder or disk of the material is compressed diametrically. A tensile stress is set up at right angles to the direction of the applied load (Fig. 4.7). The tensile strength is calculated from the formula:

$$TS = 2P/\pi td$$

where P is the load to fracture the material and t and d are the thickness and diameter of the specimen. The material must be Hookean up to fracture for this formula to be valid.

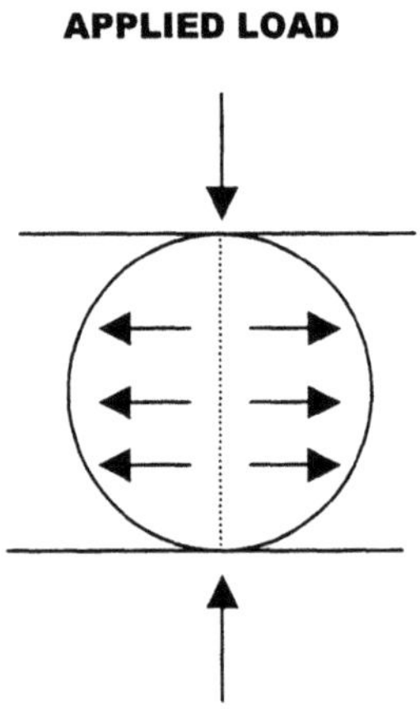

Figure 4.7. Diametral compression test - a tensile stress is set up at right angles to the direction of the applied load.

Compressive and tensile strength tests are easy to perform. However, they are poor predictors of clinical performance and are mostly used as quality control tests in regulatory standards and industrial dental materials.

4.4.10 Resilience and toughness

The *modulus of resilience* is the maximum amount of energy a material can absorb without undergoing permanent deformation. It is measured by the area of the triangle OAD in Figure 4.3, and can be expressed by the formula:

$$R = P^2/2E,$$

where P is the proportional limit and E the modulus of elasticity. R is expressed in terms of energy per unit volume, e.g. J/m^3.

The *toughness* of a material is its ability to absorb energy without fracture. The total area under a stress-strain graph measures it. This can also be expressed in the units J/m^3.

4.5 IMPACT STRENGTH

In the previous section we have been considering the effects of applying a gradual increase in load to a material until fracture occurred. In practice, it is also desirable to know the effects of the application of a sudden force to a material because under these conditions materials are often more brittle.

This can be measured by making a specimen of known dimensions, clamping it firmly in position and breaking it with a swinging pendulum. The resulting reduction in amplitude of swing of the pendulum is measured. From this the energy to break a material can be calculated.

Two types of impact tester are available. In the Charpy tester the specimen is supported horizontally at the ends, and in an Izod instrument the material is clamped at one end and held vertically.

A problem of impact testing is that inconsistent results can be obtained, because specimens break in different places. In order to ensure more consistent results, specimens are notched. The material fractures at the notch, since this is its weakest part (Figure 4.8). A notch also makes the material more brittle hence this is a severe test of the toughness of a material. Impact strength varies markedly with the angle of the notch.

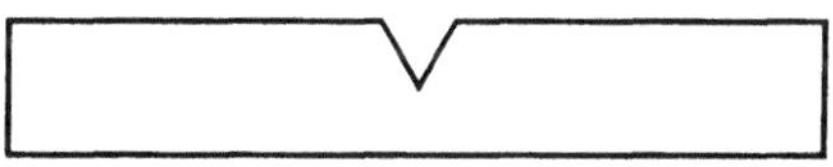

Figure 4.8. Notched specimen for impact testing.

4.6 FRACTURE TOUGHNESS

Fracture toughness determines the resistance of a material or tooth substance to the propagation of a crack. Enamel is easily prone to fracture. Large restorations without cuspal coverage may weaken teeth sufficiently to cause cusp fracture.

The fracture toughness test measures the resistance to propagation of a crack in a specimen in which the crack has already been initiated. Many different forms of specimen are possible. However one common measurement of fracture toughness is called the *critical stress intensity factor* (K_{Ic}). When the K_{Ic} value is exceeded at the crack tip the material will then fracture spontaneously leading to complete failure. Below the K_{Ic} value the crack can still grow slowly. Because the K_{Ic} value is measured as a stress intensity and not just as a stress, its units are $MN/m^{1.5}$.

The fracture toughness test is very efficient and other parameters can also be derived from it including modulus of elasticity and the plasticity of the material. Fracture toughness is closely related to fatigue, as discussed below.

4.7 FATIGUE STRENGTH

Fracture toughness measures the failure of a material after one continuous application of a load. In contrast, in *fatigue strength* experiments the crack in the material is propagated by a repeated application of a small cyclic load. This is the situation in clinical practice when the occlusal surface of the tooth is subjected to a repeated biting or chewing force. Typically this load will be in the elastic region of the stress-strain curve, when the test is referred to as *high cycle fatigue.*

It is tested in the laboratory by giving many bending or twisting movements to a specimen, and counting the number of cycles (N) a material can withstand at a known stress (S). A graph of S versus log N is plotted, as in Figure 4.9. From the graph the *endurance limit* can be found; stresses below this limit will not cause fatigue fracture. N may be as high as 10^7 cycles, so this type of test is clearly a service longevity test. This test is useful, but it is difficult to perform, because of a long time commitment.

A very important point of both the fracture toughness and fatigue tests is that materials may fail catastrophically well below the limits of fracture described by both tensile and compressive strength tests. Thus these latter tests are poor predictors of clinical experience.

A variant of this test is the *low cycle fatigue test,* in which the load exceeds the elastic limit so that a small amount of plastic deformation is involved. This brings on failure much more quickly, with N being between 5×10^3 and 100×10^3. This test is more convenient than high cycle fatigue, but may be less realistic.

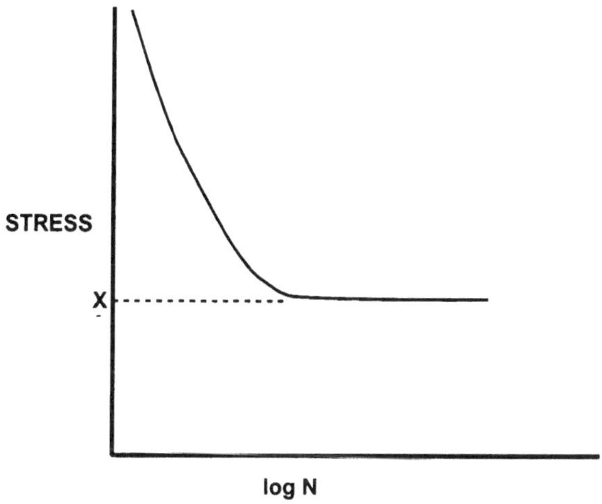

Figure 4.9. *S-N* curve for a material, where *S* is the stress and *N* the number of cycles. X is the endurance limit (observed mainly for ferrous alloys; the *S-N* curves does not necessarily have a horizontal portion).

4.8 HARDNESS

Hardness is the ability of a material to withstand indentation. An indenter of known dimensions is pressed into a material under a known load for a measured length of time. The hardness is calculated either from the depth or area of indentation. A small indentation indicates a hard material, and *vice versa*. Several types of tester are available (Table 4.2 and Figure 4.10). With metals, the indentation is permanent, and the hardness number is related to the yield stress in compression. However, some problems are encountered with the use of steel ball indenters. They may shatter a brittle material; they may be deformed by a hard material, and may cause elastic deformation rather than indentation.

Hardness is a convenient and easy test to perform. More than other tests it has spatial resolution. This means that properties can be determined at a point as opposed to integrating over the whole sample size as in most other tests. Spatial resolution is important in measuring properties of hard tissues because the properties change significantly at different anatomical locations.

Table 4.2. Hardness testers

Test	Indenter	Measurement	Results expressed as:
Brinell	Steel ball	Area of indentation	Brinell Hardness Number (BHN)
Knoop	Diamond	Area of indentation	Knoop hardness Number (KHN)
Rockwell	Steel ball or diamond point	Depth of indentation	Rockwell*
Vickers	Diamond	Area of indentation	Vickers Hardness Number (VHN)

*Rockwell hardness is expressed as a letter and a number, e.g. M95. The letter indicates the condition of testing, such as the load in the indenter, and the number indicates the hardness. For other test methods only a number is quoted.

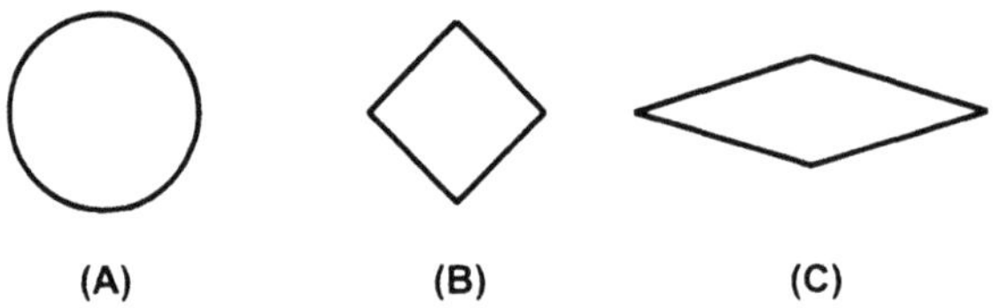

Figure 4.10. Shapes of indentations produced by hardness testers: (A) Brinell (B) Vickers (C) Knoop.

4.9 ABRASION RESISTANCE

Abrasion or *wear* refers to the loss of anatomic form from the surface of the restoration or tooth. It may be measured as a volume loss or a depth loss. The appropriate wear test requires an antagonist (often a tooth) which slides against the test material. With fixed conditions, such as the load and the distance of the slide, comparative wear numbers can be achieved. Most wear machines in dentistry are empirical. This means that the force, slide and geometric arrangement are arbitrary. These values are then fixed to produce a predetermined amount of wear which is used for comparative purposes. There is usually very little effort to reproduce the occlusal relationships between the treatment sample and the antagonist. However, it is possible to improve relevance of dental wear testing by resynthesizing biomechanical conditions in the dental laboratory (Section 9.5).

In clinical terms, wear due to tooth to tooth contact is often called *attrition*. Wear due to a third body such as a toothbrush is referred to as *abrasion*. Loss of contour due to chemical dissolution, from drinks of low pH or gastric reflux, is called *erosion*.

Mechanisms of loss of tooth substance such as attrition, abrasion, erosion and abfraction are defined and described in Chapter 10.

4.10 TIME-DEPENDENT PROPERTIES (VISCOELASTICITY)

In some materials, particularly polymers, application or removal of a load produces a deformation, the magnitude of which is time-dependent. The apparent modulus of elasticity will depend on the time at which the strain is measured. The elastic modulus measured after a short time is relatively high compared with the modulus at infinite time, owing to the relaxation, which can occur over a period of time. This phenomenon is termed *viscoelasticity*, because of the similarity of the behavior of such a solid to a viscous fluid, and is considered further in Sections 5.6 and 5.7.

Time dependency in properties reveals itself in the phenomenon of hysteresis. An example would be the application of the occlusal load to enamel cusp of an amalgam filling. The cusp will deflect outwards at the rate of application of the force. But when the force is removed the cusp will recover much more slowly. Thus the outward and returning curves are different, which is called *hysteresis*.

Time dependent properties are used biologically to modify occlusal forces that may be otherwise unhealthy for the supporting tissues. The most time dependent of the dental tissues is the periodontal ligament. Dentin is less time dependent. Enamel, which is almost perfectly elastic, with only a very small viscous component, is the least time dependent biological material in terms of its properties.

FURTHER READING

Horath, L (1995). *Fundamentals of Materials Science for Technologists*. Prentice Hall, Englewood Cliffs, New Jersey, pp 255-274.

Chapter 5

Rheological Properties

Summary: A study of the flow and deformation properties of matter.

Dental significance: The ability of clinical material to flow and adapt to a required shape is important. For example, direct filling materials must be able to flow to adapt to the shape of a tooth cavity, and impression materials must flow to record the shape of the oral tissues. The deformation of solids (for example, tooth fillings and dentures) is also important.

5.1 INTRODUCTION

The science of the study of flow and deformation of matter is termed *rheology*. This is of importance in dental biomaterials in many practical situations. Often materials are mixed to form fluid pastes that then undergo a setting reaction. For example, impression materials are applied to the mouth in a fluid state, and it is important to know how well the material will flow to record all the necessary detail of the oral tissues. Likewise, many tooth-filling materials are applied to the tooth as pastes that set *in situ*. It is essential that the material will be able to flow to be readily adapted to the shape of the tooth cavity. It is also important to know the change of viscosity with time. Analysis of such changes enables working time and setting time to be determined. The *working time* is the period during which the material can be manipulated, ideally with no thickening occurring (Figure 5.1). The *setting time* is the time when the material has reached a given degree of rigidity.

Flow and deformation of solids is also important. In Chapter 4 the deformation of solids is presented as being either plastic or elastic. In practice, some solids are *viscoelastic*. Such materials combine both viscous flow and elasticity, and their properties are time-dependent.

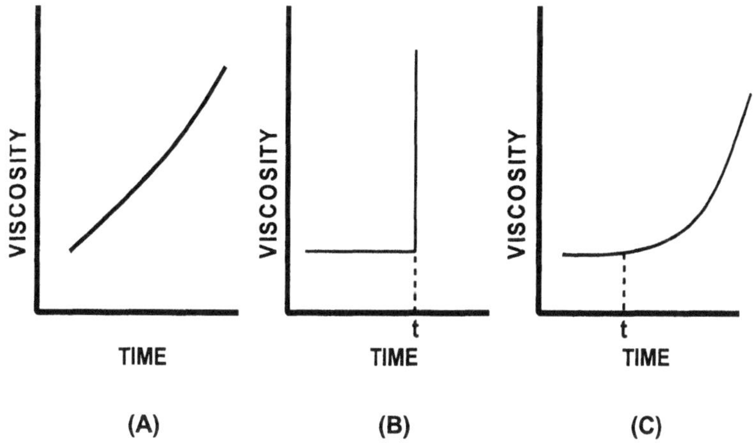

Figure 5.1. Change in viscosity with time for setting materials.
(A) poor rheological characteristics; no well defined working time.
(B) ideal properties – a well defined working time *t* followed by sudden setting.
(C) good properties; a working time *t* followed by gradual setting.

5.2 VISCOSITY: NEWTONIAN BEHAVIOR

The *viscosity* of a fluid is its resistance to flow. Consider a liquid as consisting of many parallel layers, or laminae, of material (Figure 5.2). A tangential force F is applied to the upper layer, of area A, in a plane perpendicular to that of the flow, so that it moves with velocity v. The layer in contact with the retaining surface is assumed to have zero velocity (stationary plane). Throughout the material there is a velocity gradient, that is, the velocity changes from one layer to another. The slope of the velocity-distance curve is the velocity gradient or shear rate, D, of the material, where $D = dv/dx$, and x is the distance from the retaining surface. D is expressed in units of velocity/distance (e.g., s^{-1}). The shear stress, τ is the force per unit area = F/A.

According to Newton's Law τ and D are proportional to each other, and the constant of proportionality is equal to the *coefficient of viscosity*, thus:

$$\tau/D = \text{constant} = \eta \text{ (coefficient of viscosity)}$$

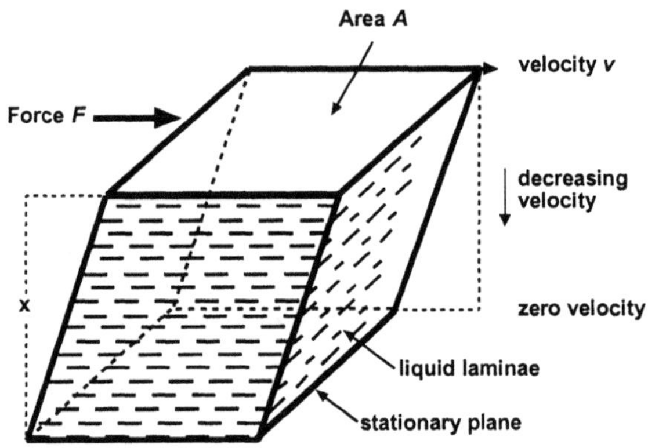

Figure 5.2. Laminae of liquid.

When τ is in dynes/cm^2 and D in s^{-1}, η will have units dyne.sec/cm^2. 1 dyne.sec/cm^2 = 1 poise. Viscosity is often expressed in centipoise, where 100 centipoise = 1 poise. In SI units, 1 Pa.s = 1 Nsm^{-2} = 10 poise.

The viscosity of a fluid depends on a number of factors, including:

- The nature of the substance;
- Temperature — the viscosity decreases with increasing temperature;
- Pressure — at very high pressures viscosity is greater;
- Shear history — for example, the structure of some materials is broken down on shearing.

Fewer than 10% of all liquids are Newtonian — that is, they do not obey Newton's Law. Thus τ/D is not a constant but varies with D. In these instances τ/D is termed the *apparent viscosity*.

5.3 NON-NEWTONIAN FLOW

For Newtonian behavior, a plot of shear stress versus shear rate is a straight line through the origin (Figure 5.3A). Non-Newtonian fluids are of the following types:

1. *Bingham flow* occurs when the shear stress - shear rate plot is linear, but has an intercept on the shear stress axis (Figure 5.3B). This is termed the *yield stress*: below this stress the material will not flow. Examples include clay suspensions in water, and some composite filling material pastes.

2. Some fluids that show a yield stress also show a curvature in their D-τ curves - this is *plastic flow* (Figure 5.3C).
3. Some materials have a non-linear relationship between D and τ, but show no yield stress. These are termed *pseudoplastic* or *dilatant* (Figure 5.3D and E). For pseudoplastic materials the apparent viscosity decreases with increasing shear rate (shear thinning) and shear thickening occurs for dilatant materials (Figure 5.4). Examples include many polymers, natural resins, blood, saliva, impression materials, fluoride gels and viscous oils which are pseudoplastic; wet sand with low water content is dilatant.

> **Dental significance**: Dental elastomeric impression pastes are often pseudoplastic – that is – their apparent viscosity is less at higher flow rates.

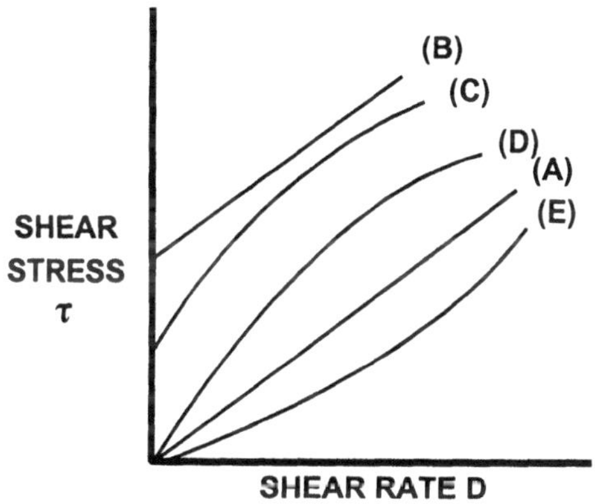

Figure 5.3. Types of flow behavior: (A) Newtonian flow; (B) Bingham flow; (C) plastic flow; (D) pseudoplastic flow; (E) dilatant flow.

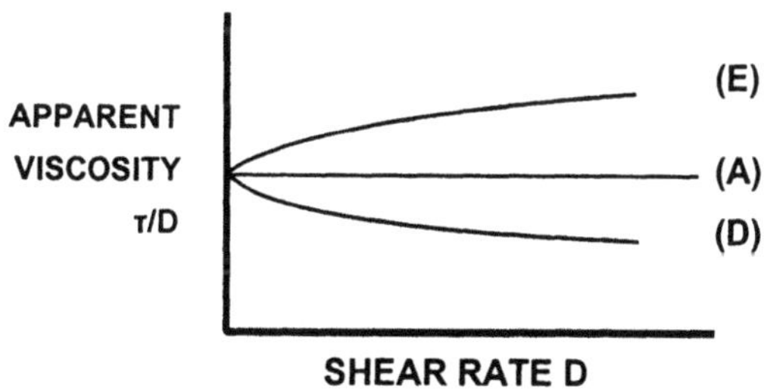

Figure 5.4. Effect of shear rate on apparent viscosity: (A) Newtonian; (D) pseudoplastic; (E) dilatant.

Some fluids have been found empirically to obey the following law:

$$\tau = kD^n, \quad \text{where } k \text{ and } n \text{ are constant.}$$

From this:

$$\log \tau = \log k + n \log D$$

Thus a plot of log τ versus log D is linear, with intercept log k, and slope n which is termed the *flow index*. If $n = 1$, the material is Newtonian; if n is less than 1, it is pseudoplastic; if n is greater than 1, it is dilatant. These are called *power law fluids*.

5.4 EFFECT OF SHEAR HISTORY

When some fluids are sheared at a steady rate, viscosity decreases with time. On standing the fluid regains its original viscosity. This is defined as *thixotropy* and is caused by structural breakdown and reformation. Gels are often thixotropic.

5.5 MEASUREMENT OF VISCOSITY

In all rheological measurements good temperature control is essential. The apparatus used may be classified into a number of various principal types.

1. Capillary viscometers can be used to determine the viscosity of Newtonian fluids by timing their flow in a capillary tube. Pressure extrusion though a capillary can also be used. Viscosity can be calculated from data for force of extrusion, volumetric flow rate through the capillary and capillary dimensions. It is important that the material should flow in laminar fashion without turbulence.
2. Falling body viscometers: viscosity can be calculated from the time taken for a sphere to fall or roll through a fluid.
3. Rotational viscometers are of a number of different types. In a coaxial cylinder viscometer the fluid is placed between two coaxial cylinders, either of which is rotated, depending on the equipment design (Figure 5.5). The shear rate is derived from the speed of rotation, and shear stress is

obtained from a meter, which determines the torque transmitted through the liquid.

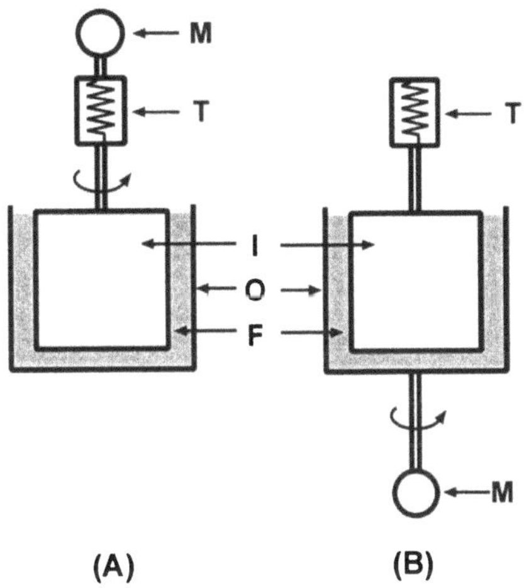

Figure 5.5. Coaxial cylinder viscometers: (A) inner cylinder driven by motor; (B) outer cylinder driven by motor. M = motor, T = torque meter, I = inner cyliner, O = outer cylinder, F = fluid.

Another type of rotational viscometer is a cone-plate instrument, in which the fluid is sheared in the gap between a stationary plate and a rotating cone (Figure 5.6). In all the viscometers described above, Newton's law is assumed in order to calculate the results. However, in the cone and plate viscometer, the shear rate is constant throughout the material, and depends only on the cone angle and speed of rotation. Shear stress can be calculated from torque and instrument dimensions. Hence shear stress and shear rate are independently measured. Thus, this instrument is very suitable for the study of non-Newtonian fluids. With an alternative instrument, the cone is fixed and the plate rotates or oscillates. Oscillatory shear tests can be used to measure elastic and viscous components of the deformation of fluids.

In rotating spindle viscometers, a spindle is made to rotate in the fluid, and viscous traction is measured.

4. A parallel plate plastometer has two discs of the same size, between which the fluid is placed. One plate is made to move towards the other, and viscosity calculated from the force applied to move the plate and rate of movement.

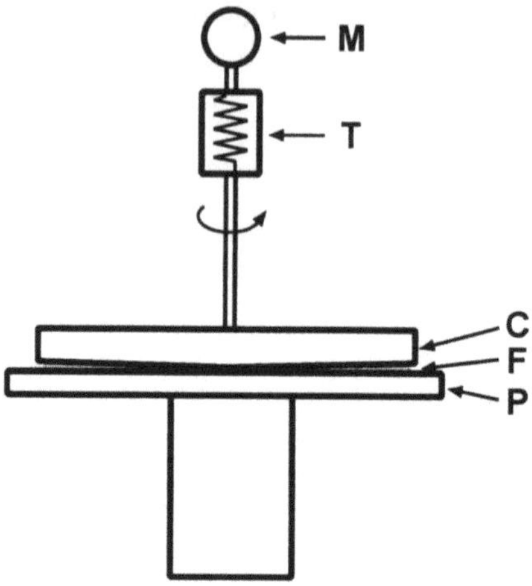

Figure 5.6. Cone-plate viscometer. M = motor; T = torque meter; C = cone; F = fluid; P = plate.

5. Qualitative instruments include orifice viscometers, consisting of a fluid reservoir and an orifice. The time for a given volume of fluid to flow through the orifice is measured. Alternatively, a penetrometer consists of a rod with a needle or cone, which drops on to a sample, and depth of penetration is measured. Oscillating or reciprocating rheometers are frequently used to assess dental materials. A platen oscillates in the material and the decrease in amplitude of oscillation is recorded as setting of the material occurs. Thus working and setting times are obtained.

5.6 VISCOELASTICITY

Dental significance: Viscoelastic properties are of major importance in, for example, creep of dental amalgam (Chapter 24), and the properties of polymers such as soft lining materials (Chapter 46) and denture base polymers (Chapter 45). In Chapter 11, structure property relationships of polymers are considered.

So far, the properties of elastic solids (Chapter 4) and viscous fluids have been discussed. In the latter case, deformation of the material is time dependent. In practice, many materials show a combination of both elastic and viscous properties. This phenomenon is termed *viscoelasticity*.

One method of representing viscoelastic behavior is by models consisting of springs and dashpots.

1. A spring will behave as shown in Figure 5.7 when deformed. At time t_0 when a load is applied, there will be instant deformation. At time t_1 when the load is removed, there is instant and complete elastic recovery.
2. A dashpot can be considered as a cylinder filled with a Newtonian fluid, with a leak-proof and frictionless piston. The fluid is in a vessel with an opening to a large reservoir of the same fluid. Figure 5.8 illustrates that application of a force at time t_0 to a Newtonian dashpot causes a time dependent deformation which stops at time t_1 when the load is removed. Permanent dcformation rcsults.
3. Combinations of springs and dashpots can be considered - see Figures 5.9 and 5.10 and Table 5.1 – include:

- Maxwell units, composed of a spring and dashpot in series;
- Voigt units comprising a spring and a dashpot in parallel.

4. Models close to the behavior of actual materials can be put forward, such as a Maxwell and Voigt unit in series - see Figure 5.11 and Table 5.1.

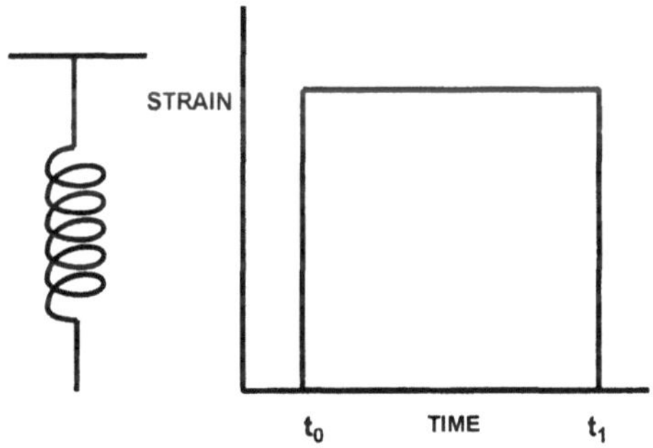

Figure 5.7. Deformation of a spring.

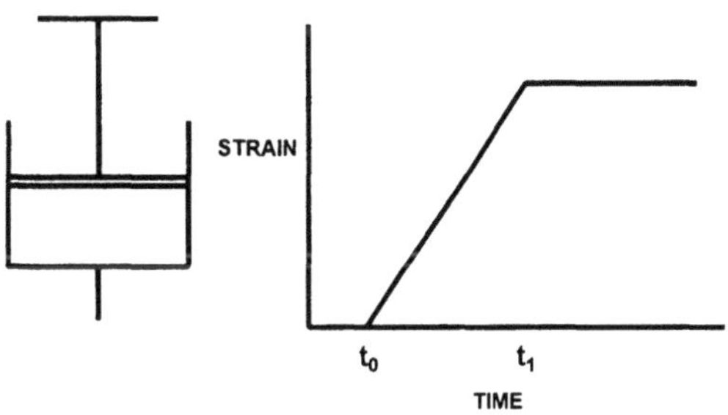

Figure 5.8. Deformation of a dashpot.

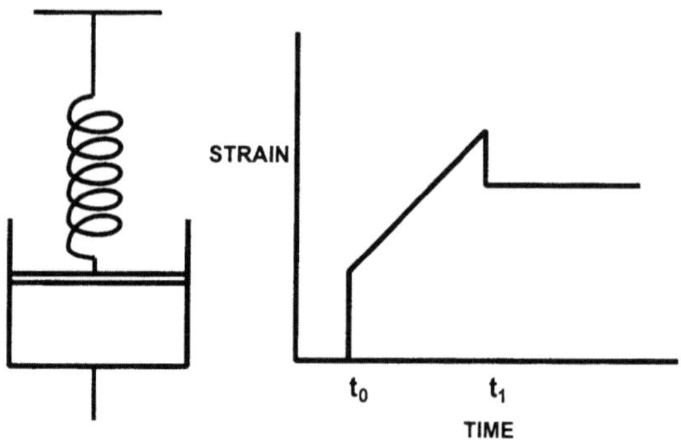

Figure5.9. Deformation of a Maxwell element, spring and dashpot in series.

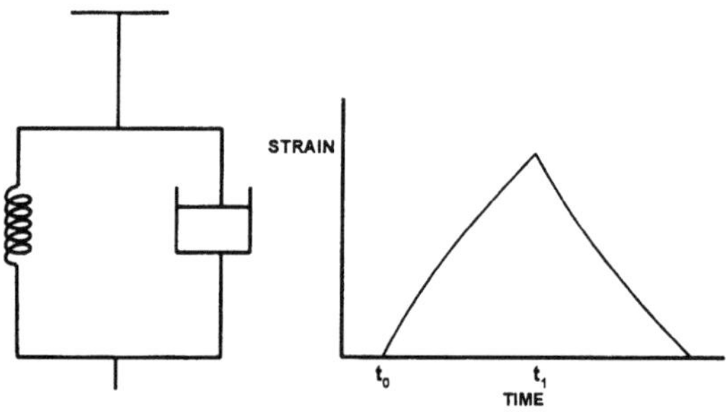

Figure 5.10. Deformation of a Voigt element, spring and dashpot in parallel.

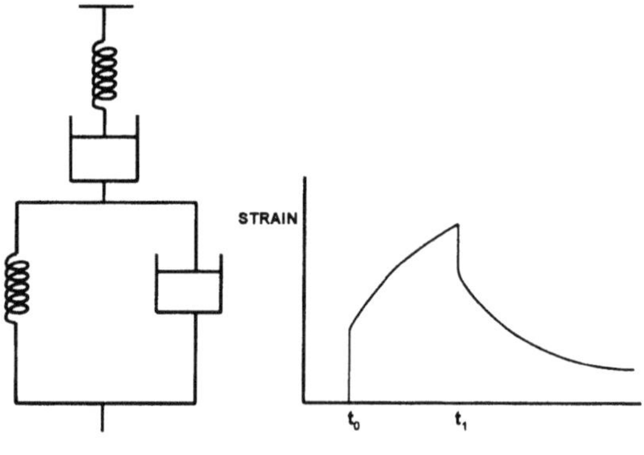

Figure 5.11. Deformation of Maxwell and Voigt elements in series.

Table 5.1. Models of elastic, viscous and viscoelastic behavior

Element	Components	Load applied at time t_0	Between time t_0 and t_1	Load removed at t_1	After time t_1	Figure number
Spring	Hookean spring	Instant de-formation	No change	Instant total recovery	No permanent deformation	5.7
Dashpot	Newtonian fluid	Beginning of gradual deformation	Time-dependent increase in deformation	No further change	Permanent deformation	5.8
Maxwell	Spring and dashpot in series	Some instant deformation of spring	Time-dependent increase in deformation due to dashpot	Elastic recovery of spring	Permanent deformation	5.9
Voigt	Spring and dashpot in parallel	Deformation begins	Gradual opening of spring with damping effect of dashpot	Recovery begins	Slow recovery of spring with damping effect of dashpot	5.10
Maxwell-Voigt	Maxwell and Voigt elements in series	Some instant deformation of spring of Maxwell unit	Gradual opening of Voigt element and dashpot of Maxwell unit	Instant recovery of spring of Maxwell unit	Slow recovery of Voigt unit and permanent deformation of dashpot of Maxwell unit	5.11

5.7 MEASUREMENT OF VISCOELASTIC BEHAVIOR

Reference has already been made to the use of oscillatory shear tests for measurement of elastic and viscous components of the deformation of fluids. For studies of the viscoelastic behavior of solids, two types of technique are of importance:

- Time-dependent techniques, including creep and stress relaxation measurement;
- Oscillatory techniques.

5.7.1 Time-dependent properties

1. *Creep* is the slow deformation of a material under constant stress. The magnitude of deformation depends on the material, the temperature, the load, and the time of application of the load. Figures 5.9 and 5.11 illustrate the strain-time behavior of material showing creep, in contrast to elastic and plastic deformations.
2. *Stress relaxation*: When a viscoelastic material is given a constant strain, a gradual reduction in stress is observed (Figure 5.12).

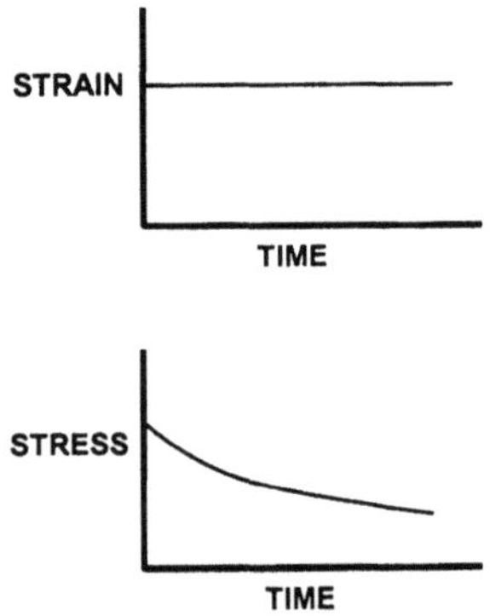

Figure 5.12. Stress relaxation at constant strain.

5.7.2 Oscillatory techniques

Applying sinusoidal stresses or strains can also make viscoelastic measurements. The techniques include the torsion pendulum (free oscillation), vibrating reed techniques and wave propagation methods (fixed vibrations). It is possible theoretically to inter-relate oscillatory and time-dependent methods.

FURTHER READING

Barnes H A, Hutton J F, Walters K (1989). *An Introduction to Rheology*. Elsevier, Amsterdam.

Chapter 6

Thermal Properties

Summary: Thermal conductivity, thermal diffusivity and coefficient of thermal expansion are defined.

Dental significance: Because there are temperature fluctuations in the mouth, it is important to know about the ability of a material to transmit heat, and also to know the effect of temperature change on the dimensions of materials. Ideally a restorative material should expand and contract at the same rate as tooth substance.

6.1 INTRODUCTION

Materials in the mouth are subjected to variations in temperature because of the intake of hot foods and drinks. It is important to know about the transmission of heat by the materials, which can have significant clinical consequences.

Dental significance: Tooth substance has low thermal diffusivity. If a restorative material with high thermal diffusivity replaces this, heat will be conducted to the dental pulp that can be damaging to the pulp and painful for the patient.

Dimensional changes associated with thermal changes are also important.

Dental significance: If there is a difference in the degree of thermal expansion between a tooth filling material and enamel and dentin, thermal changes can cause stresses at the interface, with resultant leakage at the margins of the restoration (Chapter 18).

6.2 THERMAL CONDUCTIVITY

Consider a lagged bar of materials, length *d*, surface area of cross-section *A*, the ends of which are kept at different temperatures, θ_1 and θ_2 (Figure 6.1). The quantity of heat passing per second, *Q*, from one end to the other is given by:

$$Q = KA\,(\theta_1 - \theta_2)/d$$

where *K* is a constant, termed the *thermal conductivity* of the material. This may be defined as the quantity of heat passing per second between the opposite faces of a unit cube when the difference in temperature is unity. Thermal conductivity is expressed in units of W/mK.

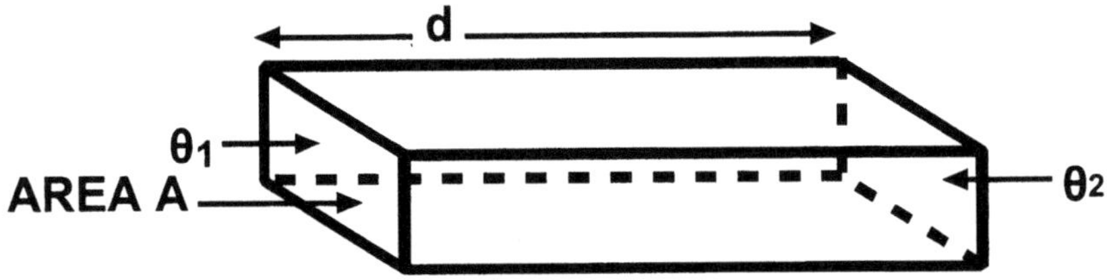

Figure 6.1. Thermal conductivity.

6.3 THERMAL DIFFUSIVITY

The above discussion assumes steady heat conditions. However, in the mouth, it is more relevant to consider transient temperature changes. To express the rapidity with which a material warms up before reaching the steady state, the *thermal diffusivity* (Δ) is important. This is defined as the thermal conductivity divided by the product of the specific heat and density, thus:

$$\Delta = K/C_P\,\rho$$

where C_P is the specific heat and ρ is the density.

The units for diffusivity are mm^2/s. Typical data for some common dental materials are given in Table 6.1.

Table 6.1. Thermal diffusivity of typical dental materials

Material	Thermal diffusivity (mm^2/s)
Gold	118
Dental amalgam	9.6
Acid-base reaction cements	0.26-0.47
Poly(methyl methacrylate)	0.124
Resin composites	0.30-0.70
Tooth enamel	0.469
Tooth dentin	0.183

Some general comments can be made, based on these data. Metals have high thermal diffusivity, in contrast to polymeric and ceramic materials. Tooth enamel and dentin have low diffusivities, indicating that they can give good thermal protection for the dental pulp. Ideally a dental restorative material should also have low thermal diffusivity.

6.4 THERMAL EXPANSION

The *linear coefficient of thermal expansion* of a material is the change in length per unit length when its temperature is lowered or raised by 1°C. This can be expressed as parts per million/°C; typical data are given in Table 6.2. As a very broad generalization, in terms of thermal expansion:

polymers and thermoplastic materials > metals > ceramics

Table 6.2. Thermal expansion coefficient of typical dental materials

Material	Coefficient of thermal expansion (parts per million per °C)	Temperature range of measurement (°C)
Tooth structure: crown	11.4	20-50
Tooth structure: root	8.3	20-50
Dental waxes	300	22-37
Elastomers:		
- Polysulfide	140	22-37
- Silicone	200	22-37
Poly(methyl methacrylate)	81	20-50
Glass-ionomer cement	35	20-50
Resin composites	26-35	0-60
Dental gold alloy	15	40-500
Dental amalgam	25	20-50
Dental porcelain	7-16	30-500

Note that tooth tissue has a low coefficient of thermal expansion, and that, of the materials represented in Table 6.2, porcelain comes closest to matching tooth tissue in this respect. It can also be seen that the expansion of resin composites is lower than that of polymeric materials; this is achieved by the incorporation of ceramic fillers.

6.5 DENTAL CONSIDERATIONS

Temperature changes in the mouth are important. It would be desirable for denture base materials to transmit some heat to the mucosal surfaces, so that denture wearers have the sensation of hot and cold foods. In contrast, filling materials should not transmit heat to the pulp of the tooth. Cements that have low thermal diffusivity are used for pulpal protection.

Dimensional changes caused by temperature changes are also of relevance. Ideally, filling materials should have similar coefficients of thermal expansion to enamel and dentin to minimize interfacial stress. Likewise, denture base materials and synthetic tooth materials should have similar coefficients to each other.

In general terms, thermoplastic materials such as waxes have high coefficients of thermal expansion. For example, it can be calculated that the percentage shrinkage of a wax of coefficient of thermal expansion 350 ppm/°C, on cooling from 55°C to 35°C is 0.7%.

FURTHER READING

Park J B, Lakes R S (1992). *Biomaterials. An Introduction.* 2nd edition. Plenum Press, New York, pp 48-52.

Chapter 7

Light, Color and Esthetics

Summary: The nature of light and its interaction with matter is discussed. Physical, physiological and psychological aspects of color perception are considered, and some objective methods of color measurement are presented.

Dental Significance: Esthetic considerations, including color matching, are of importance in contemporary dentistry.

7.1 INTRODUCTION

In contemporary dental practice there is considerable emphasis on esthetic dentistry. The appearance of teeth can be improved by the use of bleaching systems (Chapter 40) or the application of veneers (Section 34.8.3). It is also important to be able to place tooth restorations that closely resemble the appearance of surrounding tooth tissue, and to supply dentures that have a 'natural' appearance. Thus it is important to appreciate the principles of color science.

7.2 THE NATURE OF LIGHT

Visible light is a very small part of the electromagnetic spectrum (Table 7.1), being that region of the spectrum of wavelength approximately 380 nm to 780 nm. White light is made up of mixtures of color (Table 7.2) as can be demonstrated by the well-known experiment of Newton, in which light is dispersed by a prism (Figure 7.1).

To characterize a source of visible light, it is essential to know how much light is emitted at each wavelength. When energy *versus* wavelength is plotted, a *spectral energy distribution curve* is obtained. Figure 7.2(A) shows a typical curve for daylight, and Figure 7.2(B) is for blue light, with a peak wavelength of about 470-480 nm (of the type used for photo-polymerization (visible light curing) of dental restorative materials, see Section 27.3).

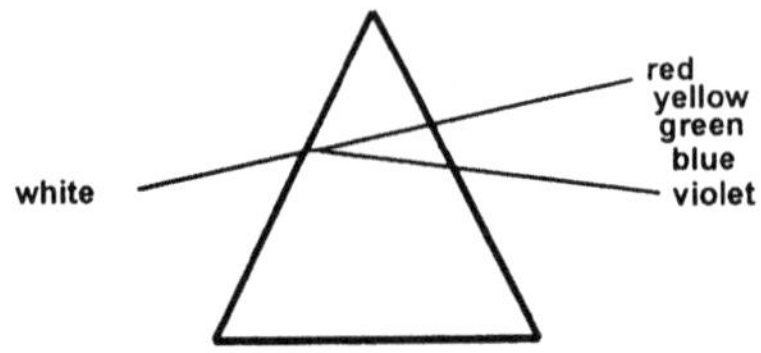

Figure 7.1. Diagram of white light as it passes through a prism.

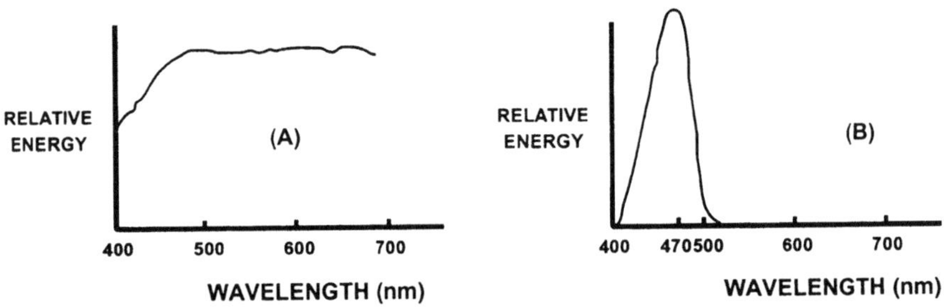

Figure 7.2. Spectral energy distribution curve for (A) sunlight, (B) blue light.

Table 7.1. The electromagnetic spectrum

Nomenclature	Frequency (Hz)	Approx. wavelength (m)
Gamma rays	$3 \times 10^{23} - 3 \times 10^{19}$	$10^{-14} - 10^{-11}$
X-rays	$3 \times 10^{19} - 3 \times 10^{16}$	$10^{-11} - 10^{-8}$
Ultraviolet	$3 \times 10^{6} - 6 \times 10^{14}$	$10^{-8} - 5 \times 10^{-7}$
Visible light	$6 \times 10^{14} - 3 \times 10^{14}$	$4 \times 10^{-7} - 8 \times 10^{-7}$
Infra-red	$3 \times 10^{14} - 3 \times 10^{12}$	$10^{-6} - 10^{-4}$
Microwaves	$3 \times 10^{12} - 3 \times 10^{8}$	$10^{-3} - 1$
Radio waves	$<3 \times 10^{8}$	>1

Table 7.2. Wavelength of different regions of the visible spectrum

Color	Approximate wavelength (nm)
Violet	380 – 430
Blue	430 – 460
Blue-green	460 – 500
Green	500 – 570
Yellow	570 – 590
Orange	590 – 610
Red	610 – 780

7.3 COLORS

There are three additive *primary colors*, namely, blue, green and red. If lights of these colors are added in the correct proportion, white light is produced. A secondary color is obtained by the addition of two primary colors, for example:

- Blue light + green light = cyan light;
- Green light + red light = yellow light;
- Red light + blue light = magenta light.

Color addition can be represented by an equilateral triangle, with the primary colors at the corners, and secondary colors at the mid-point of the sides (Figure 7.3). Two colors are said to be *complementary* if they combine to produce white. For example, the following combinations of colored lights will produce white light: blue + yellow; green + magenta; red + cyan (Figure 7.3).

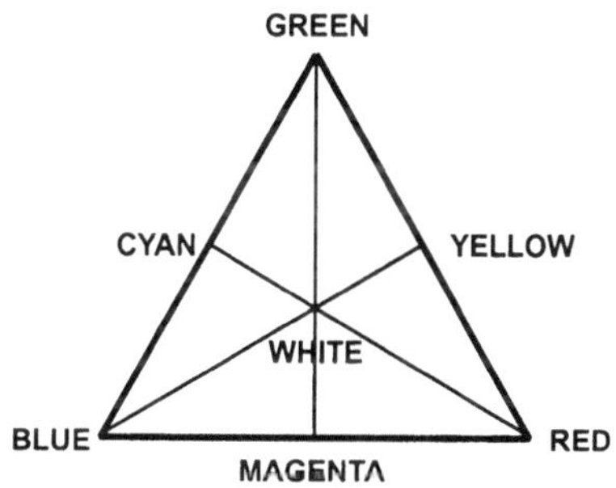

Figure 7.3. Representation of color addition.

Different principles apply when colored paints or pigments are mixed. In this case, a pigment absorbs light; that is, it subtracts out certain wavelengths of light and reflects the rest of the light. On mixing pigments, color subtraction occurs, so that:

- Yellow pigment + cyan pigment = green;
- Cyan pigment + magenta pigment = blue;
- Magenta pigment + yellow pigment = red.

7.4 LIGHT AND MATTER

When a beam of light strikes an object, one of three things can happen: transmission, absorption or scattering of the light.

7.4.1 Transmission of light

Substances, which are transparent, can transmit light. A beam of light changes direction at the boundary between materials, unless the angle of incidence is 90°. The *refractive index n* of a substance is given by:

$$n = \sin i / \sin r$$

where i is the angle of incidence of light entering the material from air and r is the angle of refraction of the light (Figure 7.4) Note that as well as refraction some light is reflected from the surface of the material.

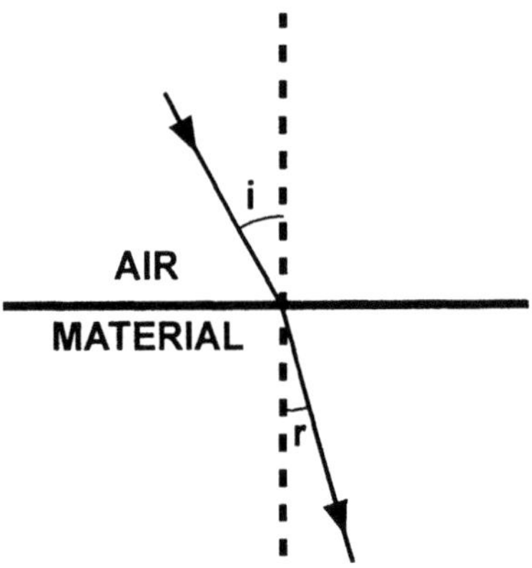

Figure 7.4. Refractive index = sin *i*/sin *r*.

7.4.2 Absorption of light

Opaque materials absorb light. Lambert's law of absorption states that each successive layer of a substance absorbs an equal fraction of the light passing through it. This may be expressed as:

$$I_x / I_o = e^{-Kx}$$

where I_o = initial intensity of light, I_x = intensity of light after passage through distance x of the material and K = the *absorption coefficient* of the material.

7.4.3 Scattering of light

In certain circumstances light can be scattered by matter. This will occur with a material that contains small particles of different refractive index from the bulk of the substance (Figure 7.5). If some light is transmitted, and some scattered, the substance is said to be translucent.

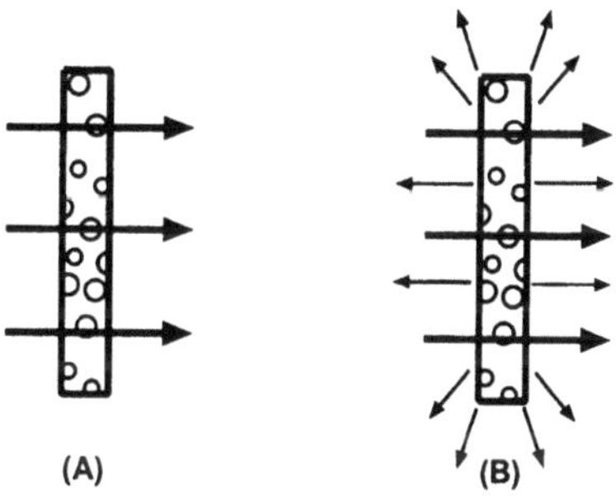

Figure 7.5. (A) Two components with same refractive index; no light scattering. (B) Two components with different refractive indices; light scattering occurs.

7.5 COLOR: PHYSICAL ASPECTS

Dental significance: Manufacturers of materials often supply shade guides, and it is important to be able to select the correct shade of material by color matching. However, in addition to color matching, a dental filling should have similar translucency and refractive index to tooth substance.

The color of an object will depend on a number of physical factors. The color of the light source is important. In particular, the spectral energy distribution curve affects the color appearance of an object. For example, materials may appear to be different when viewed under different conditions, e.g. fluorescent light *versus* daylight. Also, the color of the surroundings may alter the light source.

The nature of the object must also be taken into consideration. If the object transmits colored light, the material absorbs some light energy. For example, a green filter absorbs blue and red light.

For objects which reflect light: if it appears white, it reflects all colors; if it is black, it absorbs all colors; if it is colored, that color is reflected and all others are absorbed by the material.

A translucent material appears lighter in color than an opaque object. A substance which appears to have a high gloss reflects a large amount of light at the surface.

Color matching is important. *Metamerism* is said to occur when objects appear to match under one light source but not another.

Some materials have the property of *fluorescence*. This is defined as the ability to absorb light of one wavelength and emit light of a different wavelength or color. For example, natural teeth absorb ultra-violet radiation (< 400 nm wavelength) and emit light of 400-450 nm wavelength.

7.6 COLOR: PHYSIOLOGICAL AND PSYCHOLOGICAL ASPECTS

The retina of the eye contains specialized cells, which are called rods and cones. Stimuli received by the cones result in detection of color. Some people have defective color vision; this is caused by cell abnormalities. The eye is not equally sensitive to all colors; the greatest sensitivity is to green (wavelength *circa* 550 nm). Color fatigue can occur; after seeing one color constantly for a long period, the response of the eye to that color is diminished.

Psychological aspects are important, since optical illusions can occur. For example, the appearance of an object depends on its background; darker backgrounds make materials appear lighter.

7.7 COLOR MEASUREMENT

To define a color unambiguously, three parameters are important. The *hue* is the color - e.g. blue, red, green. *Value* is the darkness or lightness of the color. *Chroma* or saturation measures the intensity of the color; e.g. low values of chroma indicate a weak color.

One frequently used method of specifying colors is the Munsell color co-ordinate system (Figure 7.6). On the vertical axis is plotted the value. A circle represents the hue. The chroma is the distance from the center.

An alternative system is to express color in the L*a*b* system designated by the Commission Internationale de l'Eclairage (CIE), where L* is the lightness factor and a* and b* are chromaticity coordinates; *chromaticity* includes both hue and chroma. (Figure 7.7).

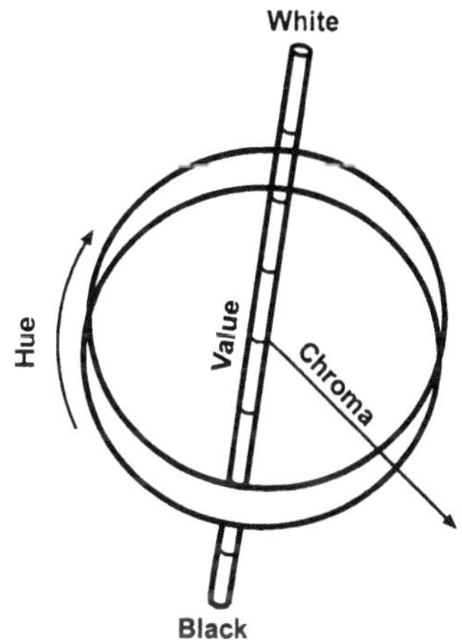

Figure 7.6. Munsell color coordinate system.

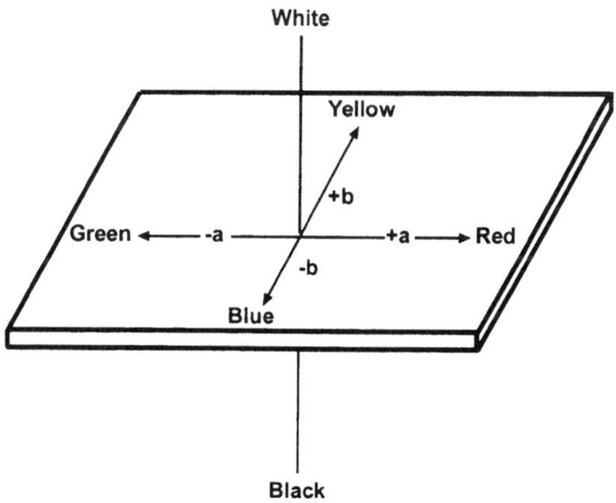

Figure 7.7. L*a*b* color measurement system.

7.8 DENTAL CONSIDERATIONS

In many aspects of restorative dentistry, esthetic considerations are important

The manufacturer pigments materials, and care should be taken in choosing a shade of material to ensure a correct match to adjacent tooth tissue. Shade guides are often provided for this purpose. It is important to match colors under appropriate conditions of lighting.

Esthetic materials should be permanent in color, neither showing staining (caused by external factors, e.g. constituents of diet) nor discoloration (caused by internal factors, such as chemical changes in components of the material).

For best esthetic effects, materials should have similar translucency to tooth tissue, unless it is necessary to mask underlying dentition.

In some instances, dental materials (e.g. dental porcelain) contain fluorescing agents to enhance esthetic appeal. Under certain lighting conditions, a restorative material that does not fluoresce will appear dark in contrast to the adjacent enamel that does fluoresce.

FURTHER READING

Billmeyer F W Jr, Saltzman M (1981). *Principles of Color Technology*, 2nd edn., Wiley, New York.

Qualtrough A J E, Burke F J T (1994). A look at dental esthetics. *Quintessence International* **25**: 7-14.

III

THE ORAL ENVIRONMENT

Chapter 8

Composition and Properties of Tooth Tissue and Saliva

Summary: In this chapter many aspects of the oral environment are considered, including the composition and properties of hard tooth tissues, the nature and function of saliva, and the nature of plaque and other accumulations on tooth surfaces.

Dental significance: It is important to know (i) the properties of tooth tissue, since an ideal replacement material should have similar properties, (ii) the effects of chemical treatments on the dental tissues and (iii) the nature of saliva and oral microflora.

8.1 RELEVANCE TO BIOMATERIALS SCIENCE

Teeth, both restored and unrestored, are being retained for longer periods of time by the population of the industrialized world and more of the population have retained significant numbers of teeth into old age. It may therefore be considered that the physical properties of tooth substance are, in general, adequate for their normal function. It follows that materials which replace lost tooth tissue should attempt to replicate (or be better than) those of enamel in terms of wear resistance and compressive strength, and that the physical properties of materials used for bases under restorations are best if they replicate the properties of dentin. Tooth substance, or its restorative replacement, must be capable of functioning in the oral environment, which is a potentially hostile environment in which forces are applied to teeth while they are bathed in saliva, foodstuffs and drinks, mouthwashes, toothpastes and, in many instances, plaque. Furthermore, teeth and restorations are often subjected to parafunctional forces as applied by bruxing and those with clenching habits and it is therefore essential that materials are available which may, if indicated, be used to restore the tooth substance lost during such parafunction.

Knowledge of the anatomy and physiology of tooth tissues and their environment is therefore essential when developing dental materials and in evaluating the potential performance of a restorative material, and assessing the compatibility of the material and tooth tissue at their interface. Furthermore, in cases where the material is placed in close proximity to the pulp, knowledge of the method by which pulp damage may occur is of relevance. In restorative and preventive dentistry, enamel and dentin are often treated with chemicals such as phosphoric acid and/or resin-based primers and conditioners. An understanding of the structure of dental tissues is therefore desirable in order to discern the potential effect of the given chemical on tooth tissue and to consider how the chemical may best achieve complete bonding at the tooth/material interface.

8.2 ENAMEL

8.2.1 Chemical composition

Enamel is an almost homogeneous, highly mineralized material, 97% inorganic substance by weight, making it the most highly calcified and hardest tissue in the human body. The inorganic content is principally apatite molecules, mainly hydroxyapatite [$Ca_{10}(PO_4)_6(OH)_2$], but with smaller amounts of other apatites such as fluoroapatite. Other minerals are present in much lower quantities along with a wide variety of trace metals. Water and organic substances make up the remaining 3%. The organic content is less than 1%, consisting of soluble and insoluble protein, peptides and citric acid. Enamel is composed of millions of calcified rods or prisms that traverse the width of the enamel in a direction roughly perpendicular to the dentin surface (Figure 8.1). The periphery of the enamel prisms, the prism sheath, is much less calcified than the rest of the prism and is rich in organic material.

8.2.2 Physical properties

It is generally accepted that enamel is the hardest of human tissues, and when measured by indentation testing, a Knoop Hardness Number of 200 to 500 KHN is achieved, the wide variability being due to the variation of the plane in which testing is carried out. Peripheral regions of the tooth are harder than deeper regions, but other factors are involved such as degree of calcification, prism orientation and distribution of metallic ions. Enamel is semi-translucent, with the color being dependent, in part, on its thickness. In places where the enamel is thin, the underlying yellow-white dentin can shine through. Hardness alone is not sufficient to withstand masticatory forces; indeed, on the contrary, hardness may make the enamel prone to splitting and chipping, but this is tempered by the cushioning effect of the underlying dentin. Enamel has a high elastic modulus (130 GPa) and a relatively low tensile strength (76 MPa). Solubility is an important clinical consideration, since exposure of enamel to acid will result in dissolution. Various ions will alter enamel solubility, for example, fluoride reduces the solubility of enamel and other substances such as silver nitrate and zinc chloride will have a similar effect. Enamel from the surface regions of the tooth is less soluble than that from deeper regions.

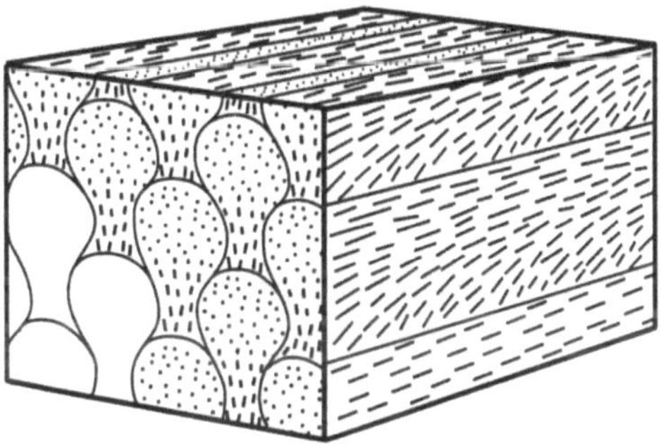

Figure 8.1. Structure of enamel showing enamel prisms which have keyhole-shaped outlines. After Mechel A H, Griebstein W J, Neal R J (1965). Structure of mature human dental enamel as observed by electron microscopy. *Archives of Oral Biology* **10**: 775-783.

8.2.3 Effect of acid etchants

As a result of the rich organic content of the enamel prism sheath, it resists the action of acids better than the prism itself or the interprismatic substance. Acids, most commonly 35-37% phosphoric acid, when applied to enamel, therefore cause preferential loss of enamel prism core material leaving the prism peripheries relatively intact, although variations on this pattern have been reported, not only from tooth to tooth but also from surface to surface. This differential loss on enamel substance produces a micromechanically retentive surface that reliably retains resin-based materials when these are placed under optimum conditions (Chapter19) — See Figure 8.2.

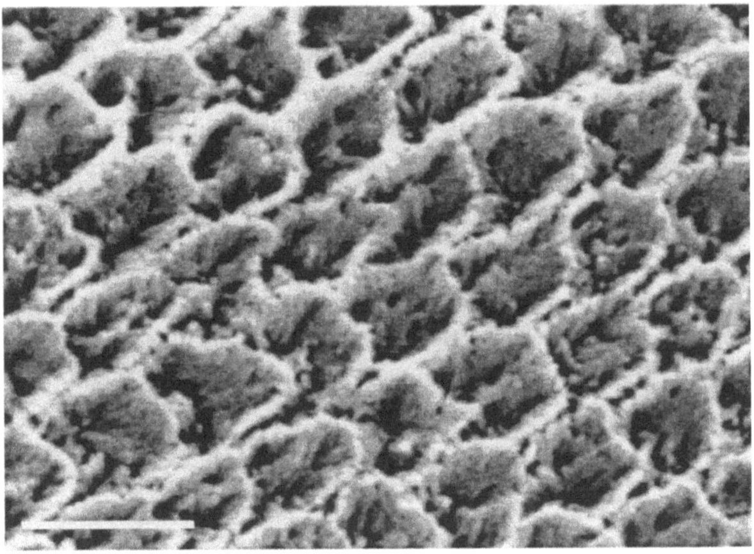

Figure 8.2. Scanning electron micrograph of etched enamel. The horizontal bar represents 10 μm.

8.2.4 Fluorides

Fluoride solutions may be applied to the enamel surface as part of a preventive routine, or may be present intrinsically following the ingestion of fluoride during tooth formation. This results in the formation of fluoroapatite rather than hydroxyapatite; the fluoroapatite is more resistant to acid dissolution, which is of relevance in the prevention of carious attack but also as an increased resistance to dissolution by acid etchants applied to the tooth.

8.3 DENTIN

8.3.1 Chemical composition and structure

Dentin, which may be considered to be a biologic composite of apatite crystal filler particles in a collagen matrix, forms the bulk of the tooth substance and gives the basic shape to each tooth. It has a considerably higher organic content than enamel (Table 8.1), with the organic material comprising 18% collagen, 1% citric acid with the remainder being protein similar to collagen which is characterized by four amino acids, glycine, alanine, proline and hydroxyproline. It is covered by enamel on the crown and cementum on the root. The internal surface of the dentin forms the walls of the pulp cavity. The inorganic content is mainly a carbonate rich, calcium deficient apatite: the calcium:phosphorus ratio is lower than in enamel. Fluoride, zinc and lead are present in trace amounts.

Table 8.1. Composition of enamel and dentin

	Enamel (wt %)	Enamel (vol %)	Dentin (wt %)	Dentin (vol %)
Mineral	97	92	70	45
Organic material	1	2	20	33
Water	2	6	10	22

Dentin is composed of cells, the odontoblasts, and an intercellular matrix which is everywhere permeated by the dentinal tubules in which contain the protoplasmic processes of the odontoblasts (Fig. 8.3). The tubules run in one direction, from the outer surface of the dentin, converging towards the pulp cavity. Each tubule is lined with a sheath of highly mineralized, collagen-poor, dentin, known as peritubular dentin.

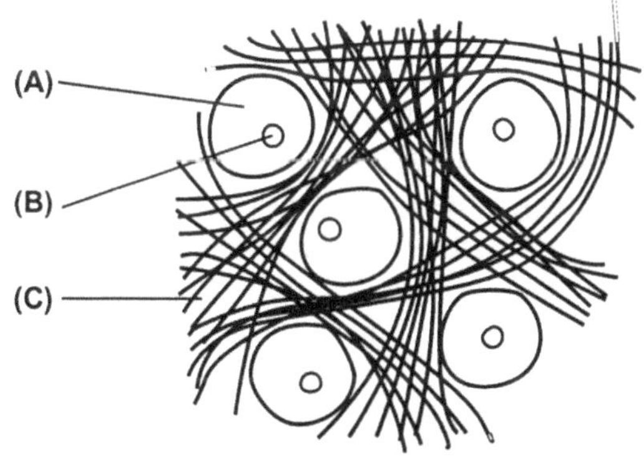

Figure 8.3. Structure of dentin: (A) peritubular dentin, (B) dentinal tubule, (C) collagen fibers of the intertubular dentin.

The tubules are separated by intertubular dentin, a network of collagenous fibrils reinforced by apatite. It consists mainly of collagenous fibers running in bundles in a mesh-like pattern between the tubules roughly at right angles to the tubules, and smaller amounts of apatite crystals. The intertubular dentin matrix is therefore less highly mineralized than the peritubular matrix and forms the principal structural component of the dentin that surrounds the lumen of the dentinal tubules. The tubules are more tightly packed towards the pulp than in the outer dentin (Table 8.2); it therefore follows that the amount of intertubular matrix varies considerably at different levels of the dentin.

Table 8.2. Dentin tubules

Distance from pulp (mm)	Number of tubules per cm^2	% area occupied by intertubular dentin	% area occupied by water-filled tubules
0.1-0.5	4.5×10^6	68.2	31.8
1.6-2.0	3.0×10^6	78.8	21.2
3.1-3.5	1.9×10^6	86.6	13.4

8.3.2 Physical properties

The apatite crystals provide strength while the collagen provides toughness. The hardness of dentin is substantially less than that of enamel (KHN 70) but nevertheless greater than either bone or cementum, with the hardest dentin being found close to the enamel-dentin junction and the lowest value at the innermost layer. As a result of the variations in the properties of dentin at different depths, conventional micro-indentation methods for measuring hardness may be considered inappropriate, with nano-indentation methods using a smaller indentation stylus being more useful. Dentin is more elastic than enamel, with a modulus of elasticity of 11.7 GPa, a compressive strength of 270 MPa and a tensile strength of 40 MPa. The shear strength of dentin may be of relevance in explaining bonding failures, with figures of 40 MPa being reported near the pulp and 130 MPa near the dentin-enamel junction. This increase in shear strength moving outwards through the dentin, in general, mirrors the increase in hardness.

The movement of substances into or across the dentin, principally due to the network of tubules is known as dentin permeability. However, this permeability is not uniform throughout the tooth, coronal dentin permeability being higher than that of root dentin. If the substance moves across the entire thickness of dentin via the tubules to reach the pulp, this is termed *transdentin permeability*. However, if the substance enters the tubules but does not travel across the dentin, this is known as *intratubular permeability*.

8.4 PULP

8.4.1 Introduction

The dental pulp is a vital connective tissue, 75% water and 25% organic, consisting of collagen fibers and ground substance which supports the cellular, vascular and nerve structure of the pulpal tissue. It receives its blood supply from the apical foramen and is otherwise rigidly enclosed within the dentin. Should inflammation occur within the pulp tissue, there is therefore no space for expansion. Dental pulp produces primary and secondary dentin, provides the blood supply to the tooth and fulfils a protective function, by removing noxious substances into the peripheral blood stream. It also has a sensory function, in that it transmits pain - its nervous tissue consists only of pain fibers. The majority of pulpal nerve fibers are either myelinated A-δ or smaller, unmyelinated C fibers. Activation of the A-δ fibers produces a sharp, intense pain while activation of the C fibers is slower, although, as these fibers are resistant to tissue hypoxia, a pain response may be obtained from these fibers even in anaesthetized, infected or non-vital teeth. The outermost component of pulp tissue is the odontoblast layer. This produces the primary and secondary dentin. Routine dental procedures may cause temporary disruption of this layer.

8.4.2 Maintaining pulpal health

Excessive heat during cavity preparation procedures (that is, without proper water cooling) has been considered to be the most damaging insult to the pulp, other than the ingress of bacteria from caries. A rise in intrapulpal temperature of 11°C may cause necrosis of more than 50% of pulpal cells. Temperature rises may also occur during over-vigorous amalgam polishing techniques. Burs which are not rotating concentrically have also been considered to cause damage to pulpal tissue. There is no evidence to show that application of acids such as those used during adhesive restorative procedures (see Chapter 28) may cause pulpal damage, provided that the dentin is bonded and 'sealed' with a dentin bonding system. Microleakage, due to the use of materials that do not bond adequately to dentin has long been considered to be a source of irritation to pulpal tissue.

8.4.3 Thermal sensitivity

Prevention of thermal sensitivity has been the rationale for placement of liners and bases beneath metal restorations. However, it is now considered that there are two reasons for such sensitivity. One is that of direct thermal shock, the other is the 'hydrodynamic' theory, which is currently more widely accepted. This theory purports that restorations have a gap between the wall of the cavity and the restoration. This permits the slow outward movement of dentinal fluid, and cold causes a sudden contraction of this fluid, and the increase in fluid flow is recorded as pain. In restorations nearer the pulp, the dentinal tubules are wider in diameter and tubules are greater in density, which both have the effect of increasing the effects of the hydrodynamic theory. The increasing acceptance of this theory has led to a change in emphasis, away from achievement of thermal insulation of the dentin, towards dentinal sealing. The need for extensive thick bases beneath amalgam restorations is therefore questionable: if such bases are to be placed, their minimum thickness need not exceed 1 mm and they should be constructed in a material which adheres to the dentin surface.

8.5 THE ORAL ENVIRONMENT

8.5.1 Saliva

Saliva is of fundamental relevance to the performance of dental materials, given that it is the principal medium in which teeth and restorative materials must coexist. It is of importance in providing a buffer for acids produced in plaque (see below) and in supplying the inorganic ions, such as calcium and phosphate, which are required to remineralize carious lesions and in diluting and washing away sugars from around the teeth. Stimulated saliva is more effective at these functions than unstimulated. Caries occurs when the chemical conditions on the tooth surface favor demineralization over remineralization as a result of pH changes in plaque. Saliva contains several proteins that may have antibacterial effects as well as digestive, lubrication and ion-binding properties. It is the latter which confers the ability of certain salivary proteins to bind to teeth and these proteins may also constitute a selective growth medium for oral bacteria. It is these properties which make it essential that tooth surfaces are thoroughly debrided before an attempt is made to bond any restorative material to the tooth surface.

Xerostomia (dry mouth) may affect as many as 30% of patients in the USA. Those patients who sip liquids to help swallowing dry foods, who may have difficulty in swallowing dry foods or who have a mouth which feels dry when eating a meal may have some degree of salivary hypofunction. In these patients, restorative materials may be subjected to drying more readily than for patients with normal salivary function. Furthermore, for these patients, the lack of normal salivary lubrication makes eating difficult and may make the mouth uncomfortable. The development of an effective saliva substitute would therefore appear to be a priority.

Saliva is a complex mixture of fluids secreted by the major salivary glands, minor (or accessory) glands and the gingival crevicular fluid. Additionally, it contains bacteria, desquamated cells and residues of food or drink. The salivary glands are under purely nervous control, the normal daily input of saliva being about 500 ml, of which about 200 ml is secreted during feeding and 300 ml as unstimulated resting saliva. Unstimulated flow peaks at about 5 p.m. in most individuals with a reduced flow during sleep. Saliva is a dilute fluid, being 99% water, with varying concentrations of dissolved solids. It contains proteins - approx. 200 mg per 100 ml. These include enzymes, immunoglobulins, mucins, antibacterial proteins and glycoproteins. Inorganic constituents include sodium, potassium, calcium, inorganic phosphorus and chloride, with the major ions (sodium, potassium, calcium, chloride and bicarbonate) being the main contributors to the osmolarity of saliva. Not all the calcium and phosphate in saliva is free in solution, part of the calcium being bound to protein.

The principal functions of saliva are:

- In digestion, with the salivary amylase initiating the digestion of starch;
- Lubrication of the intra-oral surfaces for speech, mastication and swallowing;
- Oral health and function, dilution of substances introduced into the mouth, neutralization and buffering (saliva has a pH of 5-8).

Saliva also has antibacterial effects, given its antibody content, and it contributes to pellicle and plaque, given that both pellicle and plaque matrices contain proteins derived predominantly from the saliva. Pellicle protects the teeth and their restorations against chemical and mechanical insult.

8.5.2 Dental plaque

The mouth is similar to other parts of the body in having its own resident microflora, and the microflora of mucosal surfaces is different from that found on teeth. Dental plaque forms naturally on teeth and is an aggregation of bacteria which are tenaciously attached to the teeth and other oral surfaces, including restorations, with a cuticle or pellicle interposed between the microbial cells. It may also contain a few inflammatory and epithelial cells. The plaque microflora also differs at different sites on the teeth, for example in the fissures, the gingival crevice, the approximal surfaces. The resident microflora can be of benefit in preventing the colonization by exogenous and/or pathogenic microorganisms. Dental plaque contains between 100 to 200 species of microorganisms such as *Streptococcus Sanguis*, but the microflora may alter depending on the prevailing conditions. For example, the frequent exposure of plaque to low pH leads to the selection of micro-organisms with an aciduric physiology such as mutans streptococci and lactobacilli. The spaces between the bacterial cells are bridged by intercellular substances, allowing the percolation of saliva, gingival fluid and liquids from the diet through the structure. After reaching a certain thickness, yellow/white dental plaque may be detected with the naked eye, often in the gingival third of the crown of the tooth or in approximal areas.

The chemical composition of dental plaque is of relevance as this may contribute to the environment in which restorations may have to exist. Chemical composition varies with age and diet, but, in general, is 80% water and 20% solids, which comprise bacterial cells and extracellular components in the ratio of 1 to 2. Microorganisms in dental plaque may produce dilute organic acids as a product of fermentation, but, in general, the dental plaque pH will vary according to the dietary factors to which it is exposed.

8.5.3 Other accumulations

Pellicle is an organic film derived principally from the saliva and deposited on the tooth surface; it initially contains few bacteria but may be colonized after a number of hours.

Materia alba is a bacterial accumulation containing bacteria, leucocytes and desquamated epithelial cells, but, in contrast to dental plaque, it is easily removed by a water spray.

Calculus is calcified plaque, which is often covered with a layer of uncalcified plaque.

All of the above deposits may stain yellow, black, green or brown depending on diet, age, smoking habits and presence of chromogenic bacteria.

FURTHER READING

Edgar W M (1992). Saliva: its secretion, composition and functions. *British Dental Journal* **172:** 305-312.

Jordan R E, Abrams L, Kraus B S (1992). *Kraus' Dental Anatomy and Occlusion*. Mosby Year Book, St Louis.

Marshall G W, Marshall S J, Kinney J H, Balooch M.(1997). The dentin substrate: structure and properties related to bonding. *Journal of Dentistry* **25:** 441-458.

Chapter 9

Aspects of Biomechanics

Summary: An account is given of the forces and movements generated between the upper and lower teeth and of the modification of the resulting stress within the different hard tissues.

Dental Significance: Forces and movements generated between the upper and lower teeth are responsible for optimal function such as mastication. They are also, along with the hostile environment of the mouth (Chapter 10), a major challenge to the longevity of restorative materials within the mouth.

9.1 FORCES BETWEEN TEETH

The forces (or stresses as forces/unit area) that are generated when teeth come together (or occlude) are ultimately generated by the muscles of mastication. The stress travels as a trajectory through the skeletal apparatus, principally in the mandibular and maxillary bones, and when the teeth meet in contact, the biomechanical loop is complete and includes bones, teeth, periodontal membrane and muscles. (Figure 9.1).

As noted, within this biomechanical loop there are many important functioning anatomical sub-units, such as the tooth itself, the periodontal ligament, and the corpus and alveolar processes of the mandible. Some of those that are germane to dental biomaterials are dealt with in this chapter.

Macroscopically the closed masticatory biomechanical loop with the teeth in contact is clinically rigid, which is shown by the facial constant height as measured by a gauge between fixed points on the chin and the nose, even when increasing forces are generated between the teeth. Conversely, when the teeth are apart and the jaws are at rest the face is flexible as measured between the nose and chin. These points become important when one considers how forces are applied between the teeth.

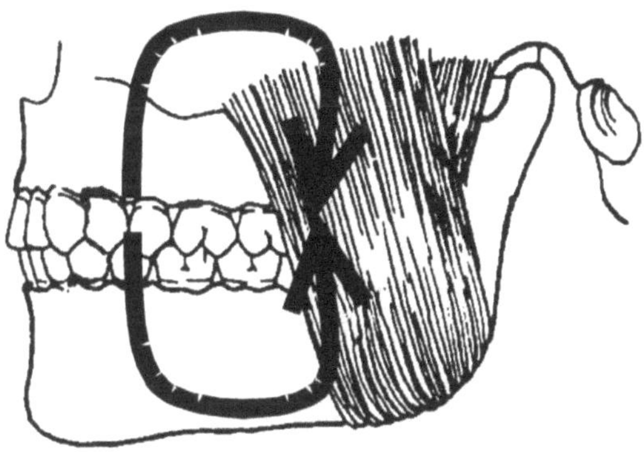

Figure 9.1. The biomechanical loop.

9.2 HOW FORCES ARE APPLIED IN THE MOUTH

When increasing occlusal forces are applied between the teeth when they are in contact, there is no palpable change in the major anatomy of the jaws in the vertical direction. This condition is referred to as *isometric* (or in engineering terms, *load control*). However when the teeth are apart and the subject is biting through a relatively soft material, clearly the jaws are moving through the material and coming closer together. This condition is referred to as *isotonic* (or in engineering terms, *stroke control*). These are two fundamental ways of applying force through teeth and it applies throughout the musculo-skeletal system. The two conditions may be mixed isotonic-isometric in which case it is called *isokinetic*.

These different methods of applying forces are of first importance in mechanical testing and in attempting to simulate the chewing forces in the mouth in the laboratory situation.

9.3 FORCE VALUES

There are two force values of immediate interest and these are the magnitude of the force in Newtons (N) and the time of force application. Two other force values are of interest. These are the area of contact that determines the instantaneous stress and the force vector that describes the direction of the force. These latter two values, while important, are extremely difficult to measure. The area of contact is continually changing and the force vector is controlled by the anatomy at the point of contact that is also continually changing.

Even force measured in Newtons is difficult to measure because measuring devices interfere with the normal function of tooth contact.

Maximum biting force is often measured. This involves putting a transducer between the teeth and asking the subject to bite as hard as possible. Typical values generated are in the region of 400 N. The value is nonfunctional and has limited value.

The habit of grinding teeth together is called *bruxism* and fits into the classification of tooth contact as parafunction as opposed to useful functional contacts. Forces generated in bruxism can be high and have been modeled as 40 N on a sustained basis. Bruxism is entirely a tooth-to-tooth contact phenomenon and can be very destructive to the hard dental tissues.

The most important functional process in the mouth is perhaps mastication. This results in the comminution of food just before swallowing. The anterior teeth are involved in incising, which also controls the bite size. And the posterior teeth are involved in comminuting or grinding the food to a smaller particle size. The average forces involved in this are suprisingly small and may be about 15 N per tooth to tooth contact. The standard deviation is expected to be large and there will be occasions when this figure is exceeded over very short time spans.

There are two other kinds of contacts, glancing contacts and contacts during swallowing. Glancing contacts are almost instantaneous, and probably have a role in guiding the movement of the mandible. Swallowing contacts stabilize the mandible just before swallowing. They can be quite long (1 second) and they have no sliding component. Neither glancing nor swallowing contacts are regarded as being detrimental to dental materials in the mouth.

Total time of tooth-to-tooth contact per day from all sources is usually less than 20 minutes.

9.4 MANDIBULAR MOVEMENT

The movement of the mandible with the open mouth position and with the teeth in contact is an extremely complex subject and is dealt with in texts on the subject of occlusion. However from the point of view of biomaterials and biomechanics some general observations may be made, especially with regard to mastication and bruxism, which are most important to the performance of dental materials in the mouth.

Both mastication and bruxism have a sliding component, which is primarily responsible for the interdental friction and wear phenomenon in both natural teeth and dental materials. The movement is mostly lateral from side to side although there is also an anterior-posterior component. When protrusive movements are made, such as when the anterior teeth are brought edge to edge, of course the movement is anterior-posterior.

In mastication the time when the teeth are in contact is approximately 0.25 seconds. The chewing cycle is approximately 1 Hz (one per second) so it appears that in chewing most of the time is spent with the teeth apart. The distance of the sliding movement in mastication varies from 1.0 mm at one extreme to almost zero with a canine guided occlusion when the teeth are almost locked in position. However a normal range of sliding movement in mastication might be considered 0.3 – 0.6 mm.

Bruxism as a grinding and sliding movement is quite different from chewing. It is a reciprocating movement with the teeth in contact throughout the process. The forces are higher, perhaps 40 N per interdigitating tooth and the sliding movement is large 1 – 2 mm or larger. It is clear why bruxing can be so destructive of the dentition. It has been considered that 20% of population may be bruxers. However in a random sample of 20 first year dental students 50% proved to be bruxers clinically.

When the teeth meet during chewing it is essentially a 'soft landing.' In other words the speed of mandible slows down on approaching contact. After contact the force increases to the 15 N mentioned above and then begins to decline at the end of the sliding movement before lifting off again. This means that the shape of the force profile is in the form a half sine wave.

The number of chewing cycles in a sequence before swallowing is about 30 – 35. Curiously, this number can be fairly constant for one individual. It was believed at one point that the teeth never touched during the chewing cycle. But it is now believed that the teeth do meet during the last half of the chewing sequence, when the food particle size is reduced and a cohesive food bolus is formed.

9.5 RESYNTHESIZING BIOMECHANICAL CONDITIONS IN THE LABORATORY

The problem of resynthesizing biomechanical conditions in the laboratory has proved difficult, especially in respect of dental wear. A number of different biomechanical configurations have been suggested. However it seems that the conditions should comply approximately with an occlusal isometric force of 15 N in form of a half sine wave with a lateral slide of 0.25 mm. Under these conditions with the appropriate lubricant (usually a high volume rate of water) about 250,000 masticatory cycles will approximate one year's clinical wear.

9.6 HOW STRESS TRAJECTORIES ARE MODIFIED WITHIN THE HARD TISSUES

As noted above when the teeth are in contact there is a complete biomechanical loop that involves the maxilla, mandible, muscles and joint and the contact areas of the teeth. As the stress trajectories move through these structures they are modified to be consistent with the health of the tissue. This means mostly a change in the stress concentration. Stress concentrations are most intense at the area of tooth contact, which typically involves the enamel-to-enamel. Enamel is a very hard and rigid material and almost perfectly elastic, and the area of contact is small, which leads to a highly localized stress intensity.

The occlusal stress must pass to the dentin, which is a more resilient and less rigid tissue. The stress trajectory spreads out in the dentin with a reduction in intensity. This is consistent with the role of dentin as the main supporting tissue. Dentin also has a greater viscoelastic component. This means that time is required for the stress intensities to build up which may be consistent with the health of dentin. This is quite unlike enamel where the build up of stress intensity, in addition to being localized, is almost instantaneous.

The occlusal stress must also pass through the radicular dentin to the periodontal membrane that forms the attachment between the root of the tooth and the alveolar process of the mandible or maxilla. The periodontal membrane is also a viscoelastic component, and time modifies the transfer of stress to the alveolar process and its subsequent build up within the bone. This again is consistent with the health of the bony alveolar process. Taken together the tooth, the periodontal membrane and the alveolar process form the dentoalveolar complex, an important sub-unit of the masticatory process. The role of the alveolar process may be secondary to that of the periodontal membrane by providing recoil, leading to fast recovery following the removal of occlusal loads.

FURTHER READING

Ahlgren J, Owall B (1970). Muscular activity and chewing force: a polygraphic study of human mandibular movements. *Archives of Oral Biology* **15**:271-280.

Delong R, Douglas W H (1991). An artificial oral environment for testing of dental materials. *IEEE Transactions on Biomedical Engineering* **38**: 339-345.

Gibbs C H, Mahan P E, Lundeen H C, Brehan K, Walsh E K, Holbrook W B (1981). Occlusal forces during chewing and swallowing as measured by sound transmission. *Journal of Prosthetic Dentistry* **46**: 443-449.

Korioth T W P, Hannam A G (1994). Deformation of the human jaw during simulated tooth clenching. *Journal of Dental Research* **73**: 56-66.

Luke D A, Lucas P W (1985). Chewing efficiency in relation to occlusal and other variations in the natural human dentition. *British Dental Journal* **159**: 401-406.

Chapter 10

Hostile Effects of the Oral Environment

Summary: Factors that are harmful to tooth tissues are considered, including the causes of tooth substance loss and discoloration.

Dental significance: It is important to understand the causes of damage to the tissues of the mouth, and ways of minimizing or preventing this occurrence.

10.1 CAUSES OF TOOTH SUBSTANCE LOSS

Tooth substance may be lost in a variety of ways, and it therefore follows that restorative materials should also resist such loss. Terminology of tooth wear varies throughout the world, from dental wear, to tooth wear and tooth surface loss. In this chapter, the term *tooth substance loss* (TSL) will be used to describe the loss of enamel and dentin.

It is likely that the increasing retention of natural teeth into older age will increase the prevalence of tooth substance loss. As a result of shortened clinical crowns and loss of interocclusal space, the dental profession and materials manufacturers face a severe challenge in respect of how restorations may be satisfactorily retained. There are many etiologic factors to TSL and the interrelationship of these factors may often be difficult to determine. However, it is rare to see all teeth in a particular mouth affected by TSL to the same degree, and indeed, TSL often affects only the anterior teeth and often only the teeth of one arch.

Reports giving current details of the epidemiology of TSL are scarce, despite the large number of published reports of tooth wear in earlier populations. It has been considered that Saudi, Eskimo and Australian Aborigine populations are particularly affected, but anecdotal reports in the

United Kingdom appear to suggest increasing incidence of TSL in both the elderly and young populations.

Traditionally the terms attrition, abrasion and erosion are used to describe non-carious pathologic loss of tooth substance, but they also reflect the particular mechanisms by which TSL may occur. These mechanisms often act concurrently, with severe progressive TSL often having a multifactorial etiology.

10.1.1 Attrition

Attrition may be defined as the gradual loss of hard tooth substance as a result of chewing activity, that is, the physical wear of one tooth surface against another. This tooth substance loss therefore occurs on the contacting surfaces of teeth, occlusally and incisally, although some slight tooth substance loss may occur interproximally. There may be varying degrees of attrition, such as physiologic, intensified and pathologic, the latter being used to describe extreme TSL. Physiologic TSL may be expected to occur throughout life, but it may be considered that the normal non-abrasive Western diet does not present much risk for attrition. Pronounced attrition-related wear may be associated with parafunctional activity, with teeth showing distinct faceting, with facets in one arch matching the facets in the opposing arch in positions of contact. Additionally, iatrogenic wear may result from contact between tooth substance and a rough hard opposing surface such as a poorly polished ceramic restoration.

10.1.2 Abrasion

Abrasion is the pathologic TSL caused by friction from a foreign body, not associated with the occlusion between the teeth, i.e., the physical wear by objects rather than teeth. Examples may include loss of tooth substance due to repeatedly biting thread, chewing a pipe stem or using a toothpick. However, the most common abrasive lesions are due to overzealous toothbrushing with abrasive toothpastes or salt.

10.1.3 Erosion

Erosion is a loss of enamel and/or dentin resulting from non-bacterial chemical attack, usually involving acids. Dietary (acidic foods or drinks), intrinsic (gastric regurgitation) and occupational (chemical installations) sources of acids may be implicated. In general, intrinsic acid affects the palatal surfaces of the upper teeth, particularly the incisors, while dietary acid may also affect buccal, occlusal and incisal surfaces. Areas affected by erosion will present as smooth, rounded areas of TSL with loss of the normal tooth surface detail. Restorations in a material such as amalgam may appear 'proud' of the remaining tooth surface for patients with severe erosive TSL, such as in bulimic patients, given that amalgam is less soluble in acid than enamel.

10.1.4 Abfraction

Non-carious loss of tooth structure has been attributed to three factors - abrasion, attrition and erosion, acting independently or together, but the cause of non-carious cervical lesions (NCCL) has been the subject of interest and debate for almost a century. Traditionally, the pathogenesis of the class V NCCL has been associated with abrasion or erosion. NCCL have been considered to be increasing in prevalence and incidence, with reports of their prevalence in varying patient and population groups ranging from 27% to 85%. NCCL have been considered to be more prevalent in older patients and gender differences have also been reported. As tooth substance loss (TSL) from erosion is a result of dissolution, it would be expected that lesions resulting from erosion would be rounded and smooth, with the TSL occurring over a wide area. However, NCCL may be wedge-shaped and limited to the cervical area of the tooth and this would tend to indicate that other factors are involved in the pathogenesis of NCCL. It has been suggested that tensile stresses resulting from occlusal overload may be involved — the so-called 'occlusal' theory for the pathogenesis of NCCL. These bending stresses may cause disruption of the surface enamel in the cervical area, resulting in increased susceptibility to dissolution and abrasion at the affected sites and in the development of wedge-shaped lesions. These NCCL have also been termed *abfractions*, this being an engineering term relating to stress corrosion and derived from the Latin 'to break away'.

In support of the occlusal theory of NCCL are the following:

- Class V non-carious lesions are seen in teeth while adjacent teeth (not subjected to lateral forces) are unaffected;
- The lesions progress around restorations;
- The lesions are rarely seen on the lingual aspect of lower teeth;
- The lesions may be subgingival;
- The lesions may be seen in animals.

Increasingly, therefore, tooth flexure is becoming accepted as a mechanism for the loss of dental hard tissue, although this is the least studied of the processes thought to cause TSL.

Other alternative etiological hypotheses for NCCL have been suggested:

- A high mucin content in saliva may prevent the precipitation of calcium phosphate which repairs minor injuries to enamel;
- Abrasion from hyperactive oral soft tissues;
- Piezoelectric effects have been implicated in the development of NCCL.

It is therefore apparent that the material chosen for the restoration of an NCCL will have to withstand the bending forces that may be present in situations of occlusal overload. That is, the bonding system and/or material employed should be of sufficiently low modulus so as not to be affected by these forces.

10.1.5 Dental caries

The total number of bacteria in the mouth has been estimated at one thousand billion (10^{12}). In health, there is equilibrium between the growth of bacteria and the host-defense mechanisms. Most of the normal bacteriological flora grow at a neutral pH, but as a result of the action of some bacteria present in plaque on fermentable carbohydrates in the diet, the ecological balance may be altered to an acidic pH and demineralization of mineralized tissues may occur. Indeed, a fall to below pH of 5 may occur in less than three minutes. This is the commencement of the process of dental caries (Figure 10.1). Repeated acid attacks may result in demineralization at a susceptible site on the tooth surface, and, ultimately, progression of the carious lesion into dentin, bacterial invasion of the pulp and its subsequent death. Not all carbohydrates are equally cariogenic. High molecular weight, complex carbohydrates such as starch are not cariogenic because they are not easily digested in the mouth, but low molecular weight carbohydrates, such as sugars, may diffuse easily into plaque and be rapidly metabolized by plaque bacteria. Sucrose is the most cariogenic sugar although glucose, lactose and fructose may also be involved. Repeated consumption of sugar will lower the plaque pH and eventually cause demineralization of teeth at a susceptible site in a susceptible patient. Susceptible sites include pits and fissures in molars and premolars, approximal smooth surfaces just apical to the contact area and the area adjacent to the cervical margin. Particular organisms involved in the carious process include mutans streptococci and lactobacilli, as these organisms can readily produce acid from fermentable carbohydrates.

The ideal restorative material must be capable of withstanding attack by microorganisms and acids at the levels of pH that may occur in the mouth. Alternatively, a 'smart' restorative material could release a caries-inhibiting substance such as fluoride when the surrounding pH falls below a certain value.

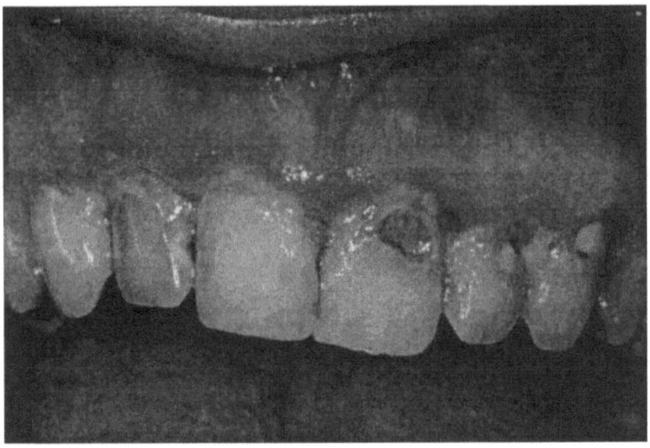

Figure 10.1. Dental caries.

10.1.6 Trauma

Trauma is a common cause of loss of tooth tissue, either directly or by traumatic occlusal forces that cause TSL or by fracture of teeth weakened by caries or restorations. Ideally restorative materials should be capable of resisting fracture or should be capable of restoring tooth fracture resistance if bonded in place. However, an alternative strategy exists, namely, that a restoration should be capable of fracturing in such a manner that the remaining tooth structure is easily restored. That is, the restoration 'protects' tooth structure and acts as a 'failsafe' mechanism, rather than fracturing synergistically with the tooth in such a way that the tooth may be rendered unrestorable.

10.2 DISCOLORATION

Tooth color results from intrinsic pigmentation that is naturally/genetically controlled. Intrinsic tooth discoloration may result from substances or medications ingested during the time of tooth formation. Most common examples are:

- Brown discoloration or mottling, due to excess intake of fluoride;
- Yellow/gray discoloration which may result from administration of tetracycline;
- Pink discoloration from porphyria.

In such instances the discoloration is intrinsic, that is, it cannot be polished off the tooth surface.

Extrinsic staining may also cause tooth discoloration due to deposition of stains on the tooth surface from, for example, tobacco or dyes from foodstuffs. Additionally, the oral microflora may contain *chromogenic* (pigment producing) microorganisms which may cause black, brown, green or yellow/orange stains which are easily removed by prophylaxis.

Restorative materials may also discolor intrinsically as a result of chemical changes occurring following initial set, but this is an undesirable factor that has largely been overcome in modern materials. Restorative materials, ideally, should have a surface morphology that resists the accumulation of extrinsic stains.

FURTHER READING

Dahl B L, Carlsson G E, Ekfeldt A (1993). Occlusal wear of teeth and restorative materials. A review of classification, etiology, mechanisms of wear and some aspects of restorative procedures. *Acta.Odontologica Scandinavica* **51:** 299-311.

Lee W C Eakle W S (1984). Possible role of tensile stress in the etiology of cervical erosive lesions in teeth. *Journal of Prosthetic Dentistry* **52:** 374-380.

Levitch L C. Bader J D, Shugars D A, Heymann H O (1994). Non-carious cervical lesions. *Journal of Dentistry* **22:** 195-207.

Kidd E A M, Joyston-Bechal S (1997). *Essentials of Dental Caries.* Oxford University Press, Oxford.

IV

MATERIALS SCIENCE BACKGROUND

Chapter 11

Polymers

Summary: An account is given of the chemistry, structure and properties of polymers of dental interest.

Dental Significance: Polymers are widely used as constituents of dental restorative, prosthodontic and impression materials.

11.1 INTRODUCTION

Polymers are long chain molecules, consisting of many repeating units. A *monomer* is the smallest repeating unit in the polymer chain. A polymer or polymer intermediate with relatively few structural units is called an *oligomer*. *Polymerization* is the reaction by which polymers are prepared from monomers. In most polymers, the chain is made up of covalently linked carbon atoms. Inorganic chains are also possible, composed of alternating silicon and oxygen atoms; these are silicones or polysiloxanes.

Many polymers are naturally occurring, some of which find dental application. These include:

- Proteins (or polyamides or polypeptides), containing an amide or peptide link, as in Figure 11.1;

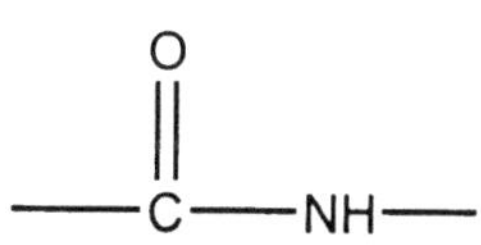

Figure 11.1. Amide or peptide link.

- Polyisoprenes, such as the isomers rubber and gutta percha;
- Polysaccharides, e.g. starch, cellulose, agar and alginates.

Many synthetic polymers are produced industrially, or in the laboratory, by chemical reactions. Many such materials have become familiar to everyone, for example 'Bakelite', 'Nylon', 'Terylene', 'Polythene', 'Perspex', poly(vinyl chloride). Not surprisingly, many of these have been used for dentures, and in other dental applications. In this chapter we are primarily concerned with synthetic polymers (including some inorganic materials), the reactions by which they can be made, how they are molded, and their structure and properties.

There are two types of chemical reaction, which result in polymers of dental interest — namely, condensation reactions and addition reactions. Each is considered in turn.

11.2 CONDENSATION REACTIONS

A *condensation reaction* is defined as a reaction between two molecules to form a larger molecule, with the elimination of a smaller molecule, which is often, but not always, water. Some well-known examples are listed.

1. Nylon. An organic acid (with a -COOH group) can react under appropriate conditions with an amine (with a $-NH_2$ group), to give a material with an amide linkage (as in proteins, see above). Figure 11.2 shows such a reaction. When a di-functional acid (with 2 -COOH groups) reacts with a di-amine (2 $-NH_2$ groups), the reaction continues in a stepwise manner to yield a polymer, called nylon.

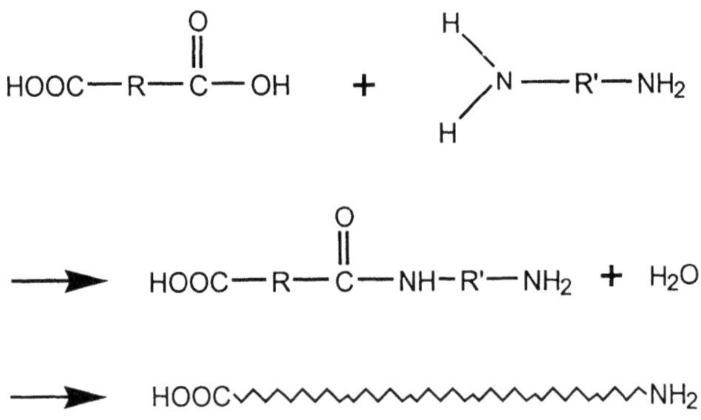

Figure 11.2. Formation of nylon.

2. Phenol can react with formaldehyde to give molecules with a complex three-dimensional network - this is the basis of 'Bakelite' polymers.
3. Polycarbonates, which are high impact resistant materials, are formed by condensation reactions.
4. Polysulfides, the basic constituents of some synthetic rubber materials, are formed as shown in Figure 11.3.

Figure 11.3. Formation of polysulfides.

5. Silicones or siloxanes are formed by the condensation of silanols, to give a chain of alternating silicon and oxygen atoms (Figure 11.4).

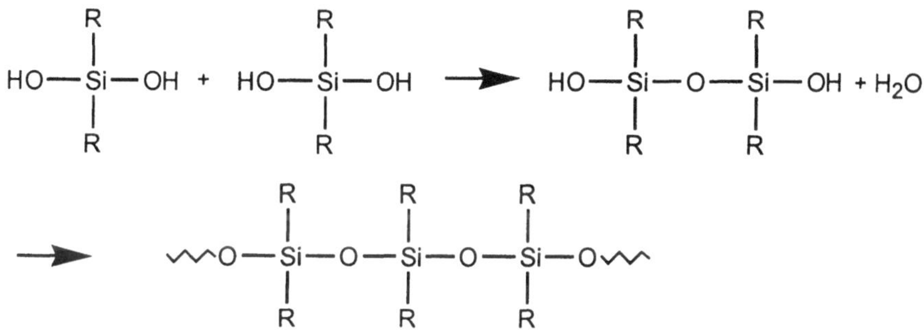

Figure 11.4. Condensation of silanols to give a silicone polymer.

11.3 FREE RADICAL ADDITION REACTIONS

An *addition reaction* occurs between two molecules (either the same or dissimilar) to give a larger molecule without the elimination of a smaller molecule such as water. Addition reactions that form polymers can be classified as free radical reactions and ionic reactions.

Free radical addition reactions take place for *vinyl compounds* - these are reactive organic compounds containing carbon-carbon double bonds. Some examples are listed in Figure 11.5. There are a number of stages in such polymerization reactions – namely: activation, initiation, propagation and termination.

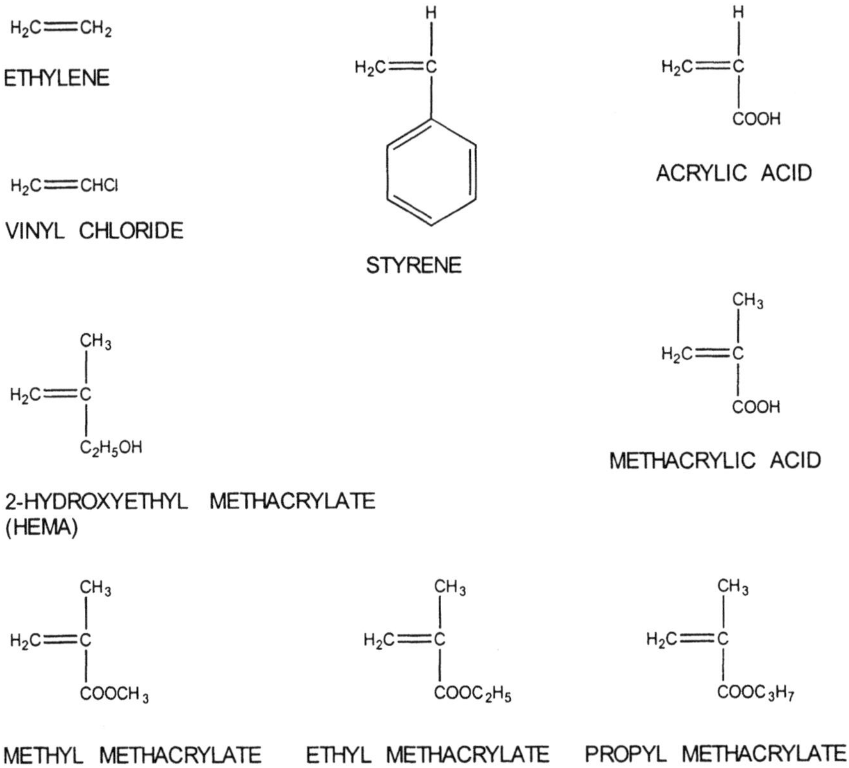

Figure 11.5. Vinyl monomers.

11.3.1 Activation and initiation

The polymerization of a vinyl compound requires the presence of free radicals - these are very reactive chemical species having an odd (unpaired) electron. Such free radicals are formed, for example, in the decomposition of a peroxide. Thus under appropriate conditions, a molecule of benzoyl peroxide can yield two free radicals (Figure 11.6). Such chemical species are able to initiate vinyl polymerization; they will be designated R•.

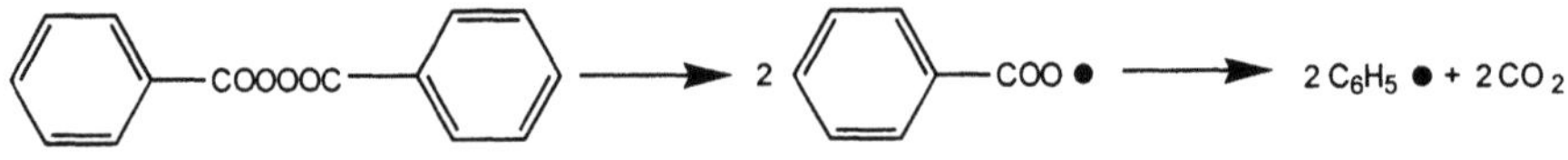

Figure 11.6. Decomposition of benzoyl peroxide to give two free radicals.

Before initiation occurs, however, the initiator requires to be activated. Activation can be achieved by decomposition of the peroxide by an energy source. This may be ultra-violet light, visible light or other electromagnetic radiation such as γ-rays. Visible light curing is often used in conjunction with polymer-containing tooth filling materials. Alternatively heat may be used to break down a peroxide, as in denture base resin materials. Chemicals, such as tertiary amines (Figure 11.7) are also activators for the polymerization reaction.

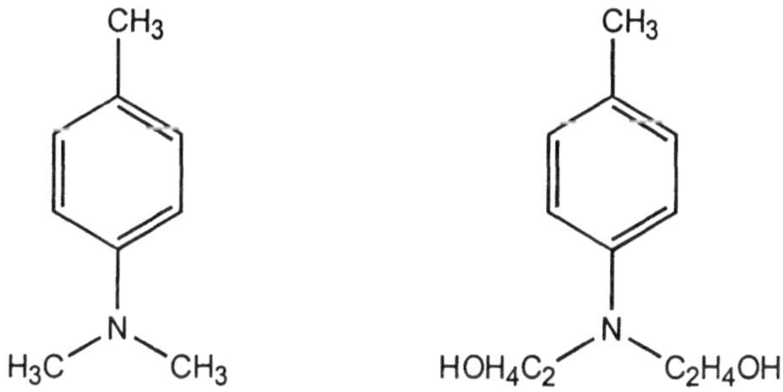

(A) (B)

Figure 11.7. Tertiary amine activators: (A) N,N-dimethyl-*p*-toluidine; (B) N,N-dihydroxyethyl-*p*-toluidine.

11.3.2 Propagation

Free radicals can react with monomer as follows to form a larger free radical (Figure 11.8).

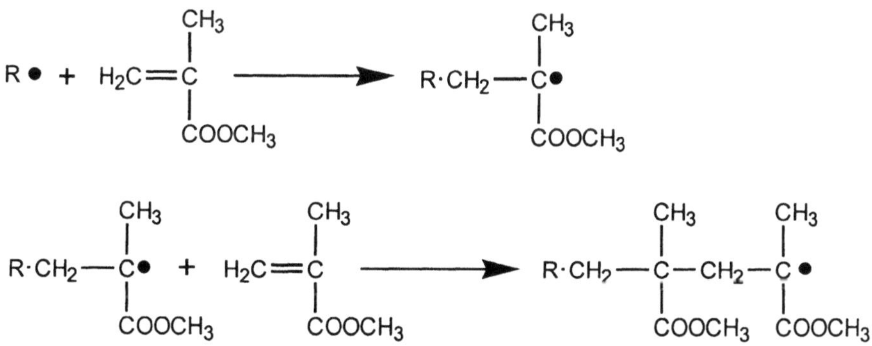

Figure 11.8. Propagation of free radical polymerization of methyl methacrylate.

This can be presented in simplified form, where M represents a monomer molecule:

$$R\bullet + M \longrightarrow R\text{-}M\bullet$$

$$R\text{-}M\bullet + M \longrightarrow R\text{-}M\text{-}M\bullet \quad \text{etc.}$$

Thus the reaction proceeds, leading to the formation of a polymer chain.

11.3.3 Termination

This occurs when two free radicals react to form a stable molecule, or by a transfer process. In simplified form these reactions may be represented as:

$$R\text{-}M_n\text{-}M\bullet + R\bullet \longrightarrow R\text{-}M_{n+1}\text{-}R$$

and:

$$R\text{-}M_n\text{-}M\bullet + RH \longrightarrow R\text{-}M_{n+1}\text{-}H + R\bullet$$

11.4 IONIC ADDITION REACTIONS

As stated above, polymerization can occur by ionic as well as by free radical mechanisms.

1. Anionic polymerization. An example of this is the polymerization of cyanoacrylates (Figure 11.9). An anion adds on to a monomer to form a larger anion, and thus the reaction propagates in an analogous fashion to the free radical reactions described above.

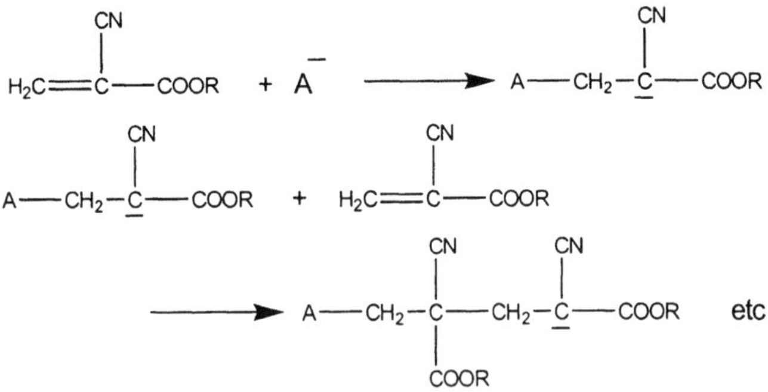

Figure 11.9. Anionic addition polymerization of a cyanoacrylate, where R may be methyl, ethyl, propyl or butyl and A^- may be OH^-, for example.

2. Cationic polymerization. Similarly, cationic reactions can lead to the formation of polymers. An example of this is an epimine compound (a compound with a 3-member ring containing nitrogen, Figure 11.10A which can react with a benzene sulfonate ester (Figure 11.10B) that can supply cations to give a ring-opening reaction (Figure 11.11).

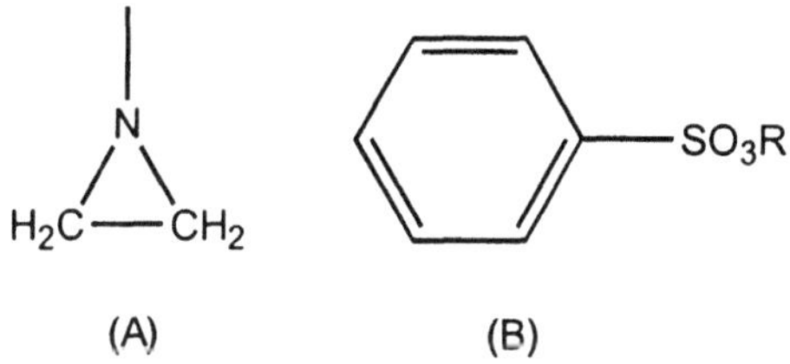

Figure 11.10. (A) Three membered ring containing nitrogen - an epimine compound; (B) benzene sulfonate ester.

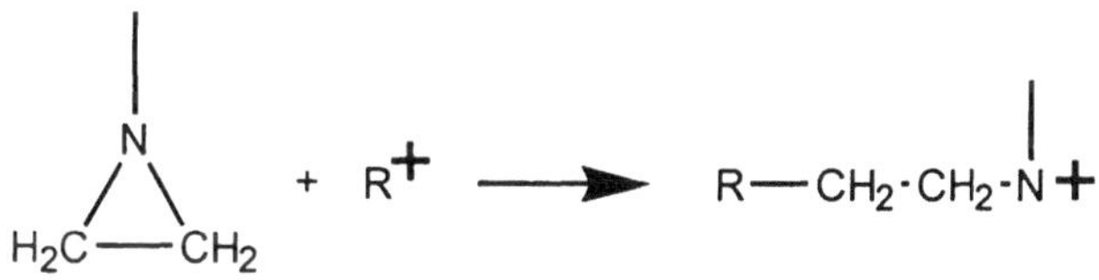

Figure 11.11. Cationic ring opening of an epimine.

11.5 POLYMER STRUCTURE AND PROPERTIES

11.5.1 Degree of polymerization and molecular weight

The *degree of polymerization* may be defined as the number of repeating units in a polymer, i.e. the number of monomer units joined together. The *molecular weight* is equal to the degree of polymerization multiplied by the molecular weight of the repeating units.

It should be noted that the growth of polymer chains is a random process - some chains grow faster than others do, some are terminated before others. Thus not all chains have the same length - that is, they have a distribution of molecular weights. The quoted molecular weight for a polymer is an average value.

11.5.2 Effect of molecular weight on properties

In many polymers the chains are held together by secondary, or Van der Waals forces, and molecular entanglement. Materials of high molecular weight have a greater degree of molecular entanglement, and have greater rigidity and strength and higher values of glass transition temperature (T_g - see below) and melting temperature than low molecular weight polymers.

11.5.3 Physical state

In terms of physical state, polymers exist as:

- Elastomers or rubbers;
- Hard amorphous polymers (organic glasses), for example, poly(methyl methacrylate);
- Hard partially crystalline polymers, for example, poly(ethylene);
- Fibers; for example, nylon can exist in this form.

The first two of the above are considered here, as they are the most relevant to dentistry. Rubbers consist of long chain molecules that are coiled and in random thermal motion. These molecules may be linked on to one another at relatively isolated points by covalent bonds (cross-linking). The specific feature of a rubbery polymer is that when the material is stretched the only work done is in uncoiling the molecules. Thus such materials are easy to deform, the deformation being largely reversible.

Although these materials are rubbery at room temperature, the effect of intermolecular forces will increase as temperature decreases, and at a reasonably well defined temperature (T_g, the *glass transition temperature*) the forces become so large as to inhibit uncoiling. Below the glass transition temperature the material will therefore be rigid.

If a rigid polymer is heated, it loses rigidity at a well-defined temperature above room temperature, and to become rubbery. In fact the difference between flexible and rigid polymers is that the former have a T_g well below room temperature, whereas the T_g of the latter is above room temperature. This is an important concept in prosthodontics, where a denture base needs to be rigid (high T_g), but may have a soft lining material, the T_g of which must be below mouth temperature (Chapter 46).

11.5.4 Cross-linking

Many reactions can be used to prepare polymers with chemical bonds between different chains. These materials are said to be *cross-linked.*

Some condensation polymers, such as phenol-formaldehyde are extensively cross-linked.

Dimethacrylate compounds can undergo similar free-radical addition reactions to methyl methacrylate, and are widely used in resin composite tooth restorative materials. These dimethacrylates may be aliphatic, such as triethylene glycol dimethacrylate (Figure 11.12), or aromatic, such as a compound known as Bis-GMA or Bowen's resin (Figure 11.13). Urethane dimethacrylates are also used dentally (Figure 11.14).

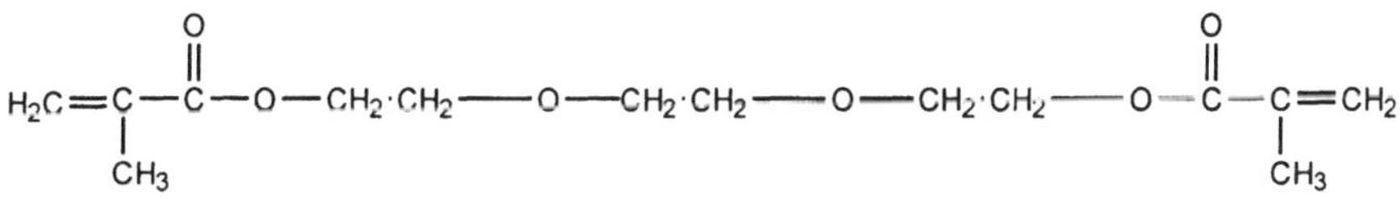

Figure 11.12. Triethylene glycol dimethacrylate.

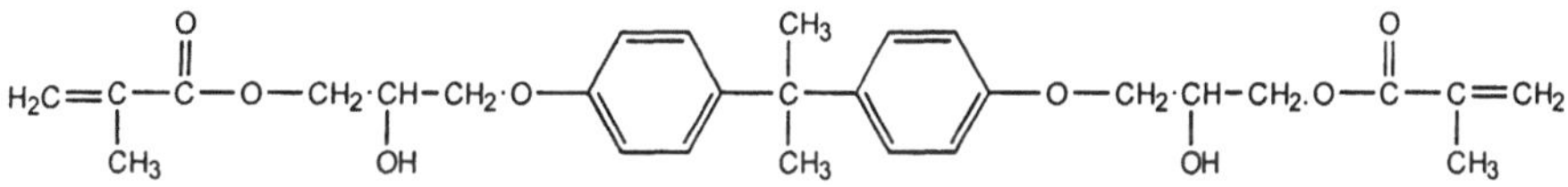

Figure 11.13. 2,2-bis[4(2-hydroxy-3-methacryloyloxy-propyloxy)-phenyl] propane. This is often referred to as Bis-GMA or Bowen's resin, and is a constituent of many resin-based filling materials and sealants.

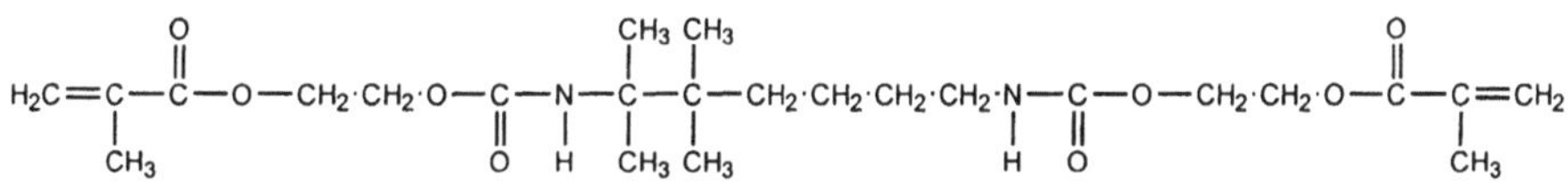

Figure 11.14. A urethane dimethacrylate.

Compounds with two epimine groups can be cross-linked by a benzene sulfonate ester (Section 11.4).

Elastomers are also cross-linked, and this is important for an understanding of elastomeric impression materials (Chapter 33).

Cross-linking affects the physical properties of a polymer. A small degree of cross-linking limits the amount of movement of the polymer chains relative to each other when the material is stressed. Thus the deformation is elastic rather than plastic. Also, the polymer may have a higher value of T_g. Extensively cross-linked polymers are harder, more brittle and more resistant to the action of solvents than non-cross-linked materials.

11.5.5 Plasticizers

Liquids are able to penetrate between the randomly orientated chains of a polymer. As a result the molecules are further apart, and the forces between them are less. Such liquids are *plasticizers*. They soften the material and make it more flexible by lowering its T_g. If sufficient plasticizer is added, a polymer, which is normally glassy at room temperature, can have its T_g depressed to below room temperature, thus making it flexible and rubbery. This principle is used in producing acrylic soft lining materials (Chapter 46).

11.5.6 Co-polymers

Polymer chains, which contain two or more different types of monomeric units, can be prepared - these are termed *co-polymers*. Several types of co-polymer are possible, including alternating, random, block and graft co-polymers (Figure 11.15). Co-polymerization processes have enabled chemists to 'tailor-make' molecules of predicted properties for special applications.

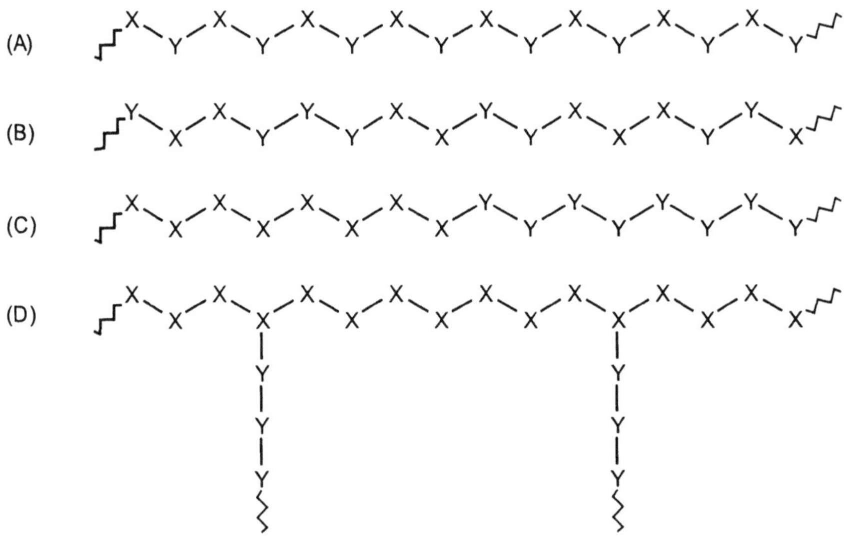

Figure 11.15. Co-polymers: (A) alternating; (B) random; (C) block; (D) graft co-polymers, where X and Y represent different monomer groups.

11.5.7 Viscoelasticity

Polymers show viscoelastic behavior. Models for this are discussed in Chapter 5. Elastic behavior (similar to that of a spring) is caused by uncoiling of the polymer molecules. Plastic behavior (equivalent to a dashpot) is caused by breaking of intermolecular Van der Waals forces. When a load is removed from a polymer, there is some instant elastic recovery with recoiling of the molecules, followed by some slow recovery during which the intermolecular bonds reform.

11.6 METHODS OF FABRICATING POLYMERS

11.6.1 Condensation polymers

When these were used dentally, they were supplied in an intermediate stage of condensation, and molded by the application of heat and pressure to the required shape; during this process the condensation reaction continued.

11.6.2 Compression molding

The products of addition polymerization are usually *thermoplastic*; that is, they soften on heating and harden on cooling, without chemical change, (contrast to *thermosetting* polymers, which do not soften, but burn or decompose on heating). Thermoplastic polymers can be molded by the application of heat and pressure.

11.6.3 Injection molding

Industrially, thermoplastic materials are often molded by heating the polymer until it is soft enough to be injected into a mold of the required shape. This method is used dentally, though not frequently, for example, for polycarbonates.

11.6.4 Dough technique

This method is widely used dentally in the molding of poly(methyl methacrylate) for dentures. A dough is formed from a mixture of the monomer (liquid) and polymer (powder); this is packed into a mold and the monomer is polymerized under the appropriate conditions of activation and initiation to give a solid material.

11.7 SUMMARY OF DENTAL APPLICATIONS

Tables 11.1 and 11.2 give a summary of the main applications of polymers in dentistry, with the main chapter references where the materials are discussed.

Table 11.1. Summary of applications of naturally occurring polymers

Classification	Application	Chapter
Polyisoprene	Gutta percha is a constituent of root canal filling materials	29
Polysaccharide	Agar is used in reversible hydrocolloid impression materials	32
Polysaccharide	Alginic acid salts are constituents of irreversible hydrocolloid impression materials	32

Table 11.2. Summary of applications of synthetic polymers

Classification	Type	Application	Chapter
Hard	Methacrylates	Denture materials	45
Polymers	Dimethacrylates	Fissure sealants	19
		Components of resin composite dental restorative materials	27
Flexible	Silicones	Elastomeric impression materials	33
Polymers	Silicones	Denture soft lining materials	46
	Polysulfides	Elastomeric impression materials	33
	Polyethers	Elastomeric impression materials	33
	Poly(vinyl acetate)	Mouth guards	42
Water-soluble	Poly(acrylic acid) and related co-polymers	Adhesive dental cements – zinc polycarboxylate and glass-ionomer cements	25,26

FURTHER READING

Horath L (1995). *Fundamentals of Materials Science for Technologists.* Prentice Hall, Englewood Cliffs, New Jersey, pp 82-122.

Chapter 12

Metals

Summary: This is an introduction to metals, including a discussion of the relationship between structure and properties.

Dental significance: This chapter forms a basis of understanding of alloys (mixtures of metals) which are widely used in dentistry, and are discussed in Chapter 13.

12.1 DESCRIPTION AND DEFINITION

Most metals have the following properties: they are usually hard, lustrous, dense, good conductors of heat and electricity, opaque, ductile and malleable. Of over 100 elements in the periodic table, some 68 are metals. A further 8 elements are *metalloids* (for example, silicon, arsenic and boron) which exhibit both metallic and non-metallic behavior. All the remaining elements are non-metals. An essential feature of a metal is that it is electropositive; that is, it gives positive ions in solution. An *alloy* is a mixture of metals. In this chapter there is a discussion of the structure and properties of metals. Chapter 13 deals with the nature of alloys and discusses some alloy systems of dental interest.

12.2 FORMING AND SHAPING

12.2.1 Casting

This involves melting the metal or alloy and shaping it in a mold. For example, steel, bronze, aluminum, etc. can be poured into molds of sand and clay. The clay bonds the sand together. Such molds are destroyed after use. Die-casting uses permanent metal molds. In dentistry investment casting is very important where an investment mold is made from a wax pattern; the principles of this are discussed in Chapter 54.

12.2.2 Cold working

In general, metals can be hammered into a sheet, extruded, or rolled. They can be pulled through dies to form wires (Figure 12.1).

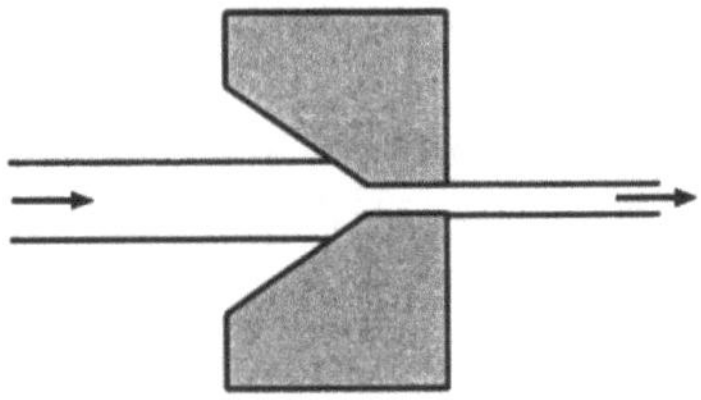

Figure 12.1. Drawing a wire through a die.

12.2.3 Powder metallurgy

A metal powder can be pressed under high pressure to produce a formed object. The product of this process is weak, as there is little adhesion between the particles. Improved strength results on sintering, in which the pressing is heated in a non-oxidizing atmosphere below the melting point, and the particles agglomerate. This technique is used to make tungsten carbide burs for cutting tooth tissue.

12.2.4 Electroforming

Using the process of electrolysis, a metal can be plated on to a conducting surface. This technique may be used for the production of dies (Section 51.3).

12.3 THE NATURE OF METALLIC BONDING

An atom of a metal can easily lose some of its outer shell electrons to give a positive ion. A solid metal may be pictured as consisting of positive ions, held together by a 'cloud' of free electrons (Figure 12.2). This gives a ready explanation for some of the characteristic properties. Electrical and thermal conductivity are due to the mobility of the free electrons to move rapidly through the metal. Metals are opaque because the free electrons oscillate and absorb the electromagnetic energy of light. Mixtures of metals to form *alloys* can readily be formed because the atoms of different metals and held together by a common cloud of free electrons.

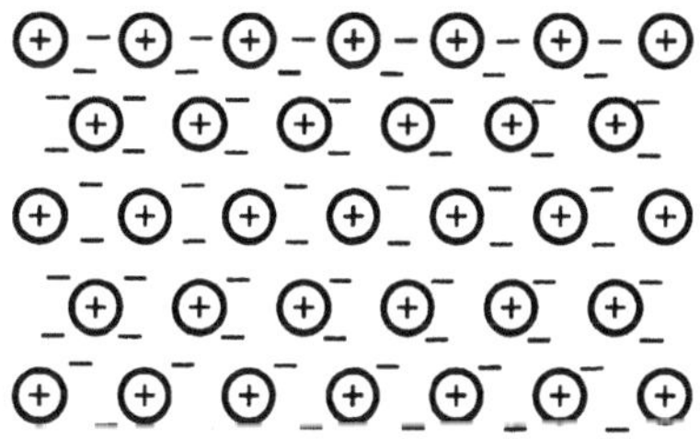

Figure 12.2 Diagrammatic representation of metallic bonding.

12.4 SPACING OF ATOMS

Two factors influence the distance between atoms in a solid (Figure 12.3):

- Forces of attraction, due to inter-atomic bonding;
- Repulsive forces occur between the electrons of neighboring atoms; these forces increase rapidly with decreasing inter-atomic distance.

When two atoms are spaced such that these forces are equal and opposite, the atoms are in their equilibrium position. Application of an external force to a solid can displace atoms from this position. At the equilibrium position, the potential energy of the system is at a minimum.

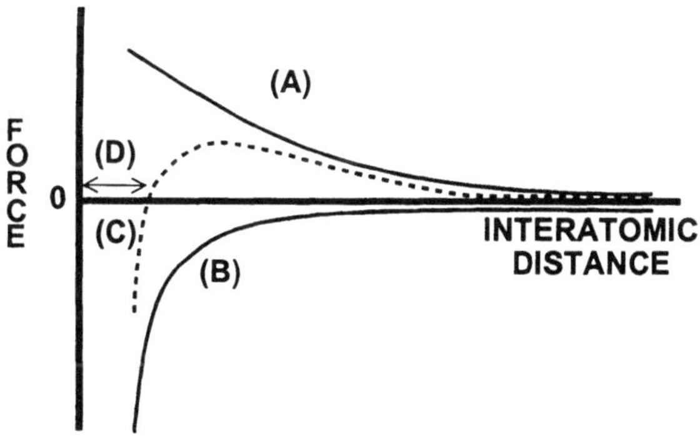

Figure12.3 Factors influencing the distance between atoms in a solid: (A) forces of attraction; (B) forces of repulsion; (C) resultant force, the sum of (A) and (B); (D) equilibrium interatomic distance.

12.5 CRYSTALLINE SOLIDS

In many solids, the constituent atoms are regularly arranged in a crystal lattice. This is true in general of metals (and also of some materials with ionic bonding such as NaCl and covalent bonding such as diamond.)

12.5.1 Types of crystal lattice

Different configurations of crystal lattices are possible, the simplest way to study these is to consider a *unit cell* - this is defined as the smallest repeating unit that is contained in a crystal. There are some 14 different possible crystal lattices; only three of dental interest are considered here:

1. Body centered cubic (b.c.c.), as in some metals, e.g. iron below 910°C. Figure 12.4 shows the unit cell, with an atom at each corner of the cube, and one in the center.
2. Face centered cube (f.c.c.), as in gold, silver, copper, platinum, and palladium; also iron above 910°C. The unit cell is a cube with an atom at each of the eight corners, and one in the center of each of the six faces, but none in the center of the cube (Figure 12.5).
3. Hexagonal close packed structure (h.c.p.), as in zinc and magnesium. This is depicted in Figure 12.6.

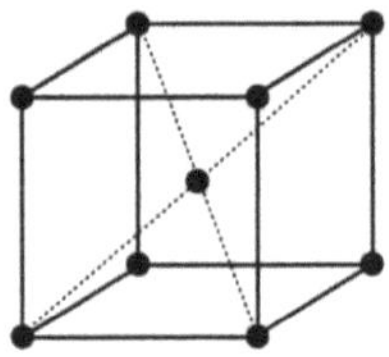

Figure 12.4 Unit cell of a body centered cubic (b.c.c.) crystal lattice.

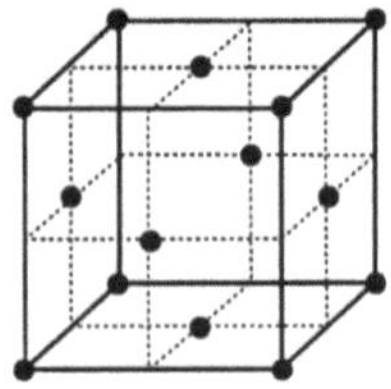

Figure 12.5. Unit cell of a face centered cubic (f.c.c.) crystal lattice.

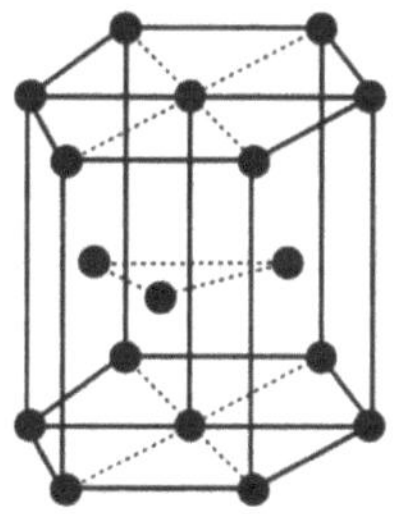

Figure 12.6. Unit cell of a hexagonal close packed structure (h.c.p.).

12.5.2 Crystal imperfections

Dental significance: Imperfections in the crystal structure of a metallic material have a significant effect on mechanical properties – for example, they can facilitate permanent (plastic) deformation.

The above are structures of ideal crystals. In practice imperfections occur, which have a considerable effect on the properties of a material. There are a number of possibilities:

1. Point defects. These include impurities, which can cause distortion of the crystal lattice (Figure 12.7). Vacancies can also occur, again leading to distortion (Figure 12.8). Vacancies provide the means whereby atoms can move in a crystal, hence solid state diffusion.

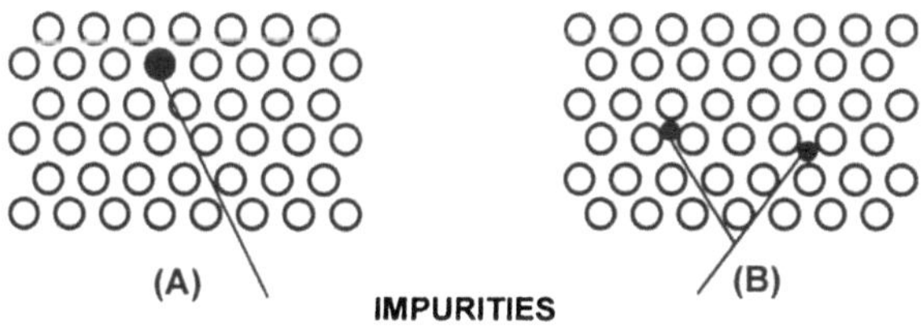

Figure 12.7. Two-dimensional representation of impurities in a crystal: (A) impurity substituted in crystal lattice; (B) impurities in interstitial positions.

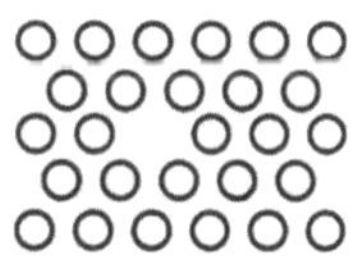

Figure 12.8. Two-dimensional representation of vacancies a crystal lattice.

2. Line defects. Dislocations can occur in a crystal lattice (Figure 12.9). These contribute to the liability of ceramic materials to fracture (Section 15.4.3). Plastic deformation in metals occurs by motion of dislocations (Section 12.7.2). Crystalline materials with few flaws and dislocations can be extremely strong.

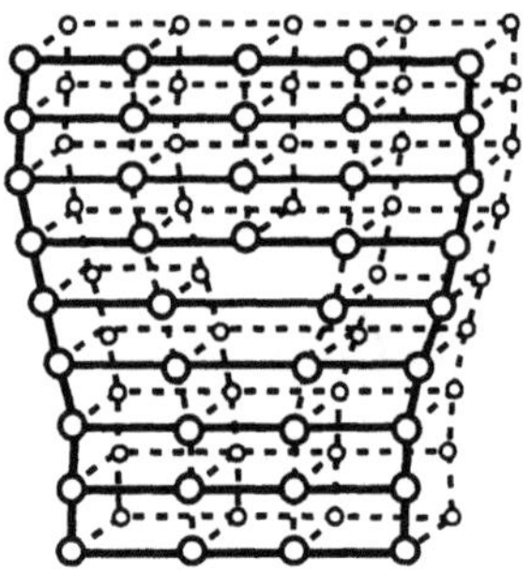

Figure 12.9. A dislocation in a crystal.

3. Planar defects. As will be shown, metals have a granular structure, and the boundaries between grains constitute planar defects.

12.6 COOLING OF A MOLTEN METAL

On cooling a pure molten metal, a temperature-time curve of the type shown in Figure 12.10 is obtained. This graph shows three portions:

- The cooling of the molten liquid (A);
- A plateau - a horizontal portion - during this time the metal is solidifying and there is evolution of latent heat of fusion which compensates for the heat loss to the surroundings (B);
- The cooling of the completely solidified metal (C).

Solidification starts at centers of crystallization called nuclei. Some of these nuclei may be impurities that exist even in a 'pure' metal, scattered throughout the material. Growth of crystals from nuclei occurs in three dimensions, in the form of dendrites or branched structures (Figure 12.11A). Growth continues until contact is made with adjacent growing crystals and solidification is complete when the pools of liquid between the dendrite arms have crystallized. Each nucleus gives rise via dendrites to one crystal or grain.

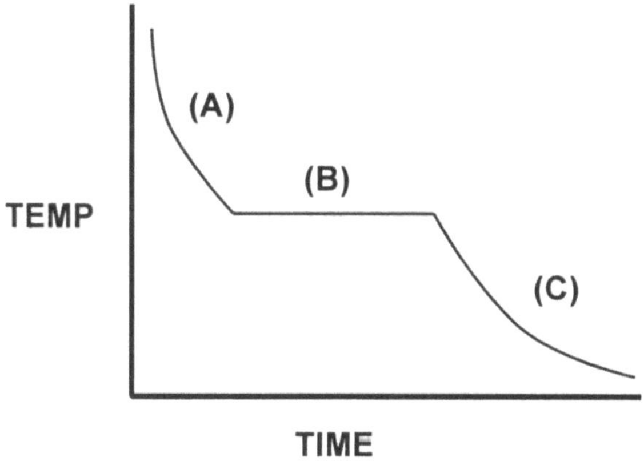

Figure 12.10. Temperature-time curve for cooling of a molten metal. (A) Cooling of the molten metal; (B) solidification of the metal; (C) cooling of solidified material.

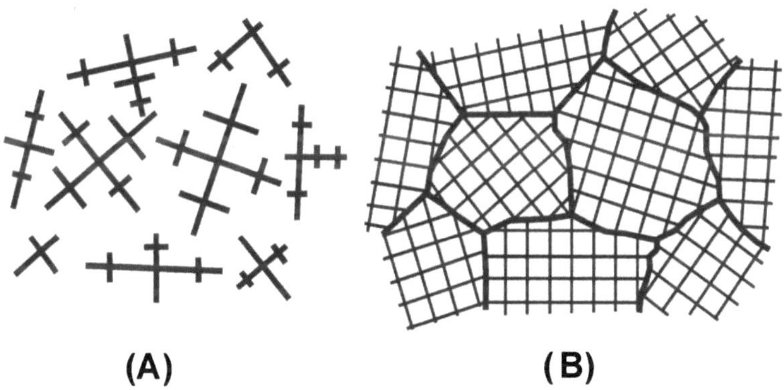

Figure 12.11. Two dimensional representation of dendritic growth.

Each crystal of a metal is termed a *grain*. Each grain has grown from a nucleus. Within each grain, the orientation of the crystal lattice and the crystal planes is uniform. Adjacent grains have different orientations, because the initial nuclei acted independently from each other (See Figure 12.11B). Thus at the grain boundary — a narrow region 2 to 3 atomic diameters wide, the atoms take up positions intermediate between those of the atoms in the adjacent crystal lattices.

12.7 RELATIONSHIP OF MICROSTRUCTURE TO MECHANICAL PROPERTIES

12.7.1 Elastic strain

Elastic strain in a metal is mainly due to a stretching of the inter-atomic bonds. The modulus of elasticity is determined by the chemical composition, and is scarcely affected by microstructure.

12.7.2 Plastic deformation

Plastic deformation involves the slip of layers of atoms over each other. Slip does not occur by the movement (or shear) of an entire plane of atoms over the next layer in a single movement - this would require an enormous stress. Instead, the slip occurs by a localized region of shear, which passes progressively through the length of the slip plane. This localized shear zone is called a dislocation (Figure. 12.9).

In general, pure metals are very ductile, because each grain has many different slip planes in various directions. Dislocation movement is easy in metals because of the nature of metallic bonding. In contrast to this, dislocations are much less mobile in non-metallic crystals.

The proportional limit, or yield stress, is a measure of the ease with which dislocations can move in a metal. The yield stress of a pure single crystal of a metal is low, but may be raised by obstructing the movement of dislocations. This may be achieved by in a number of ways.

1. Grain boundaries hinder the movement of dislocations. Thus a polycrystalline metal will have a higher yield stress than a single crystal. The yield stress is higher for a material of finer grain size, which has more grain boundaries.
2. If a metal is cold worked, large numbers of dislocations accumulate internally. As a result, there is an increase in hardness and yield stress — hence the phenomenon of *work hardening*.
3. Mixing metals to form alloys can also lead to materials of higher yield stress (Chapter 13).

In general, obstruction of the movement of dislocations results not only in an increase in yield stress and hardness, but also in a lowering of ductility and impact resistance.

12.8 FACTORS AFFECTING GRAIN SIZE AND STRUCTURE

Dental significance: The properties of a metallic material depend on (i) its composition, (ii) its mechanical history and (iii) its thermal history.

12.8.1 Rate of cooling

Slow cooling results in the formation of a coarse grain structure, whereas rapid cooling usually gives a fine structure. Rapid cooling produces more nuclei of crystallization; thus there are more grains in a given volume of material, so that each grain is smaller. The structures in Figure 12.12 are equiaxed - that is, the grains are not elongated (compare Figure. 12.13).

Rapid cooling of a molten metal is obtained in the following cases - when a mold of high thermal conductivity is used, if the bulk of the casting is small, and if the metal has been heated to only just above its fusion temperature.

After solidification the metal can then be cooled either slowly in air, or rapidly by quenching it in a cooling liquid such as water or oil.

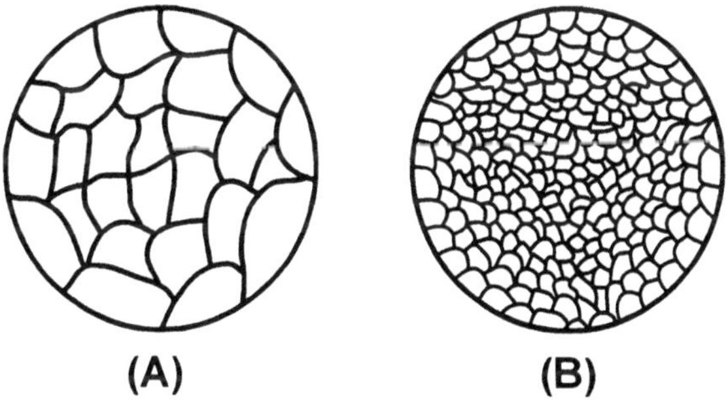

Figure 12.12. Grain structures: (A) coarse equiaxed structures (B) fine equiaxed structures.

12.8.2 Nucleating agents

Either impurities or additives can act as nucleating agents, so refining the grain structure.

12.8.3 Cold working

Hammering, rolling or drawing into a wire transforms the equiaxed structure into a fibrous structure (Figure 12.13)

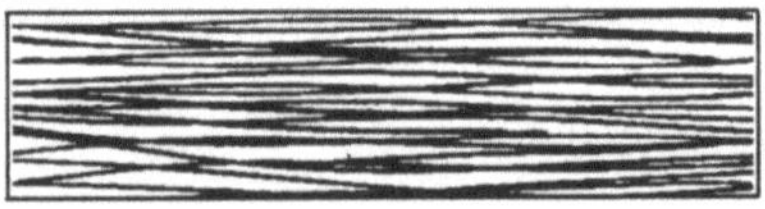

Figure 12.13. Fibrous grain structure of wire.

12.8.4 Stress relief anneal (recovery)

After cold working, there are internal stresses in a metal - these can cause cracking or distortion. A *stress relief anneal* can overcome these - it is a low temperature heat treatment which has little effect on the fibrous grain structure.

12.8.5 Recrystallization

Further heating of a cold worked materials can alter its grain structure, the new structure consisting of small equiaxed grains. In this case the metal is said to have been *recrystallized.* The *recrystallization temperature* is that temperature at or above which a metal will recrystallize rapidly. *Cold working* is defined as working below this temperature.

12.8.6 Grain growth

If a metal is overheated, or heated for too long during recrystallization, grain growth occurs. This results in a material of coarser grain structure.

Both grain growth and recrystallization occur by means of diffusion or movement of the metal atoms across grain boundaries.

12.8.7 Practical points

On the basis of the above discussion, a number of general practical points are important. Cooling a molten metal should be done rapidly, to get a fine grain structure, if strength and hardness are important. Cold working increases hardness and strength; this is known as *work hardening.* However, this reduces the percentage elongation, so the material becomes more brittle. It becomes liable to fracture if further cold work is carried out, because the potential for further slip has been lost. The internal stresses of a cold worked metal can be removed by a heat treatment at a temperature well below the recrystallization temperature. Recrystallization gives a fine grain structure. Sometimes cold working followed by heat treatment is used to obtain a fine structure, to improve the properties of the material. Overheating, causing grain growth must be avoided if properties such as high yield stress and hardness are desired.

12.9 APPLICATIONS OF METALS

There are very few applications for pure metals in dentistry. Some exceptions to this are:

- The use of pure gold for tooth restoration (Section 13.5.1);
- The application of platinum foil in laboratory procedures with dental porcelain (Sections 34.4.6 and 36.6);
- The use of 'commercially pure' titanium in prosthodontics (Chapter 47) and for implants (Chapter 50).

In general, most metals are too soft and ductile for dental usage. Better mechanical properties are often obtained by using mixtures of metals (*alloys)*. In Chapter 13 the theory of alloys is discussed, with examples of a number of alloy systems that find application in dentistry.

FURTHER READING

Horath L (1995). *Fundamentals of Materials Science for Technologists*. Prentice Hall, Englewood Cliffs, New Jersey. pp 25-80.

Chapter 13

Alloys

Summary: The theory of alloy systems is considered, followed by a discussion of some systems that are used in dentistry.

Dental Significance: Metallic materials are widely used (i) in the cast form for inlays, crowns, bridges and removable partial dentures, (ii) in the wrought form as orthodontic wires, (iii) in direct tooth filling materials such as dental amalgam and (iv) in implants.

13.1 INTRODUCTION

An *alloy* is defined as a mixture of metals. It has been shown that the properties of a metal depend on its thermal and mechanical treatments (Chapter 12). The properties of an alloy depend not only on these factors, but also on its composition. The mechanical properties of an alloy can be very different from those of the component metals. For example, an alloy of 50% gold and 50% copper has an ultimate tensile strength greater than that of either pure gold or copper.

Alloys may be classified as *binary* (2 constituents), *ternary* (3 constituents), *quaternary* (4 constituents), etc. The greater the number of constituents, the more complex becomes the structure of the alloy. For simplicity, the theory of binary systems will be considered here. More complex systems as used in dental practice are studied in terms of binary combinations. An *alloy system* refers to all possible percentage compositions of the alloy. For example, the gold-silver system refers to all combinations of the two from 100% gold to 100% silver.

When two molten metals are mixed, they usually form a solution. A *solution* is defined as a perfectly homogeneous mixture. On cooling such a solution, one of four things may happen:

- A solid solution can be formed;

- The two metals may be completely insoluble in the solid state, though this is rare;
- There may be partial solid solubility;
- Additionally or alternatively intermetallic compounds may be formed. These possibilities are considered in turn.

13.2 TYPES OF ALLOY

13.2.1 Solid solutions

In a solid solution there is only one phase present. A *phase* is defined as any physically distinct, homogeneous, mechanically separable part of a system. Solid solutions may be of two types:

1. Substitutional solid solutions. These are formed where two different types of atoms occur in different positions in the same crystal lattice (Figures 13.1, 13.2). This type of solid solution is more likely to be formed between two metals if they are similar in terms of atomic size (no more than about 15% difference in atomic diameter), type of crystal lattice (for example, f.c.c., b.c.c., h.c.p.), and chemical valency. Also there should be no reaction to form intermetallic compounds. Table 13.1 presents data for gold, and for some metals which form substitutional solid solutions with it.

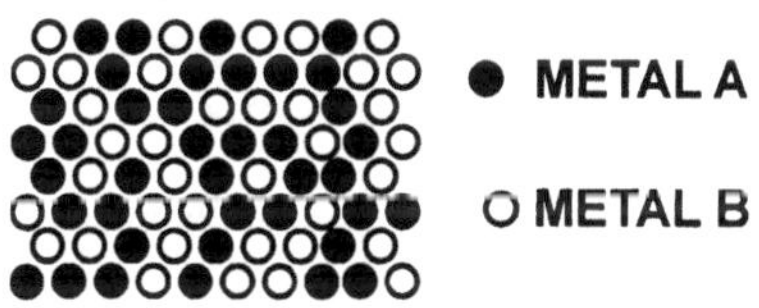

Figure 13.1. Random or disordered substitutional solid solution.

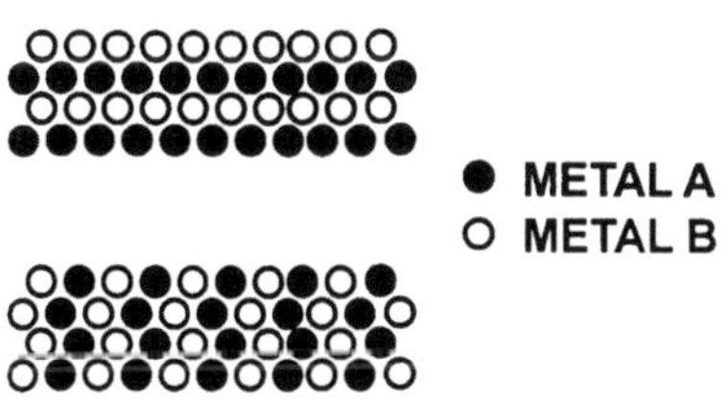

Figure 13.2. Two examples of ordered substitutional solid solutions.

Table 13.1. Properties of some metals

Metal	Atomic diameter (Å)	Approximate percentage difference in size from gold	Crystal lattice	Usual valencies
Gold	2.88	-	f.c.c.	1, 3
Copper	2.55	11.5	f.c.c.	1, 2
Silver	2.92	1.4	f.c.c.	1, 2
Platinum	2.77	3.8	f.c.c.	2, 4
Palladium	2.74	4.9	f.c.c.	2, 4

Substitutional solid solutions may be either disordered (Figure 13.1) with a random distribution of the atoms of the two metals, or contain regions where there is an ordered structure (Figure 13.2).

2. Interstitial solid solutions (Figure 13.3) are formed where very small atoms can be accommodated in the interstices or spaces between larger atoms, for example, carbon in iron.

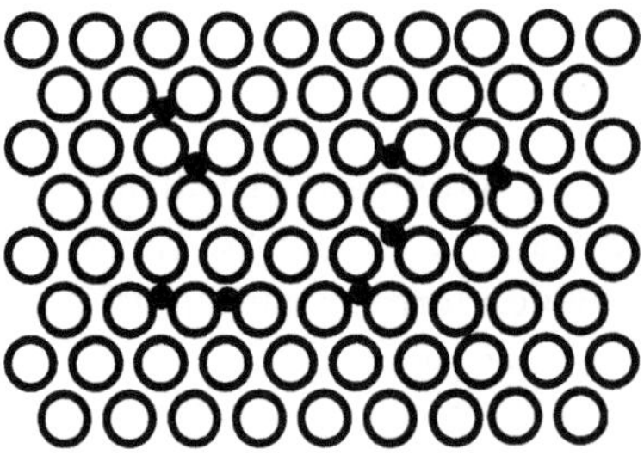

Figure 13.3. Two-dimensional representation of an interstitial solid solution.

13.2.2 Insolubility in the solid state

Complete insolubility in the solid state is rare, and occurs when very dissimilar metals are mixed. (The bismuth-cadmium system is one example, but this is not of dental relevance.)

13.2.3 Partial solid solubility

Quite frequently, partial solid solubility occurs. In the silver-copper system, for example, silver will form a solid solution with a small amount of copper, and likewise copper with a small amount of silver, resulting in a single phase material. But if, for example, equal amounts of these two metals are mixed, a two-phase structure will result. The lead-tin system provides another example of partial solid solubility.

13.2.4 Intermetallic compounds

Metals with chemical affinity for each other can form intermetallic compounds. For example, the compound Ag_3Sn can be formed between silver and tin - this is an essential constituent of dental amalgam alloys (Chapter 24). In the formation of these compounds the normal chemical valency of the metals does not always apply.

13.3 PHASE DIAGRAMS (THERMAL EQUILIBRIUM DIAGRAMS)

Dental significance: From these diagrams one can determine the composition of an alloy at any temperature, derive data for melting temperatures, and also interpret the effect of thermal history on structure and on mechanical properties such as yield strength, tensile strength, hardness and ductility.

13.3.1 Derivation

Phase diagrams are composition-temperature graphs. They can be derived from cooling curve data. Figure 13.4 is the cooling curve of a binary alloy - it has no horizontal plateau like that of a pure metal (though, for one exception to this see Section 13.3.3), but two points X_L and X_S, where there are observed changes in the rate of cooling. Above temperature T_L the alloy is completely molten; between T_L and T_S the material is solidifying; at temperatures below T_S the alloy is completely solid.

To obtain the phase diagram for an alloy system (metals A and B), mixtures of different known compositions are prepared (e.g. 90% A and 10% B; 80% A and 20% B, etc.) and values of T_L and T_S determined for each. For the pure metals A and B, since the cooling curve has a horizontal plateau (Figure 12.10), $T_L = T_S$.

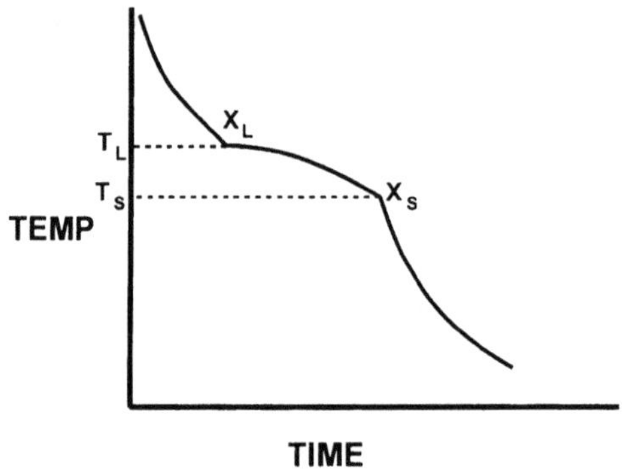

Figure 13.4. Cooling curve of an alloy.

All the results are plotted on a graph such as Figure 13.5, which is the phase diagram. There are two lines on this diagram. The upper line is obtained by joining up the plotted points of T_L values for the various compositions. It is called the *liquidus*; for any composition and temperature above this line, the alloy is completely molten. Similarly the lower line is obtained by joining up the plotted points of T_S. This line is called the *solidus*; below this the material is completely solidified. The area between the two lines represents the range of temperature and composition for the partially solidified alloy.

It should be noted that phase diagrams are obtained when there are equilibrium conditions in a system; this does not apply if an alloy is cooled rapidly.

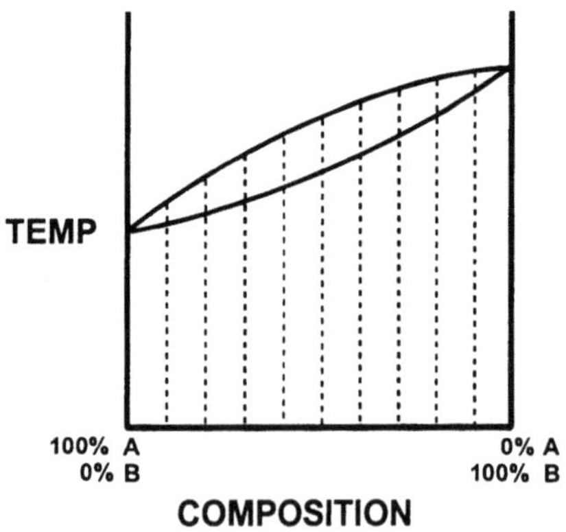

Figure 13.5. Phase diagram for a binary solid solution.

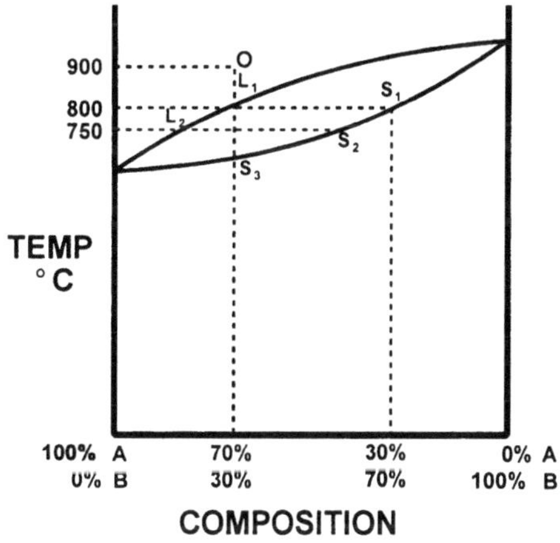

Figure 13.6 Phase diagram for a binary solid solution.

13.3.2 Binary solid solutions

Dental significance: Many casting alloys, particularly those based on gold, contain metals that form solid solutions.

Figures 13.5 and 13.6 are examples of phase diagrams for solid solutions. Consider in Figure 13.6 an alloy of 70% A and 30% B, at 900°C (point O) - it is completely molten. On cooling to 800°C (point L_1) it begins to solidify. With a solid solution alloy the composition of the solid that forms is not the same as that of the liquid from which it forms. The composition of the solid that does form can be found by drawing a horizontal line through L_1 to the point where it intersects the solidus at S_1. In this instance, the solid forming will have a composition of 30% A and 70% B, in distinction to the liquid from which it formed, which had a composition of 70% A and 30% B.

As soon as any solid is formed, this means that the composition of the liquid remaining will be different from that prior to the onset of solidification. At any temperature below L_1, but above the solidus, the composition of the liquid remaining, and of the solid formed, will be found by drawing a horizontal line at that temperature to intersect the liquidus and solidus. For example, at 750°C in Figure 13.6 the composition of the total solid which has formed is S_2 and that of the liquid remaining is L_2. The solid forming becomes progressively richer in A as solidification proceeds as does the composition of the remaining liquid. The material completely solidifies at S_3.

The consequence of this is that, provided the alloy is rapidly cooled after solidifying (see below), the composition of each grain of the alloy is not uniform — this is called *coring*. In the example above, the first material to solidify (that is, in the center of the dendrites) is richer in B than the rest of the alloy, whereas the last material will be richer in metal A. Such a cored structure can be undesirable, particularly in relation to the corrosion resistance of the alloy.

If the alloy had been cooled slowly, or reheated then cooled slowly, there would have been little or no coring - the latter process is called *homogenization.*

Homogenization depends on the movement, or diffusion of metal atoms. The greater the temperature, the greater is the thermal energy of the atoms, so they can diffuse more readily. At room temperature, the rate of diffusion in metallic materials is negligible, so no homogenization can occur. Thus rapid cooling to room temperature does not permit much diffusion to occur.

The phenomenon of order hardening can occur in substitutional solid solutions - this is discussed in Section 13.4.4.

13.3.3 Solid insolubility

A phase diagram for a binary system where there is complete solid insolubility is shown in Figure 13.7. CEF is the liquidus, and CDEGF is the solidus. At E the liquidus and solidus coincide. A material of this particular composition is called a *eutectic alloy,* which is the lowest melting alloy of the system. The temperature-time curve for this alloy has a horizontal plateau (like that of a pure metal, Figure 12.10).

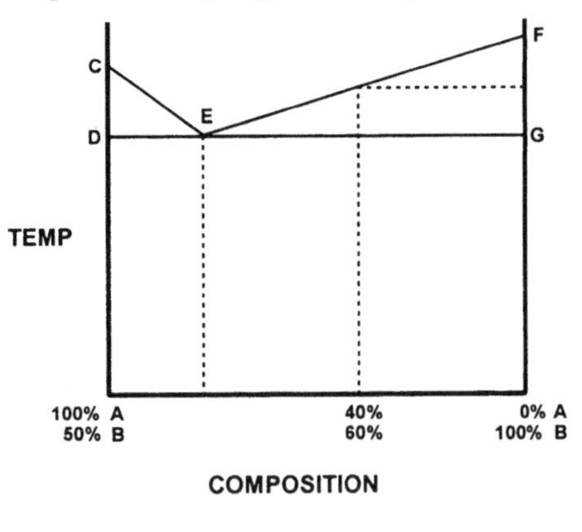

Figure 13.7. Phase diagram for a binary system where there is complete solid insolubility.

On solidifying an alloy of composition E, there is simultaneous crystallization of metals A and B, side by side, to form two phases. On cooling an alloy of composition 40% A and 60% B (Figure 13.7), with more of metal B than the eutectic composition, pure B crystallizes until the remaining molten liquid has the same composition as E, at which point A and B crystallize together.

Similarly on cooling an alloy of composition 80% A and 20% B, with more of metal A than the eutectic composition, pure A crystallizes until the remaining liquid has the composition at E, when A and B crystallize together.

13.3.4 Partial solid solubility

Dental significance: A number of systems with partial solid solubility are important, particularly spheres of silver-copper eutectic alloy that are present in some dental amalgam alloys (Chapter 24) and also low melting alloys which are the basis of solders (Chapter 54).

Figure 13.8 is the phase diagrams for systems with partial solid solubility. CEF is the liquidus and CDEGF the solidus, as before. Below this latter line, the material is completely solid. Two lines are drawn in this area, namely, AD and BG. These represent the limits of the solubilities of B in A and A in B respectively at various temperatures. From the form of these lines it will be apparent that as temperature falls the solubility of B in A and A in B also falls. To the left of AD, B is soluble in A (called the α-solid solution) and to the right of BG, A is soluble in B (the ß-solid solution). The structure of the alloy under the line ADEGB is a mixture of α- and ß-solid solutions.

If a molten alloy of composition I in Figure 13.8 is solidified (the eutectic mixture), the α- and ß-solid solutions crystallize independently. For alloy II in Figure 13.8 the ß-solid solution crystallizes first, followed by a mixture of α- and ß-solid solutions.

Alloy III forms the α-solid solution when it solidifies, but on further cooling can exceed the solid solubility of metal B in A. One of two things can happen in this case:

1. On slow cooling, some of the ß-solid solution may precipitate from the solid solution - this is the basis of precipitation hardening, discussed in Section 13.4.5.

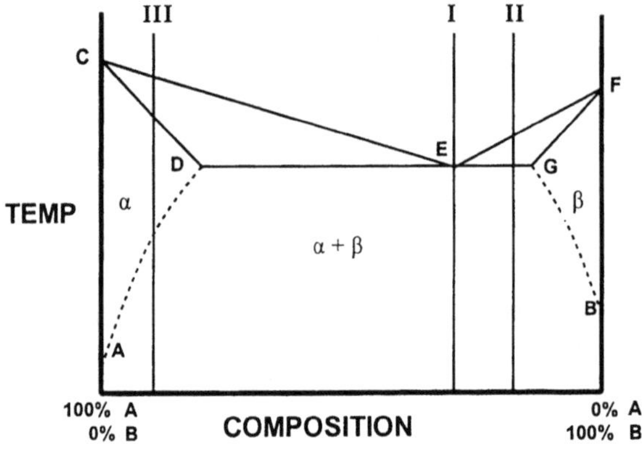

Figure 13.8. Phase diagram for a binary system where there is partial solid solubility in the solid state.

2. With rapid cooling, the alloy may not be at an elevated temperature for sufficient time to allow precipitation, which requires diffusion of metal atoms. Thus a supersaturated solid solution is the result.

Figures 13.9 and 13.10 give the phase diagrams of two systems that are of dental interest, which show partial solid solubility. Figure 13.9 is for the silver-copper system; silver-copper eutectic alloys are incorporated in some dental amalgam alloys (Chapter 24). Figure 13.10 is for the lead-tin system, which is a basis for low melting point solders (Chapter 54).

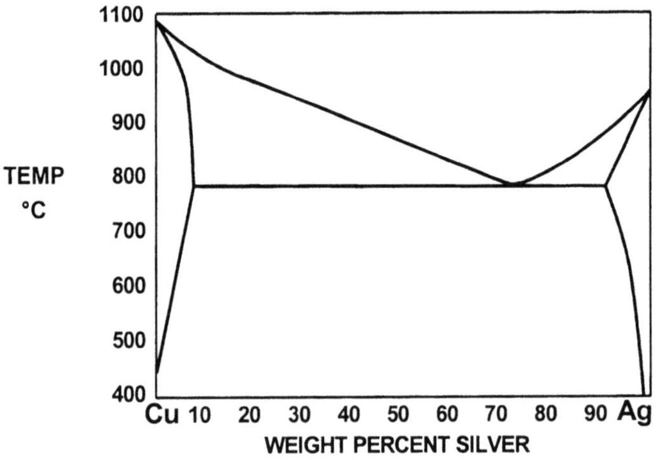

Figure 13.9. Phase diagram for the silver-copper system.

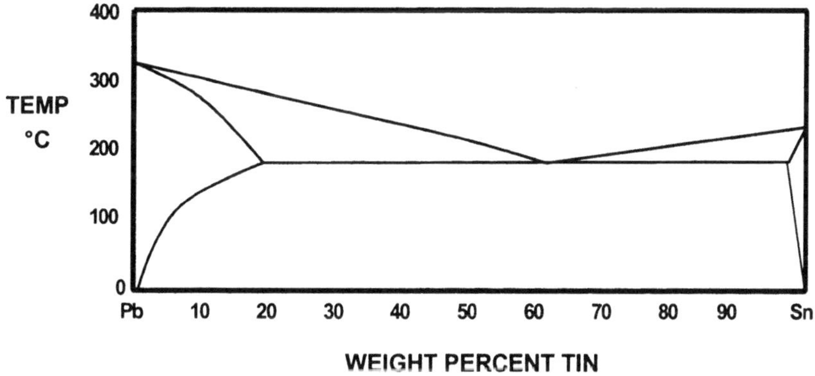

Figure 13.10. Phase diagram for the lead-tin system.

13.4 MECHANICAL PROPERTIES

Dental significance: The mechanical properties of an alloy depend on composition, mechanical history and thermal history. It is sometimes possible to achieve better mechanical properties by the application of an appropriate heat treatment (see, for example, Section 47.2)

13.4.1 Introduction

When an alloy is given a hardening heat treatment, it has the following effects on mechanical properties:

- Increase in hardness;
- Greater yield stress;
- Greater ultimate tensile strength;
- Less ductility (lower percentage elongation);
- Little change in modulus of elasticity.

13.4.2 Work hardening

The properties of an alloy can be altered by cold working, as for a metal, as described in Section 12.7.2.

13.4.3 Solution hardening

In a binary substitutional solid solution, the atoms of two constituent metals are of different sizes (examples are given in Table13.1), though the size difference is usually less than 15%. Consequently the crystal lattice of such as alloy is distorted by the presence of either smaller or larger atoms. These distortions hinder the movement of dislocations, so raising the yield stress. Thus, for example, gold alloys containing copper, silver, etc. are harder, stronger and less ductile than pure gold.

13.4.4 Order hardening

This is best illustrated by the gold-copper system, for which Figure 13.11 is a simplified phase diagram. Below the solidus, there are two areas designated (1) and (2). These represent conditions of temperature and composition where reactions can occur in the solid state, provided that the alloy is maintained at an elevated temperature for sufficient time to permit diffusion of atoms.

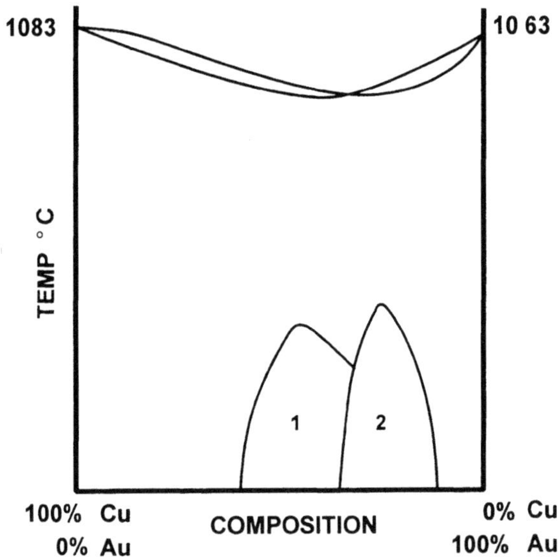

Figure 13.11. Phase diagram for the gold-copper system.

The reaction occurring in this system is called *ordering*. If an alloy of say 50% gold and 50% copper is cooled rapidly from 450°C, the lattice structure is random or disordered (Figure 13.1). But slow cooling permits the formation of regions of an ordered substitutional solid solution (Figure 13.2). In area (1) of Figure 13.11, the ordered lattice has three copper atoms to each gold atom (Cu_3Au), and in area (2) there are equal numbers of atoms of the two metals in the lattice (CuAu).

Such an ordered structure is termed a *superlattice*. The unit cell of the CuAu superlattice is face-centered tetragonal - this differs from a face-centered cubic structure in that only two of the three axes of the unit cell are equal in length.

The formation of a certain volume of a tetragonal lattice within a cubic structure involves contraction on one of the crystal axes; this sets up strains that interfere with the movement of dislocations. Hence the yield stress, ultimate tensile strength and hardness are raised, and this is termed *order hardening.*

13.4.5 Precipitation hardening

When precipitation occurs (Figure 13.8), as in the Ag-Cu system (Figure 13.9), the precipitated phase reduces the mobility of dislocations, thus increasing strength and hardness, and reducing the ductility.

13.4.6 Eutectic alloys

In general, eutectics are hard but brittle, have low melting points, and as has been noted, can be useful as solders (Chapter 54). However, their resistance to corrosion may be poorer than alloys with more homogeneous structures.

13.5 GOLD AND ITS ALLOYS

Dental significance: Cast gold alloys are used extensively in dentistry – see Chapters 35, 36 and 47.

13.5.1 Pure gold

Pure gold is soft and ductile. It has been, and occasionally is, used for restoring teeth. In this application, the gold is welded and work hardened in the tooth cavity. Pure gold does not have suitable mechanical properties for cast dental restorations and prostheses. Thus casting gold alloys for inlays, crowns, bridges and partial dentures contain alloying elements, the most common being copper, silver, platinum, palladium and zinc.

13.5.2 Effect of alloying elements

1. Copper. From Figure 13.11 a number of observations can be made. Gold and copper form a solid solution in all proportions. The liquidus and solidus are close together, and coincide at one point; such an alloy shows little tendency to form a cored structure. When copper is alloyed with gold, the melting point of the alloy is less than that of gold. Solution hardening occurs, and order hardening can occur for alloys containing approximately 40 to 88 % gold, if the correct heat treatment is given. Copper also imparts a red color to the alloy if present in sufficient quantity. It also reduces the density of the alloy.

Only a limited amount of copper can be used in a dental alloy, since corrosion may result. In general, a dental gold alloy should have at least 75% noble metals (gold, platinum and palladium) to ensure complete corrosion resistance, though alloys with lower gold content are now being used (Chapter 35).

2. Silver forms a solid solution with gold in all proportions, and there is partial solid solubility in the silver-copper system (Figure 13.9). Silver slightly increases the hardness and strength by solution hardening. Precipitation hardening can occur with copper present in the alloy under the appropriate thermal conditions. Silver can allow tarnishing to occur. Molten silver can dissolve gases such as oxygen, leading to porosity in a casting. Silver also tends to whiten the alloy, and overcome the reddening effect of copper.

3. Platinum forms a solid solution with gold, but increases the tendency for coring to occur. Precipitation hardening can occur by reaction with copper. Platinum increases the melting point and helps the corrosion resistance of the alloy.

4. Palladium is similar to platinum in its effects on dental gold alloys, and is a less expensive metal.

5. Zinc is included as a scavenger. When the alloy is being melted prior to casting, oxidation of some of the constituents (e.g. copper) can occur. The presence of an oxide of copper in the casting is undesirable, since it embrittles the alloy. Zinc oxidizes more readily than all the other constituents of a gold alloy. Zinc oxide can be removed as a slag from the molten alloy.

6. Other constituents such as nickel and iridium may be present; the latter metal helps to refine the grain structure of the alloy.

13.6 STEEL

Dental significance: Various forms of steel are used for dental instruments.

Steel is an alloy of iron and carbon, with up to 2% carbon. Alloys with greater quantities of carbon are *cast iron* or *pig iron*.

Iron can exist in two forms: face-centered cubic above 910°C, and body-centered cubic below this temperature. Carbon is practically insoluble in body-centered cubic iron (soluble up to 0.02%), but is more soluble in face-centered cubic iron; this interstitial solid solution is called *austenite*.

Part of the simplified phase diagram for the iron-carbon system is shown in Figure 13.12. It can be seen that on cooling austenite, transformations occur as the solubility of carbon reduces with decreasing temperature.

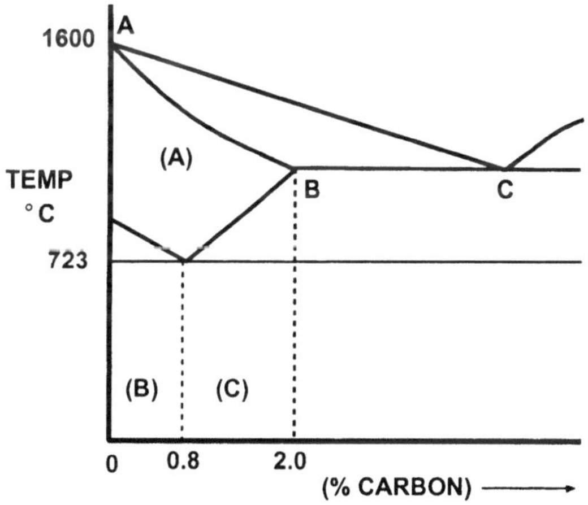

Figure 13.12. Part of the simplified phase diagram for the iron-carbon system. AC is the liquidus; ABC the solidus; (A) austenite (solid solution); (B) ferrite and pearlite; (C) pearlite and cementite.

A mixture containing 99.2% iron and 0.8% carbon produces a structure similar to that of a eutectic, since after cooling austenite slowly below a well-defined temperature (723°C), the solid material may be observed metallographically to have transformed to an intimate mechanical mixture of two components. One of these components is *cementite*, an intermetallic compound, Fe_3C, which comes out of solution as the iron changes from f.c.c. to b.c.c. The other component is *ferrite*, which is an extremely dilute solid solution of carbon in body-centered cubic iron. This mixture of constituents is called *pearlite*.

This mixture (0.8% C, 99.2% Fe) is not a eutectic, since the transformations occur in the solid state. It is called *eutectoid steel*, since the structure produced is similar to a eutectic. Alloys with less than and greater than 0.8% carbon are called *hypo-eutectoid* and *hyper-eutectoid* steels respectively.

If austenite is cooled rapidly, there may not be sufficient time for the carbon to diffuse out of the solid solution to form cementite. In this case the alloy consists of a distorted b.c.c. lattice containing carbon; this material is called *martensite*. Because of the distortion of the lattice, martensite is an extremely hard and brittle material. (Note — contrast this to gold alloys, where more rapid cooling produces a softer alloy.)

Rapidly cooled steel would be too brittle for some applications, particularly for the cutting edge of burs or other dental instruments. Such materials can be tempered, that is, heated to between 200° to 450°C, held at a given temperature for a known length of time, and cooled rapidly - see Figure 13.13. This procedure permits diffusion of carbon atoms from the crystal lattice to occur; in this way some cementite is formed.

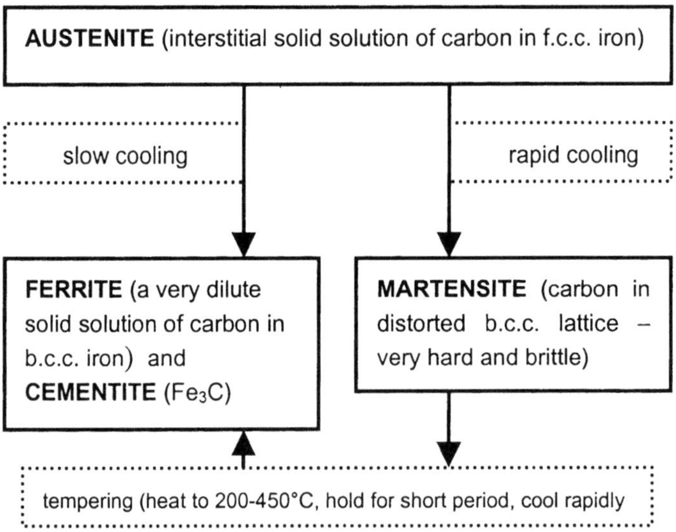

Figure 13.13. Heat treatment of steels.

In addition to iron and carbon, steels have small quantities of other constituents (stainless steel is a special case, and is discussed in Section 13.7). Chromium may be added in small quantities to improve the tarnish resistance (stainless steel has much larger quantities of chromium). Manganese may be used as a scavenger for sulfur, analogous to the effect of zinc on oxygen in gold alloys. Molybdenum, silicon, nickel, cobalt, etc may also be present.

13.7 STAINLESS STEEL

Dental significance: Stainless steel wires are used in orthodontics.

In addition to iron and carbon, stainless steel contains chromium, and often nickel. Chromium, if present in sufficient quantities, renders the alloy resistant to corrosive attack. The mechanism of this is discussed in Chapter 14. Chromium and nickel both reduce the *critical temperature* — the temperature at which the austenitic structure breaks down on cooling. Nickel also helps the corrosion resistance and strength of the alloy.

Two types of stainless steel are of importance:

1. Austenitic stainless steel which contains so much chromium and nickel that the austenite structure — a solid solution — remains even on cooling to room temperature. Such alloys may have 18% chromium and 8% nickel (often called '18/8 stainless steel') or 12% of each of these constituents ('12/12 stainless steel'). These materials can be hardened by cold working, but not hardened by heat treatment, and so are not suitable for cutting instruments. 18/8 stainless steel can be used for orthodontic wires (Chapter 41).
2. Martensitic stainless steel may contain 12 to 13% chromium, a small amount of carbon, but no other major constituents. These alloys can be hardened by heat-treatment — contrast to the above.

13.8 CHROMIUM-CONTAINING CASTING ALLOYS

Dental significance: Casting alloys based on cobalt and/or nickel that contain chromium are used for cast partial dentures (Chapter 47) and bridges (Chapter 35). Wires of cobalt/nickel/chromium are used in orthodontics (Chapter 41). Some surgical implants are made of a cobalt-chromium alloy (Chapter 50).

13.8.1 Cobalt-chromium alloys

These are hard, rigid, corrosion resistant alloys. Because of their high corrosion resistance at high temperatures they have been used for car spark plugs and turbine blades. These materials are often referred to as *stellite alloys*.

A typical composition is given in Table 13.2, together with the major effects of each constituent. Note that cobalt is the principal constituent, hence they are termed *cobalt-chromium alloys* in preference to chromium-cobalt, chrome-cobalt or chrome alloys.

Table 13.2. Constituents of cobalt-chromium alloys

Constituent	Percentage	Function
Cobalt	35-65	Hard rigid metal
Nickel	0-30	May be a partial replacement for cobalt
Chromium	20-35	Gives corrosion resistance, because of its passivating effect (Chapter 14)
Molybdenum	0-7	Reduces grain size and improves alloy properties
Tungsten, manganese, silicon	Small quantities	Improve mechanical properties
Carbon	≤ 0.4	Invariably present; forms carbides that can make the alloy too brittle

13.8.2 Nickel-chromium alloys

These contain about 75% nickel and 20% chromium, and have good corrosion resistance, similar to the cobalt-chromium alloys. They have been used for cast bridges and for porcelain bonding techniques (Chapter 36). There is some concern that nickel is an allergen.

13.9 TITANIUM AND ITS ALLOYS

Dental significance: Titanium-containing materials are sometimes used for cast partial dentures (Chapter 47), wires (Chapter 41) and as implant materials (Chapter 50).

13.9.1 Pure titanium

Titanium exists in two different forms, depending on temperature. At room temperature the metal has an h.c.p. structure (α-Ti) and it changes to a b.c.c. structure at 833°C. The melting point is around 1700°C. The rate of solidification of the metal is important, because this will determine the ratio of α- and β-phases present. A greater quantity of the β-phase gives a stronger material but with less ductility.

An attractive feature of these metals is their resistance to corrosion (Chapter 14). However, titanium is a difficult material to handle, because of its high melting point, and its reactivity with oxygen at high temperatures.

13.9.2 Titanium casting alloys

A number of titanium alloys have been developed and used for dental applications. One of the best known is Ti-6Al-4V (that is, titanium with 6% aluminum and 4 % vanadium), which is being suggested for prosthodontic use (Chapter 47). This alloy is composed mainly of α-Ti.

13.9.3 Beta-titanium

An alloy in which the β-form of titanium is stable is available for use as an orthodontic alloy (Chapter 41). This contains nearly 80% titanium with added molybdenum, zirconium and tin.

13.9.4 Nickel-titanium

Nickel and titanium form an intermetallic compound (45% Ni, 55% Ti). This alloy is also used for orthodontic wires. An interesting feature is the 'shape-memory effect,' and this is discussed further in Section 41.4.2.

13.10 SUMMARY OF DENTAL APPLICATIONS

Metallic materials are liable to corrode in the mouth, and Chapter 14 deals with this phenomenon. In later chapters, there are many examples of the use of metallic materials – for example:

- Dental amalgam filling materials (Chapter 24);
- Alloys for inlays, crowns and bridges (Chapter 35);
- Alloys for bonding to porcelain (Chapters 36);
- Wires, brackets and bands for orthodontic appliances (Chapter 41);
- Implant materials (Chapter 50);
- Steel dental instruments.

Also covered are laboratory aspects of handling alloys:

- Casting procedures (Chapter 54);
- Associated investment materials (Chapter 53);
- Joining of metals (Chapter 54).

FURTHER READING

Horath L (1995). *Fundamentals of Materials Science for Technologists.* Prentice Hall, Englewood Cliffs, New Jersey. pp 25-80.

Chapter 14

Corrosion in the Oral Environment

Summary: corrosion is defined, and factors relating to the tendency for corrosion to occur and the rate at which this occurs are discussed.

Dental significance: the mouth is an ideal environment to cause corrosion, so care must be taken in choice and application of any metallic materials for oral use.

14.1 INTRODUCTION

Corrosion can be defined as a physicochemical interaction between a metal and its environment to form metallic compounds. The resultant changes in the metal can lead to an impairment of its function and can also change the environment in which the metal is situated. It has already been stressed that the mouth is a hostile environment into which to place synthetic materials (Chapter 10).

Many metals can react spontaneously with either a gaseous or aqueous environment. The compounds thus obtained are thermodynamically more stable than the metals from which they have been formed. Corrosion reactions can occur aided by the presence of moisture, fluctuating temperatures, and changes in pH because of the nature of foods and liquids taken into the mouth. Furthermore, debris may adhere to metallic surfaces, and under certain circumstances this can accelerate the corrosion breakdown process.

Corrosion is obviously undesirable, as it can spoil the esthetics of an alloy, and in extreme cases can severely weaken the material, as in the rusting of iron. Corrosion products may also be harmful to the body.

To avoid this in both dental and implant alloys only a few types of alloy can be used, and conditions that favor corrosion must be avoided as far as possible.

Corrosion reactions can be classified into two types. Firstly, there is *non-aqueous corrosion*, when metals can react to form compounds such as oxides and sulfides. Examples include the tarnishing of brass due to formation of sulfides, discoloration of the surfaces of alloy castings caused by oxidation, and oxidation of metal surfaces during soldering and heat treatment procedures.

Secondly, *aqueous corrosion* can occur in the oral environment; this occurs by electrochemical reactions, and is the main subject of discussion of this chapter.

14.2 ELECTROCHEMISTRY

14.2.1 Conductors of electricity

Conductors of electricity are of two main types:

- *Electronic conductors*, such as metals, where the movement of electrons causes conduction;
- *Electrolytic conductors*, or electrolytes, for example, fused salts and aqueous solutions of acids, bases and salts, where conduction of electricity is accompanied by the movement of ions.

14.2.2 Current-consuming (electrolytic) cells

Consider an electrolyte containing cations M^+ and anions A^-. If two electronic conductors, or electrodes, are placed in this electrolyte and an electrical potential difference established between them by a battery, then movement of ions will occur. Cations, M^+, move to the negatively charged electrode or cathode and anions move to the anode or positively charged electrode (Fig. 14.1A). Such a process is called *electrolysis*.

For the above, the following reactions can be written, where e^- represents an electron:

At the cathode: $M^+ + e^- \longrightarrow M$
At the anode: $A^- \longrightarrow A + e^-$

An *anodic reaction*, then, is one that produces electrons, whereas a *cathodic* process consumes electrons. This process can be used for *electroplating*, or *electrodeposition*, in which the material to be coated is made the cathode of an electrolytic cell, and the anode is made of the metal to be deposited onto the cathode. The electrolyte serves to transport ions from anode to cathode.

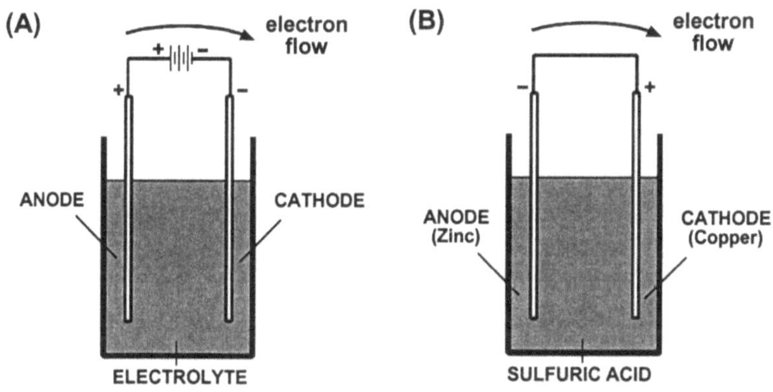

Figure 14.1. (A) Current-consuming (electrolytic) cell; (B) Current producing (galvanic cell).

14.2.3 Current-producing (galvanic) cells

Consider now two electrodes of different metals, e.g. copper and zinc, immersed in an electrolyte of sulfuric acid (Fig. 14.1B). When electrical contact is made between the electrodes, a current will flow.

The following reactions occur:

At the anode: $Zn \longrightarrow Zn^{2+} + 2e^{-}$
At the cathode: $2H^{+} + 2e^{-} \longrightarrow H_2$

As in the previous section, electrons are produced at the anode and consumed at the cathode. This is an example of a *galvanic* or *corrosion cell.* Zinc atoms are being converted to zinc ions (essentially an oxidation reaction), and passing into solution. Thus the zinc is being corroded.

14.2.4 Electrode potential

Consider the reversible reaction:

$$M \rightleftharpoons M^{n+} + n\,e^{-}$$

The forward reaction liberates electrons, and the reverse one consumes them. When electrons are produced, this causes a potential on the electrode. This *electrode potential* is therefore a measure of the extent to which the above reaction proceeds from left to right, so indicating the tendency for the metal to corrode.

The standard potential of an electrode is usually expressed relative to that of the reaction:

$$H_2 \longrightarrow 2H^+ + 2e^-$$

The above reaction is arbitrarily given the value zero. Some standard electrode potentials are given in Table 14.1.

Table 14.1. Electrode potentials of some metals*

Metal	Reaction	Electrode potential (volts)
Gold	Au^+ + 1 electron → Au	+ 1.50
Platinum	Pt^{2+} + 2 electrons → Pt	+ 0.86
Palladium	Pd^{2+} + 2 electrons → Pd	+ 0.82
Silver	Ag^+ + electron → Ag	+ 0.80
Mercury	Hg^{2+} + 2 electrons → Hg	+ 0.80
Copper	Cu^+ + 1 electron → Cu	+ 0.47
Copper	Cu^{2+} + 2 electrons → Cu	+ 0.34
Hydrogen	$2H^+$ + 2 electrons → H_2	0.00
Iron	Fe^{3+} + 3 electrons → Fe	- 0.045
Lead	Pb^{2+} + 2 electrons → Pb	- 0.12
Tin	Sn^{2+} + 2 electrons → Sn	- 0.14
Iron	Fe^{2+} + 2 electrons → Fe	- 0.44
Chromium	Cr^{2+} + 2 electrons → Cr	- 0.56
Zinc	Zn^{2+} + 2 electrons → Zn	- 0.76
Aluminum	Al^{3+} + 3 electrons → Al	- 1.70
Sodium	Na^+ + 1 electron → Na	- 2.71
Calcium	Ca^{2+} + 2 electrons → Ca	- 2.90
Potassium	K^+ + 1 electron → K	- 2.92

* These were measured at 25°C in a molar solution of the metal. Sometimes an opposite sign convention is used – that is – the electrode potential of Au is given as –1.50 volts.

Two things can be derived from this standard *electrochemical series*. A greater difference in electrode potential between two metals indicates a greater tendency for an electrochemical reaction to occur. Also, the metal that is lower in the series (as written in Table 14.1) forms the anode. The anode is the metal, which corrodes and goes into solution.

It should be noted that different electrolytes such as saline solutions and seawater could sometimes cause changes in the relative position of metals in the series. For any given electrolyte it is possible to produce a *galvanic series* which gives the potentials for metals in that electrolyte.

14.2.5 Polarization

The tendency of materials to corrode has been discussed above, but this does not tell us about the rate at which corrosion reactions occur. The extent to which corrosion proceeds in a given time depends mainly on a phenomenon called *polarization*, which is a combination of at least three factors:

1. Activation polarization results from the potential difference needed to enable the electrode reactions to proceed at a finite rate.
2. Concentration polarization, due to the accumulation of reaction products, can occur. For example, around a zinc anode, there may be a high concentration of zinc ions, which will reduce the current until they diffuse away from the anode. Evolution of hydrogen at a cathode can occur in some cells.
3. Polarization due to the formation of a film on the surface of the electrode can reduce the rate of an electrochemical reaction. This film may be composed of adsorbed gases or metallic oxides.

14.2.6 Anode and cathode polarization

Figure 14.2 illustrates anode and cathode polarization. Curves such as this are obtained by measuring the potential of each electrode for a given controlled current. As the current from the cell increases, the apparent electrode potential of the anode rises and that of the cathode decreases. The current at the point where these curves intersect, I_c, is called the *corrosion current*, and is a measure of the maximum current from the cell. Ideally, to reduce corrosion it is important to increase the polarization of either or both electrodes to decrease the value of I_c. This may be achieved by metals that passivate (Section 14.2.7).

14.2.7 Passivity

For a metal capable of forming an oxide that is stable in the presence of an electrolyte, a curve such as Figure 14.3 is obtained. At point X there is a discontinuity in the curve and the potential suddenly increases form X to Y. The metal is said to be passivated, or rendered passive, as potentials above X, when it is covered by an oxide film.

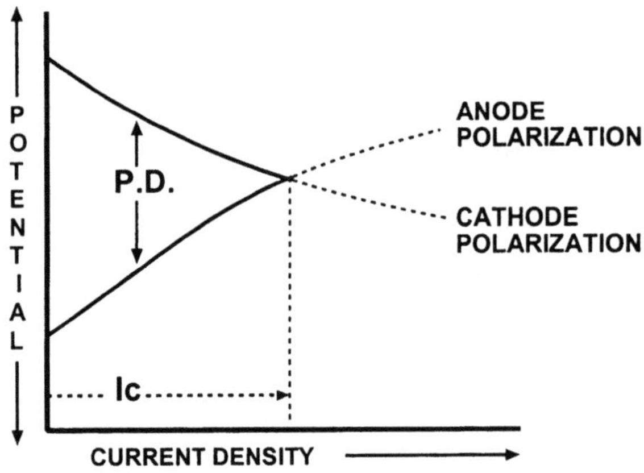

Figure 14.2. Polarization curves for a corrosion cell. P.D. marks the potential difference between anode and cathode. I_c is the maximum current density.

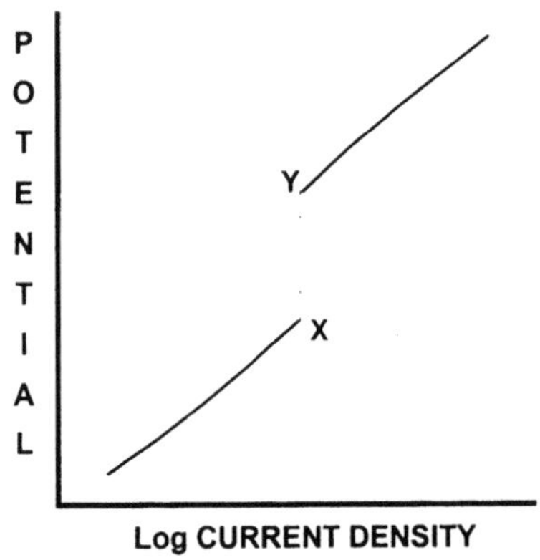

Figure 14.3. Anodic polarization curve for a metal, showing passivity at potentials between X and Y.

14.2.8 Potentiostatic measurements

To obtain experimental data on passivity, potentiostatic techniques can be used. These can yield data on the behavior of the metal in the region of the discontinuity X·········Y in Figure 14.3. Instead of measuring potential for a given controlled current as above, the potential is controlled and the current to maintain a given potential is measured. A curve such as Figure 14.4 is obtained for a passive metal. Point X is the potential for which the minimum current density is obtained.

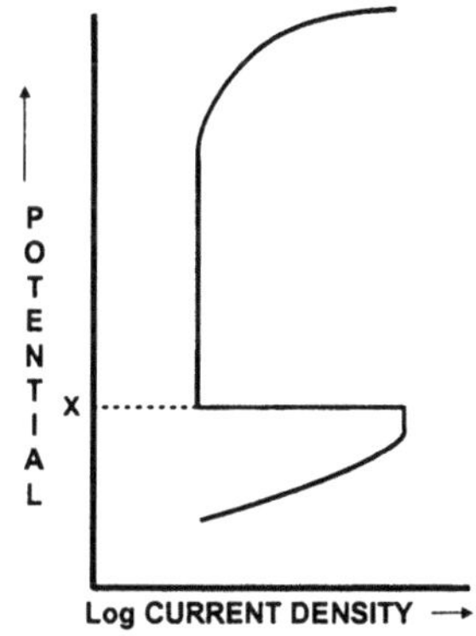

Figure 14.4. Potentiostatically determined anodic polarization curve, showing passivation of the metal.

Metals such as titanium and chromium are easily passivated. Likewise, alloys containing chromium, such as stainless steel, can form passive layers.

It should be noted that the establishment of passivity depends on the nature of the electrolyte as well as the composition of the metal or alloy. For example, in the presence of chloride ions passivity is more difficult to achieve. The corrosion characteristics of dental alloys are often assessed in saline solutions, and Figure 14.5 illustrates such data for some alloys of dental interest.

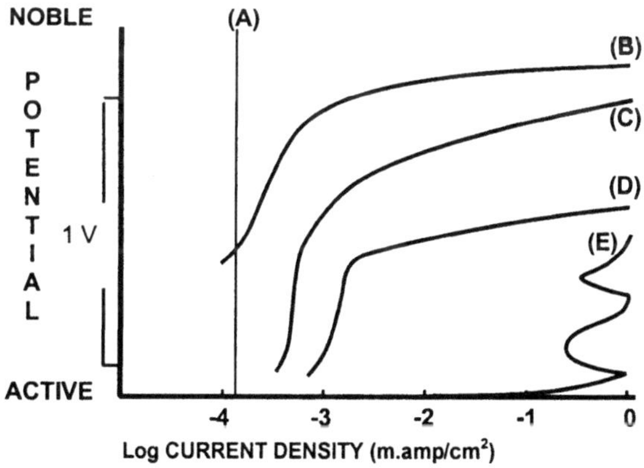

Figure 14.5. Potentiostatically determined anodic polarization curves of alloys in saline solutions. (A) titanium alloy; (B) dental inlay gold alloy; (C) cobalt-chromium alloy; (D) stainless steel; (E) dental amalgam.

14.3 EXAMPLES OF ELECTROLYTIC CORROSION

14.3.1 Differences in composition of materials

Some examples of dental situations where corrosion can occur may be cited.

1. If a gold inlay comes into contact with an amalgam restoration, the amalgam can form the anode of an electrolytic cell, and thus corrode.
2. Within an amalgam restoration there are a number of intermetallic compounds; corrosion of anodic phases with the material can occur, with significant consequences for the longevity of the restoration (Chapter 24).
3. A soldered appliance or denture may corrode, since the composition of the solder differs from that of the alloys it joins.
4. In a cored structure, differences in the composition within the alloy grains are found. Thus part of a grain can be the anode, and part the cathode, in a galvanic cell. Consequently, homogenization can help to improve the corrosion resistance of an alloy.
5. Where there is solid insolubility or precipitation in an alloy with partial solid solubility, different grains have different compositions. Again, this favors electrolytic corrosion.

14.3.2 Differences in composition of electrolyte

A homogeneous metal or alloy can undergo electrolytic corrosion where there is a difference in electrolyte concentration across the specimen. Three examples are noteworthy.

1. Consider the case of a metallic restoration that is partly covered by food debris. The composition of the electrolyte under this debris will differ from that of saliva, and this can contribute to the corrosion of the restoration.
2. Where there are differences in the concentration of oxygen in an electrolyte, an oxidation-type concentration cell is formed. Corrosion is greater at portions of the metal or alloy with lower concentrations of oxygen. This can happen in an unpolished metallic restoration. The surface concavities become filled readily with food debris; this lowers the concentration of oxygen at those parts, which corrode, and lead to pitting of the filling.
3. There can obviously be differences in the composition of the electrolyte in contact with different portions of a semi-buried dental implant.

14.3.3 Differences in stress

A metal that has been stressed by cold working becomes more reactive at the site of maximum stress. If stressed and unstressed metals are in contact in an electrolyte, the former will become the anode of a galvanic cell, and will corrode.

An example occurs in orthopedic surgery, when stainless steel plates and screws are frequently embedded in tissues. Any differences in the extent of cold working between screw and plate must be avoided. Similarly, different portions of the same piece of steel may be stressed to different extents, so favoring corrosion.

14.3.4 Stress corrosion

A combination of corrosion and stress conditions can cause failures of a metal by stress corrosion. At an anodic portion of a surface, electrolytic action can form a minute crack. This can increase in size as a result of stress concentration. More corrosion can occur in the enlarged crack, and so on, until eventual failure occurs.

14.4 CORROSION AND GALVANIC PAIN

In addition to corrosive attack on dental alloys, electrolytic corrosion can cause galvanic pain. People may experience this when a piece of metal foil wrapping has inadvertently been taken into the mouth. If the foil contacts an amalgam restoration, an electric circuit is set up, with saliva as an electrolyte. The current causes painful stimulation of the tooth pulp.

Galvanic pain is occasionally encountered in the mouth, when dissimilar metal restorations come into intermittent contact. Long-term contact is unlikely to give severe galvanic pain, because polarization can occur (Section 14.2.5).

One of the claimed functions of a cement lining under a metal is to give electrical insulation of the pulp (Section 23.2).

14.5 PREVENTION OF CORROSION

14.5.1 Choice of alloy

Alloys for long-term use in the mouth must be either noble or passive. Noble metals are those such as gold, platinum and palladium (Table 14.1). Dental gold alloys contain some copper, which has poorer corrosion resistance; however, such alloys should ideally contain at least 70-75% noble metals.

Passive alloys, such as those containing chromium, are widely used dentally. Examples include stainless steel, cobalt-chromium and nickel-chromium. Titanium and its alloys also show passivity.

14.5.2 Use of alloy

In addition to choosing suitable materials, alloys must be used correctly, and situations which are likely to lead to corrosion, as in Section 14.3, must be avoided as far as possible.

FURTHER READING

Mattson E (1996). *Basic Corrosion Technology for Scientists and Engineers*. The Institute of Materials, London.

Chapter 15

Ceramics

Summary: Ceramics are defined and a wide range of ceramic materials is described in terms of structure and properties.

Dental significance: Ceramic materials find wide use as esthetic restorative materials. Three important ceramic materials (zinc oxide, fluoroaluminosilicate glasses and silica) are discussed in detail and a list of dental applications is included.

15.1 DEFINITION AND EXAMPLES

The word ceramic is derived from the Greek word *keramos* which means 'potter's clay.' *Traditional ceramics* that are made from clay, silica and feldspar (Table 15.1) are used for pottery, porcelain, refractories (heat-resistant materials) and abrasives. The forming and burning of clay suspensions has been carried out since about 5000 B.C. Despite the antiquity of the materials, many new types of material are becoming available and ceramics are finding new industrial uses — for example, uranium dioxide as a nuclear fuel, and glass-ceramics for many industrial applications.

Ceramic substances are often considered to be composed of compounds of metallic and non-metallic elements. Examples include oxides, nitrides and silicates. Ceramics differ from metals in that they contain ionic and/or covalent bonds. In contrast to metals, they are usually electrical insulators, because they have few free electrons. They are very often transparent or translucent to light and are usually chemically stable under a wide range of environmental conditions.

It is not surprising that ceramics find many uses in dentistry. A dental porcelain, used for jacket crowns and veneers, consists essentially of a glass prepared from a high purity feldspar, sometimes containing a crystalline phase to give increased strength. Silica (SiO_2) is used as a constituent of refractory investment materials in metal casting, and as an abrasive. Ceramics can be combined with polymers to form composites (Chapter 27) which are widely used as dental restorative materials.

It has been stated above that ceramics are usually unreactive materials. Two exceptions to this are important in dentistry, namely zinc oxide and synthetic fluoroaluminosilicate (FAS) glasses. The powder of these materials can react with acids to give materials that set, and this is used in some cements and some dental restorative materials (Chapters 25 and 26).

Ceramic raw materials, and some of their major dental applications, are listed in Table 15.1

Table 15.1. Ceramic materials

Material	Formula	Dental Applications
Alumina	Al_2O_3	Glassy intermediate Abrasive Used in preparation of aluminosilicate glasses Incorporated in some dental porcelains
Boric oxide	B_2O_3	Glass former Ceramic flux – reduces fusion temperature
Calcium oxide	CaO	Glass network modifier Flux
Feldspars		Naturally occurring anhydrous aluminosilicates, used as constituents of dental porcelain
- Potash feldspar	$K_2O.Al_2O_3.6SiO_2$	
- Soda feldspar	$Na_2O.Al_2O_3.6SiO_2$	
- Lime feldspar	$CaO.2Al_2O_3.2SiO_2$	
Kaolin (china clay)	$Al_2O_3.2SiO_2.2H_2O$	Naturally occurring hydrous aluminosilicate; used in traditional pottery
Leucite	$KAlSi_2O_6$	Constituent of some dental porcelains
Potassium oxide	K_2O	Glass network modifier Flux
Silica	SiO_2	Constituent of porcelain Used in refractory investment materials Abrasive
Silicon carbide	SiC	Abrasive
Sodium oxide	Na_2O	Glass network modifier Flux
Zinc oxide	ZnO	Constituent of dental cements

15.2 METHODS OF FORMING

A wide range of techniques can be used to produce ceramics, such as porcelain jacket crowns.

1. Powder-slurry ceramics. A traditional method of forming is to prepare a plastic ceramic-water mixture that is molded to the required shape on a die. The resultant product is fired at an appropriate temperature to give a solid ceramic.
2. Some materials such as glasses can be molded by casting, blowing, drawing, pressing or rolling.
3. Injection molding can be used, in which the material is injected at high temperature under pressure into a mold.
4. Machinable ceramics are available, and CAD-CAM (computer aided design – computer aided manufacture) techniques are now available for dental use.
5. Glass-infiltration techniques are now used in which sintered alumina is in-filled with a molten glass.
6. A glaze can be applied to the surface of a fired ceramic. This is essentially a glassy material, which is fired on to the surface.

Another important dental technique is the combination of a metallic casting to which a ceramic facing is bonded. This porcelain-fused-to-metal technique (PFM) attempts to combine the strength of an alloy with the esthetic appeal of a ceramic (Chapter 36).

15.3 CRYSTALLINE AND NON-CRYSTALLINE CERAMICS

15.3.1 Crystalline ceramics

These may have ionic or covalent bonds. Compounds of metals with oxygen usually have ionic bonding. Covalent crystals, for example, silicon carbide (SiC), are usually very hard and have high melting points.

15.3.2 Non-crystalline ceramics

A *glass* may be defined as a product of fusion that has cooled to a rigid condition without crystallizing. Glasses are composed of silica (SiO_2) with other oxides, such as those of sodium, potassium, calcium, barium, etc. The silica is a network former. Alumina, though not on its own network-forming, is often used in conjunction with silica; for this reason it is termed a *glassy intermediate*. The alkali and alkali earth metal oxides disrupt the glassy network and modify glass properties. Thus the composition of a glass can be controlled to give specific properties in respect of refractive index, color, viscosity of molten material, thermal expansion coefficient, etc.

The *fictive temperature* is the temperature at which a glass is transformed from a supercooled liquid into a vitreous (i.e. non-crystalline) solid. At this temperature there is a measurable change in thermal expansion coefficient.

Crystallization of a glass can sometimes occur - this is called *devitrification*. For this to happen in a controlled fashion a nucleating agent is required; this is a material on which crystal growth can occur. To achieve this in practice, an agent such as titanium dioxide or magnesium fluoride is dissolved in the molten glass. On cooling, the agent precipitates, and crystals of glass grow on it during subsequent heat treatment. Such materials are *glass-ceramics*, and they can have greater hardness and strength than the parent glass.

15.4 GENERAL PROPERTIES OF CERAMICS

Dental significance: Ceramics are widely used for dental restorations. Their excellent biocompatibility, thermal properties and esthetic appeal make them attractive. Much research has been carried out to obtain materials with improved mechanical properties (Chapter 34).

15.4.1 Biological properties

Ceramic materials often have superb biocompatibility, which is of importance in their use dentally and as implant materials.

15.4.2 Chemical properties

Ceramics in general are extremely resistant to attack by chemicals (though note the exceptions in Sections 15.5 and 15.6) a property that is of great advantage in dental applications. To dissolve a ceramic, chemicals such as hydrofluoric acid are required.

Because ceramics are often inert, it can be difficult to obtain adhesion to them. Ceramic restorations may be roughened by etching with hydrofluoric acid/or by sandblasting to improve the retention of a cement to the internal surface of a restoration.

15.4.3 Mechanical properties

One of the problems associated with ceramics is their liability to fracture in tension. They exhibit little plastic deformation, because dislocation movement requires high energy, and the impact resistance of many ceramics is low. Stresses within the material can cause internal cracks, which can propagate rapidly through a material until fracture occurs. A number of factors are important:

1. Dislocations in crystals can cause stresses.
2. Cooling of the sample from its firing temperature, due to differences in the coefficient of thermal expansion between different phases in the material, is a significant source of stress.
3. Abrasion of the surface, or porosity within a material, can cause stress concentration to occur — the stress is concentrated where there is any irregularity of contour.

In some cases, a reinforcing agent such as alumina can be incorporated into a ceramic to improve its mechanical properties; this can act by inhibiting the propagation of cracks.

15.4.4 Thermal properties

The thermal conductivity and thermal diffusivity of these materials is very low (Table 6.1). This is because there are no free electrons, as in metals. The coefficient of thermal expansion is also low; for example, the figure for porcelain is closer to that of enamel and dentin than other restorative materials (Table 6.2).

15.4.5 Optical properties

From the dental viewpoint, these are excellent; dental porcelains are translucent because there are no free electrons (in contrast to metals), and can be colored by pigments such as metallic oxides, to match the shade of teeth.

15.4.6 Comparison of ceramic with metallic materials

It is not always possible to make a sharp distinction between these two classes of materials. For example, compounds between metals and metalloids, such as carbides, may be considered to be either ceramics, or intermetallic compounds. Nevertheless, it is useful to compare and contrast typical metals and ceramics:
1. Chemical properties. Many metals and alloys can corrode whereas ceramics are usually very resistant to chemical attack.
2. Mechanical properties. Metals have values for tensile and compressive strength that are of a comparable order of magnitude. On the other hand, ceramics are considerably stronger in compression than in tension. They are also usually much more brittle than metals, and have low impact strengths.
3. Thermal and electrical properties. Metals are good conductors; ceramics are good insulators.

15.4.7 Comparison of ceramic with polymeric materials

1. The stability of polymers at high temperature is usually less than that of ceramic materials.
2. Mechanical properties. Generally polymers are less rigid and more readily capable of plastic deformation than ceramics.
3. Crystallization. Polymers and ceramics in general crystallize less readily, and have more complex structures than metals and alloys.

15.5 ZINC OXIDE

Dental significance: Zinc oxide is widely used as a constituent of dental cements (Chapter 25).

Zinc oxide occurs as the mineral zincite. It can be prepared by the direct oxidation of zinc:

$$2Zn + O_2 \longrightarrow 2ZnO$$

or by the decomposition of the sulfate, nitrate, hydroxide or carbonate, for example:

$$ZnCO_3 \longrightarrow ZnO + CO_2$$

A number of reactions of zinc oxide are of dental interest.

1. Reaction with phosphoric acid. Zinc oxide can react with phosphoric acid to give zinc phosphate. This reaction is the basis of the zinc phosphate cements (Chapter 25).

2. Reaction with eugenol. Under certain conditions, particularly in the presence of moisture, zinc oxide can react with eugenol to give a chelate compound, zinc eugenolate (Figure 15.1). This reaction is important in zinc oxide - eugenol cements and impression materials (Chapters 25 and 31).

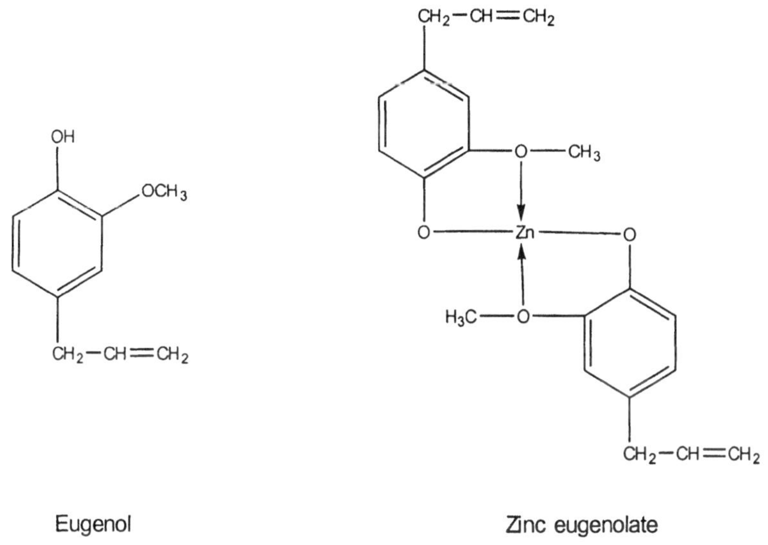

Figure 15.1. Eugenol and zinc eugenolate.

3. Reaction with other *ortho*-substituted phenols. Similar to the above, zinc oxide can react with, for example, guaiacol (2-methoxyphenol), 4-methylguaiacol, etc.

4. Reaction with *ortho*-ethoxybenzoic acid (EBA, Figure 15.2). This reaction is similar to the above, and is important in the EBA cements (Section 25.4.6).

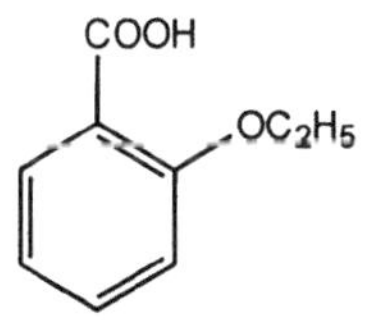

Figure 15.2. Ortho-ethoxybenzoic acid (EBA).

5. Reaction with aqueous poly(acrylic acid). In this reaction, zinc polyacrylate is believed to be the main product; this reaction is employed in adhesive polycarboxylate cements (Chapter 25).

15.6 FLUOROALUMINOSILICATE (FAS) GLASSES

Dental significance: FAS glasses are widely used in fluoride-releasing dental cements – see Chapter 26.

Fluorine-containing aluminosilicate glasses are of particular interest. The chief constituents are SiO_2, Al_2O_3, CaO, Na_2O and fluorides. The detailed composition of such materials is given in Table 26.1. The constituents of these glasses are fused together at temperatures up to 1400°C, the fluorides acting as fluxes. The fused material is plunged into cold water which cracks it (this process is termed *fritting*); this facilitates the subsequent grinding to a fine powder.

The aluminosilicate glass contains approximately equal numbers of Al and Si atoms, arranged as shown in Figure 15.3. Each aluminum ion has a net negative charge that is balanced by the Na^+ and Ca^{2+} ions which are present.

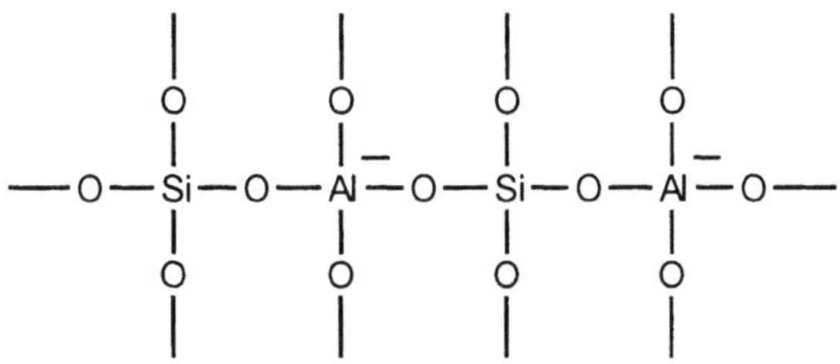

Figure 15.3. Aluminosilicate glass.

These glasses can react with, for example, phosphoric acid. Hydrated protons (H_3O^+) from the liquid attack the aluminum sites with a negative charge, so decompose the surface of the glass. Forms of aluminosilicate glass can also react with weaker acids, such as aqueous solutions of poly(acrylic acid). Further details of the dental applications of these reactions are given in Chapter 26.

15.7 PROPERTIES OF SILICA

> **Dental significance**: Silica is an important constituent in mold materials for casting alloys; their expansion characteristics are important in compensating for the shrinkage of an alloy on cooling after casting – see Chapter 53.

15.7.1 Polymorphism

Polymorphic materials are those that can exist with more than one crystal structure. Silica is an example of such material in which changes of structure can occur. There are two types of structural transformation:

1. *Displacive transformations* can take place where atoms become displaced, but no interatomic bonds are broken, when there is a temperature change. The following factors are characteristic of such processes:
   - They occur at specific temperatures;
   - The transformations are rapid;
   - The high-temperature form has a greater specific volume thus the formation of the high-temperature material is accompanied by an expansion.
2. *Reconstructive transformations* of silica involve the breaking and remaking of Si - O bonds. These processes need more energy than the preceding type, and so usually occur more slowly.

15.7.2 Forms of silica

Quartz, with a hexagonal structure, is the most stable form of silica. When quartz is heated to 867°C, a reconstructive transformation to tridymite occurs. At 1470°C, another reconstructive transformation takes place, to form cristobalite. At over 1700°C, cristobalite melts, and fused quartz, which is amorphous, is produced (Figure 15.4). It should be noted that if fused quartz, cristobalite or tridymite are cooled rapidly, there is not sufficient time for the comparatively slow transformations to take place; so all four forms can exist at room temperature.

Quartz (hexagonal structure)
867°C
Tridymite (rhombohedral structure)
1470°C
Cristobalite (cubic structure)
1713°C
Fused quartz (amorphous)

Figure 15.4. Forms of silica.

15.7.3 Displacive transformations

These can occur for quartz, tridymite and cristobalite, as follows, as illustrated in Figure 15.5.

low quartz (alpha-quartz) $\xrightleftharpoons{573^{0}\text{C}}$ high quartz (beta-quartz)

low tridymite (alpha-tridymite) $\xrightleftharpoons{105^{0}\text{C}}$ middle tridymite $\xrightarrow{160^{0}\text{C}}$ high tridymite (beta-tridymite)

low cristobalite (alpha-cristobalite) $\xrightleftharpoons{200\text{-}270^{0}\text{C}}$ high cristobalite (beta-cristobalite)

Figure 15.5. Displacive transformations.

15.7.4 Dimensional changes

During displacive transformations, dimensional changes occur (Figure 15.6). Cristobalite and quartz both expand more than tridymite; this expansion is an important property of dental investment materials (Chapter 53). Fused quartz undergoes no such transformations, and has little thermal expansion.

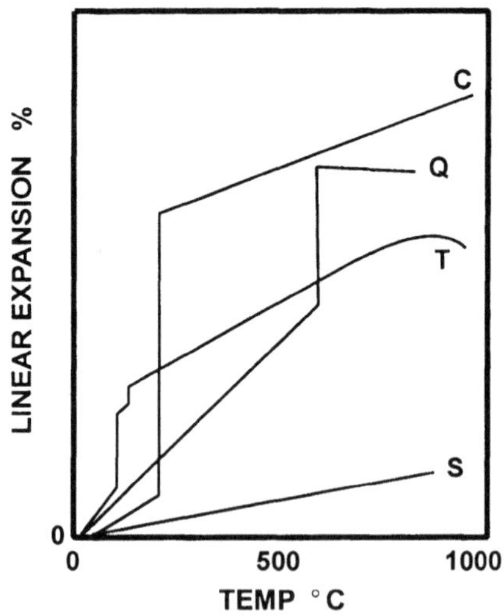

Figure 15.6. Thermal expansion of the allotropes of silica. C: cristobalite; Q: quartz; T: tridymite; S: fused silica.

15.8 DENTAL APPLICATIONS

These are summarized in Table 15.2.

Table 15.2. Dental applications of ceramics

Material	Application	Chapter number
Zinc oxide	Constituent of cements	25
Fluoroaluminosilicate glass	Constituent of cements	26
Silica, barium glass etc	Inorganic constituents of resin composites	27,37
Dental porcelain	Crowns, inlays, veneers, porcelain-fused-to-metal restorations	35,36
Silica	Constituent of refractory investment materials	53
Silica, alumina etc.	Abrasives	54

FURTHER READING

Horath L (1995). *Fundamentals of Materials Science for Technologists.* Prentice Hall, Englewood Cliffs, New Jersey. pp 149-182.

McLean J W (1979). *The Science and Art of Dental Ceramics: Volume I: The Nature of Dental Ceramics and their Clinical Use.* Quintessence, Chicago.

Park J B, Lakes R S (1992). *Biomaterials. An Introduction.* 2nd edition, Plenum Press, New York. pp 117-140.

Chapter 16

Theory of Composites

Summary: Techniques of combining materials to produce materials with enhanced properties are discussed.

Dental significance: Composite materials are widely used as dental restorative materials.

16.1 INTRODUCTION

A *composite material* is defined as a unified combination of two or more materials, and is designed to have superior properties over the individual components. Some composite materials have already been referred to in earlier chapters of this book. For example, dentin contains a protein constituent, collagen, and a mineral material, apatite (Chapter 8). In the discussion on metallurgy (Chapter 13) it was shown how some alloys are heterogeneous in structure, where there is some degree of solid insolubility. Regarding ceramics, composite structures containing a reinforcing agent to hinder crack propagation, have been mentioned (Chapter 15).

Composite materials occur widely in nature, including dentin as already discussed. Wood is also a composite, consisting of strong and flexible cellulose fibers held together by lignin, which makes the material stiff. It is not surprising that development of materials has imitated nature by combining two materials to produce a composite, either to improve the properties of one constituent, or to create a material with properties quite different from either constituent. Neither is it surprising that composites are finding applications in dentistry, owing to the need to meet the very exacting conditions of the oral environment.

The following is a note of the dentally relevant methods of combining materials.
1. Alloying - any two-phase alloy system can be considered to be a composite - for example, eutectic alloys, as in solders (Chapter 13).
2. Powder compacting can be used in the fabrication of tungsten carbide burs. Fine particles of the carbide are embedded in a matrix of cobalt.
3. Composite structures can be fabricated by fusing a ceramic coating onto a cast alloy structure. The aim of this procedure is to combine the good mechanical properties of the alloy with the good esthetics of the ceramic constituent (Chapter 36).
4. Polymer-ceramic compositions are finding widespread use in dentistry as dental restorative materials (Chapters 27 and 37), and the theory of these materials is the focus of this chapter.

16.2 POLYMER-CERAMIC COMPOSITES

Polymers can be reinforced by the inclusion of fibers and/or particulate materials. This is the most frequent use of the term 'composite.'

16.2.1 Fiber reinforcement

Perhaps the best known industrial example of this is the use of glass fibers to reinforce polymers. Fiber-reinforcement is beginning to find application in dentistry, including tooth restoration and denture materials. The degree of reinforcement that is achieved is dependent on many factors:

- The polymer (the matrix) to be reinforced should be a material capable of plastic deformation (not brittle);
- The fiber should have a higher modulus of elasticity than the matrix;
- There should be adhesion between the fibers and the matrix;
- Ceramic fibers should not be flawed by surface cracks, which will weaken them;
- The quantity of fibrous material is important;
- Fiber alignment should be noted. Fibers can be aligned in the matrix, or can have random orientation, or can be incorporated in a woven form.

Consider the case of a polymer with aligned fibers, to which a tensile load parallel to the fibers is applied. When such a composite structure is under stress, there is an associated strain; the components of the material act together to equalize their strains. This is the *principle of combined action.* The matrix flows plastically, and if the fibers are stiffer (higher modulus of elasticity), they will take a higher stress than the matrix for a given strain – compare point B with point A in Figure 16.1. In this way the fibers can significantly contribute to the strength of the composite. Note that there will not be significant reinforcement of such a fibrous composite if the load in a direction perpendicular to the fiber orientation. Note also that fiber inclusions do not improve compressive properties substantially. In practice, it is quite common to have random orientation of fibers in a matrix so that the mechanical properties of the composite are *isotropic* - that is, the same in all directions.

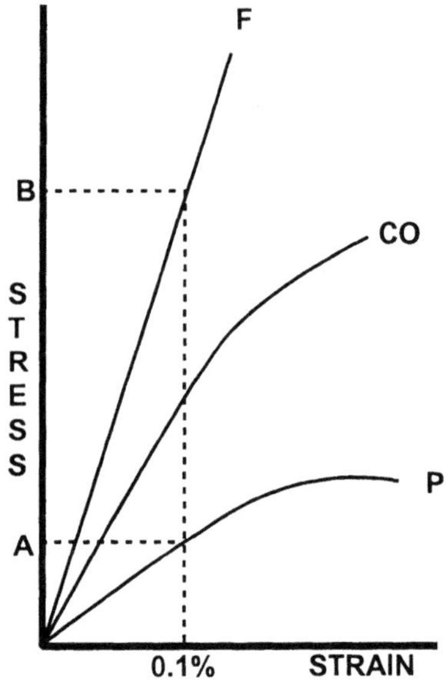

Figure 16.1. Stress-strain curves: P = polymer; F = high modulus ceramic; CO = composite material.

16.3.2 Particulate ceramic fillers

Ceramic-filled acrylics and other polymers are used dentally as restorative materials. In contrast to fibers, particulate fillers can improve compressive properties, but have less effect on tensile properties. In other respects, the principle of reinforcement is similar to that discussed above. The principle of combined action applies, provided that the filler is more rigid than the polymer, and that there is adhesion between the two phases. In dental formulations a coupling agent (a silane compound) is used for this purpose.

Ceramic particulate fillers in a resin can have other benefits as well as improving some mechanical properties. They may reduce the setting shrinkage of a polymer, and give a set material with a lower coefficient of thermal expansion (Table 6.2). If care is taken in matching refractive indices of polymeric and ceramic phases, an esthetic translucent material can be produced.

16.4 REINFORCED CERAMICS

The propagation of a crack through a ceramic, such as dental porcelain, can lead to its fracture. However, if a stronger constituent, such as alumina (Al_2O_3) is present, it may hinder the progress of cracks and so strengthen the material. This principle has been used in aluminous porcelain.

FURTHER READING

Gordon J E (1976). *The New Science of Strong Materials*, 2nd edition. Princeton University Press, Princeton, New Jersey. pp 173-205.

V

INTERFACES BETWEEN MATERIALS

Chapter 17

Surfaces and Interfaces

Summary: A discussion of surfaces of materials and interfaces between materials.

Dental significance: It is important to understand the nature of the interfaces between biomaterials and tissues, between different materials and within a material. Many problems relating to the biocompatibility and durability of biomaterials are related to surfaces and interfaces.

17.1 SURFACES

The surface atoms or molecules of a solid and liquid differ in properties from those in the bulk of a material. Consider first the case of a liquid. Its molecules are acted on by strong forces of attraction from neighboring molecules. In Figure 17.1, (A) represents a molecule inside the liquid, with equal forces in all directions. In contrast, molecule (B) on the surface is being pulled downwards perpendicular to the surface. This gives rise to the phenomenon of *surface tension.* This may be defined as the force of attraction exerted on surface molecules of a liquid by the molecules beneath the surface. This parameter has traditionally been expressed in units of dyne/cm. In SI units, 1 mN/m is numerically equal to 1 dyne/cm.

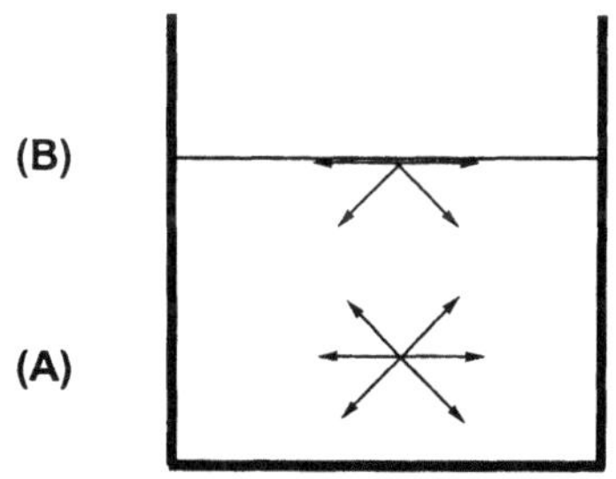

Figure 17.1. Illustration of surface tension.

In the case of solids, the surface atoms or molecules also have higher energy than the bulk of the material, again because they are not completely surrounded by atoms or molecules. Consequently, solid surfaces are reactive, and can attract atoms or molecules. This is termed *adsorption*, and may be of one of two types:

- *Chemisorption*, where a chemical reaction has taken place; this reaction is not readily reversible;
- *Physical adsorption*, where Van der Waals forces operate. In this case these forces involved are not as strong as primary chemical bonding, and such adsorption is more readily reversible.

Thus the composition of the surface of a solid may differ from that of the bulk of the material. This can have wide-ranging implications in the dental application of a material. It may influence:

- Biocompatibility – it is obviously the surface of a material that is in contact with the oral tissues;
- Interfacial properties such as the ability to adhere (see Chapter 18);
- Chemical or electrochemical reactivity – for example the passive coating on chromium-containing alloys (Section 14.2.8);
- Mechanical properties, such as ability to resist abrasion;
- Esthetics.

17.2 INTERFACES

An *interface* is a surface that forms a common boundary between two substances. There are many different types of interface that are of importance in dentistry, as classified and listed in Table 17.1.

Table 17.1. Examples of interfaces in dentistry

Interface between:	Dental example	Chapter reference
Biomaterials and tissues		
- Biomaterial/soft tissues	Dentures	45
- Biomaterial/hard tissues	Tooth filling materials and cements	24-28
- Biomaterial/pulp	Pulp capping agents	25, 43
Biomaterial and biomaterial		
- Polymer/polymer	Denture base and polymeric denture teeth	45, 48
- Polymer/ceramic	Denture base and ceramic teeth	45, 48
- Polymer/metal	Cast alloy partial denture framework with acrylic components	47
- Ceramic/ceramic	Porcelain jacket crown	34
- Ceramic/metal	Porcelain fused to metal (PFM)	36

Interface between:	Dental example	Chapter reference
- Composite/cement	Indirect composite restoration	37
- Metal/cement	Inlays, crowns and bridges	35
- Metal/metal	Solder based on eutectic alloy	54
- Ceramic/cement	Ceramic crowns, inlays and veneers	34
Within a biomaterial		
- Polymer/ceramic	Resin composite tooth filling materials	27,37
- Metal/metal	Numerous phases within a dental amalgam restoration	24
Biomaterial and fluid		
- Biomaterial/saliva	Tooth filling and denture materials	24,26,27,34-
- Biomaterial/constituent of drinks	Tooth filling and denture materials	38,45-48
- Biomaterial/dentifrice	Tooth filling materials	24,26,27,34-38
- Biomaterial/denture cleanser	Denture materials	45-48

17.3 LIQUID-SOLID INTERFACE

The ability of a liquid to wet a surface can be measured by the contact angle of a drop of liquid on the surface (Figure 17.2).

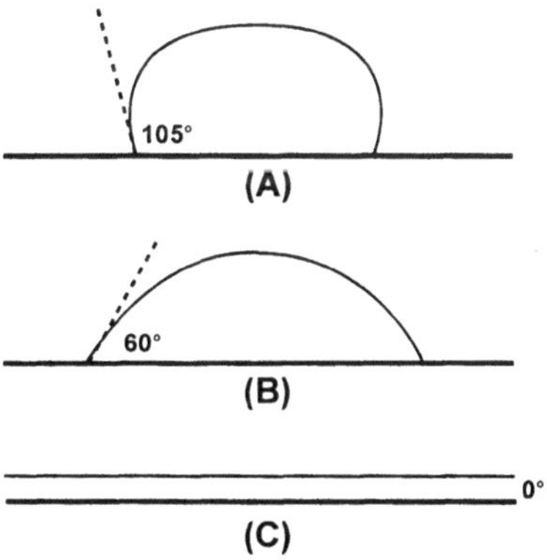

Figure 17.2. Surface wetting. (A) contact angle 105° - poor wetting; (B) contact angle 60°; (C) contact angle 0° - excellent wetting.

Contact angle measurements can be used to obtain quantitative information about the reactivity of a surface. Liquids of different surface tensions are applied to a surface, and the contact angle of each liquid on the surface is measured. Plots of cosine θ *versus* γ, where θ is the contact angle and γ the surface tension, are often found to be linear (Zisman plots). Extrapolation of the graph to cosine $\theta = 1$ (that is, $\theta = 0°$, indicating perfect wetting) gives the *critical surface tension* of the solid (γ_C) (Figure 17.3). As a general principle, good wetting occurs if the critical surface tension of a solid is greater than or equal to the surface tension of the liquid that is applied to the surface. As will be discussed, good wetting is very important in obtaining good adhesion. Table 17.2 gives some typical data for γ_C values for tooth tissue and a selection of dental biomaterials.

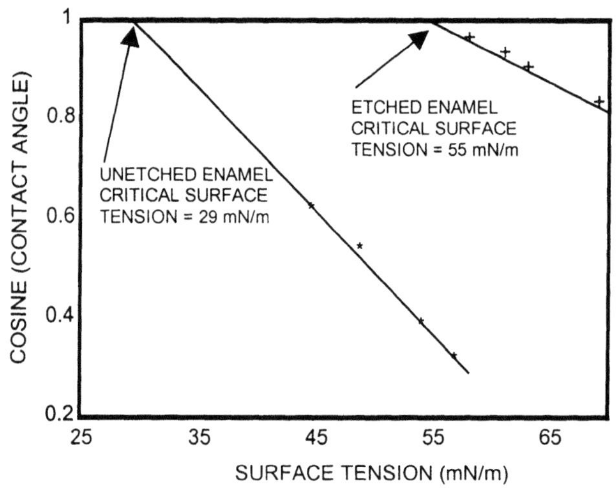

Figure 17.3. Zisman plots for enamel.

Table 17.2. Critical surface tension data for solids

Material	Critical surface tension , γ_C (mN/m)
Enamel (unetched)	29
Enamel (acid etched)	55
Poly(methyl methacrylate)	38
Silicone polymer	28
Polytetrafluoroethylene (PTFE)	18

The degree of surface roughness is a factor to be taken into account. If the surface contains capillaries, the ability of a fluid to penetrate these crevices is proportional to its surface tension, proportional to cosine θ, and inversely proportional to the fluid viscosity.

17.4 DENTAL SIGNIFICANCE

A summary of some of the principal areas of importance in relation to interfaces in dentistry is now given.

17.4.1 Interfaces between biomaterials and tissues

1. In some cases, problems can occur when a material is in contact with soft tissues. For example, denture base materials, if improperly processed, may cause irritation (Chapter 45).
2. A major area of interest relates to the interface between a tooth restoration and enamel and dentin. As defined and discussed in Chapter 18, harmful microleakage may occur, and adhesion is desirable.
3. Materials are available for pulp capping, where there has been either cariogenic or iatrogenic exposure of the pulp. This is currently an area of controversy (Sections 25.6 and 43.4.6).

17.4.2 Interfaces between biomaterials

There are many instances where a restoration or prosthesis is fabricated from a combination of different materials, and good adhesion between phases is required for durability. The principles of adhesion are given in Chapter 18.

17.4.3 Interfaces within a biomaterial

These occur in composite materials. The importance of bonding between phases has already been stressed (Section 16.2), and the application of this to dental restorative materials is discussed in Chapter 27.

17.4.4 Interfaces between biomaterials and fluids

In the mouth materials come into contact with saliva, constituents of foods and drinks, and dentifrices and mouth washes. As a result, corrosion, erosion or staining may occur.

FURTHER READING

References on the whole area of surfaces, interfacial phenomena and adhesion are given at the conclusion of Chapter 18.

Chapter 18

Adhesion to Tooth Substance and Microleakage

Summary: The principles of adhesion to tooth substance are presented, and an outline of current approaches is given. Microleakage is defined and discussed.

Dental significance: There are considerable clinical benefits in being able to bond a restorative material to tooth substance.

18.1 ADHESION TO TOOTH SUBSTANCE

Adhesion in dentistry is important in many different clinical situations. Chemically adhesive cements are available, which contain poly(acrylic acid) or a related co-polymer, which can undergo some form of ionic bonding with the mineral component of enamel and dentin. Micromechanical bonding is also widely used, following treatment of enamel and dentin with an acid etchant, which is often based on phosphoric acid.

The ability to bond to tooth tissue is used in a wide range of clinical situations, such as:

- The placement of pit and fissure sealants to prevent decay (Chapter 19);
- The placement of tooth restorations, to reduce the dependence on mechanical retention, thereby reducing the amount of tooth preparation required, in attempts to eliminate microbial microleakage (see below), to seal the dentinal tubules to eliminate postoperative pain and to reinforce the tooth;
- Cementation of ceramic restorations and veneers, and of cast alloy restorations and fixed prostheses.

18.2 PRINCIPLES OF ADHESION

18.2.1 Definitions and mechanisms

Adhesion occurs when two unlike substances join together on being brought into contact, because of forces of attraction between them. Distinguish this from *cohesion*, which results from attraction between like molecules. An *adhesive* is a material used to produce adhesion. The *adherend* is the substance to which the adhesive is applied.

Two mechanisms of bonding are possible, either or both of which may operate:
1. Chemical adhesion occurs if chemisorption occurs.
2. Micromechanical adhesion or attachment occurs when a liquid flows into pores or crevices in the adherend surface. When the fluid sets, micromechanical interlocking occurs producing a potentially strong bond.

18.2.2 Requirements for good bonding

To obtain good adhesion, a number of factors are important. Good wetting of the adherend by the adhesive is important. Surface texture must be suitable; micromechanical adhesion requires a roughened surface on the adherend. The adherend surface must be clean and free of debris. Contaminated surfaces usually have lower critical surface tension (γ_C) values, so will not be capable of being wetted as easily as clean surfaces.

The adhesive must have a suitable viscosity to enable it to flow readily over the surface of the adherend. Air pockets between adhesive and adherend should be avoided (Figure 18.1).

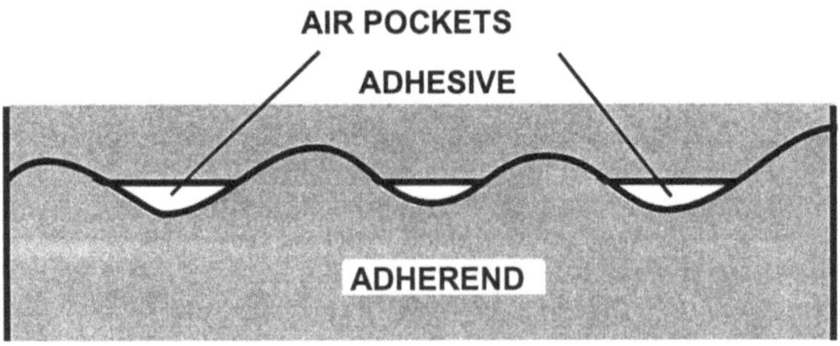

Figure 18.1. Air trapped between adhesive and adherend.

The adhesive must be converted from a liquid to a solid, to achieve mechanical strength and reasonably high rigidity in the adhesive. Solidification may be achieved by various means, such as polymerization or by the evaporation of a solvent. Ideally on setting there should be minimal dimensional change, otherwise there may be unacceptably high stresses at the interface, causing breakdown of the bond. Too great a thickness of the layer of adhesive may give weaker bonding.

Some requirements of bonding systems are especially important in the dental context. Since the hard dental tissues contain water, a dental adhesive should be *hydrophilic*; that is, it should have a strong affinity for water. A *hydrophobic* (water repelling) material would not spread well on a dentin surface, because it would have a high contact angle. It is also obvious that a dental adhesive should be suitable in terms of biocompatibility, and that the set material is stable and durable under oral conditions.

18.2.3 Measurement of adhesion

Adhesion can be measured in tension (Figure 18.2) or in shear. Bond failure can occur in a number of ways:

- *Adhesive failure* may occur, where the adhesive is removed from the adherend;
- *Cohesive failure* where the adherend itself fractures;
- A mixture of adhesive and cohesive failure may take place.

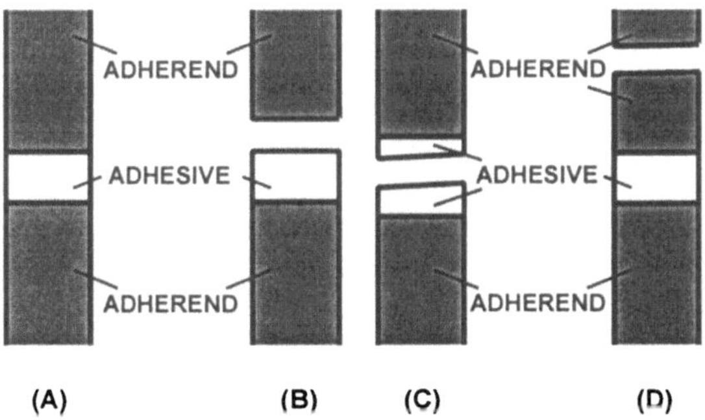

Figure 18.2. Adhesion testing (A) adhesive bond in tension; (B) adhesive failure; (C) cohesive failure of adhesive; (D) cohesive failure of adherend.

18.3 MICROLEAKAGE

18.3.1 Definition and description

The interface between a synthetic material and tooth tissue has been described as: "Dynamic micro-crevices which contain a busy traffic of ions and molecules."* The resulting *marginal microleakage* may be defined as: "The passage of bacteria, fluids, molecules or ions between a cavity wall and the restorative material applied to it."†

This microleakage can have potentially serious effects. Penetration of acids and microorganisms can result in the patient's experience of sensitivity and ultimately the occurrence of secondary caries. Pulpal damage can result from toxic products liberated by microorganisms. Staining can occur at the margin of the restoration resulting from accumulation of debris.

Clearly marginal microleakage should be avoided or minimized. This has been one of the reasons for the development of dental adhesives. However it should be noted that the attainment of adhesion does not necessarily mean that there is no leakage.

Stresses at the interface can break down bonding to tooth tissue, and can increase the amount of microleakage. These interfacial stresses can come from a number of sources:

1. Dimensional changes in the material can stress the interface. They may be the result of continued reaction of the materials (example: contraction accompanying polymerization) or absorption of water.
2. Problems can be caused by thermal stress. In the mouth there are temperature fluctuations, and if a tooth restorative material has a different coefficient of thermal expansion from tooth tissue, stresses can result.
3. Likewise, mechanical loading can cause stresses. This will occur if different materials differ in their moduli of elasticity. The material with the lower modulus will deform more.

18.3.2 Measurement

There is not a standard method of measuring microleakage, and the available data in the literature do not necessarily correlate with each other.

* Myers H M (1966). In *Scientific Bases of Dentistry* (edited by Shapiro M), Saunders, Philadelphia, p. 285.

† Kidd E A M (1976). Microleakage: a review. *Journal of Dentistry* **4**: 199-205.

Methods have included measurement of the penetration of bacteria, radioactive isotopes, chemical tracers and dyes. In addition, air pressure and electrochemical techniques have been employed. Quite often leakage is measured in samples that are thermocycled (for example, between 5°C and 60°C), in attempts to simulate temperature changes in the mouth.

FURTHER READING

Park J B, Lakes R S (1992). *Biomaterials. An Introduction,* 2nd edition. Plenum Press, New York. pp 56-58.
Taylor M J, Lynch E (1992). Microleakage. *Journal of Dentistry* **20**: 3-10.

VI

MATERIALS FOR THE PREVENTION OF DENTAL DISEASE

Chapter 19

Pit and Fissure Sealants

Summary: Techniques and materials for sealing pits and fissures of teeth are reviewed. Sealants are playing an increasing role in caries prevention.

19.1 RATIONALE FOR PIT AND FISSURE SEALING

Pits and fissures are sites on teeth that may be difficult to clean, with the risk of plaque stagnation and consequent possible onset of caries. Clinical studies continue to demonstrate continuing caries attack of permanent molars in children, despite the reduction in caries incidence reported in many areas of the developed world. Fluoride in its various forms (Chapter 20) appears to be more effective in reducing caries on proximal surfaces than on occlusal surfaces, and pit and fissure caries may account for up to 90% of the total caries experience in some child populations. Accordingly, the concept of sealing pits and fissures with resin applied to an etched enamel surface, known as fissure sealing, was developed in the 1960s shortly after the introduction of the acid-etch technique (discussed in Section 8.2.3). Such treatment could be of benefit to patients at risk to occlusal caries, given that the sealant will protect the susceptible pits and fissures from plaque accumulation and substrates that may be metabolized into acids. Not everyone will develop occlusal caries and fissure sealants are unlikely to be cost effective if applied to all teeth, in particular in patients with low caries history.

19.2 DIAGNOSIS

Difficulties may be experienced in diagnosis because a carious lesion may be hidden on the walls of the fissure and not clinically visible, and probing is not recommended because of the potential for damage to the enamel of the fissure. The formation of a cavity in the enamel is likely to occur relatively late in the progression of the caries and is likely to be related to a fairly large dentin lesion. It has also been considered that occlusal caries has become more difficult to diagnose since the advent of fluoride treatments such as fluoride-containing toothpaste. It is therefore important to develop criteria for the selection of teeth that should be sealed. These criteria include:

- Patient selection;
- Tooth selection;
- Radiographic evidence (Table 19.1).

Table 19.1. Criteria for selection of teeth for the application of sealants

Factor	Criteria for selection
Patient selection	- Children with special needs such as the medically compromised, mentally or physically handicapped or from a socially deprived background - Children with extensive caries in their primary teeth - Patients who are manageable, to allow for isolation and moisture control
Tooth selection	- Occlusal surfaces of permanent molar teeth, when the tooth has erupted sufficiently to permit moisture control - Children with occlusal caries in one first permanent molar should have the remaining first molars sealed - Children with occlusal caries in first permanent molar teeth should have the second molars sealed as soon as they have erupted sufficiently - Teeth to be sealed should be free from proximal caries. Lesion formation and progression may take many years, so there is no limit in the time from eruption for treatment by fissure sealing
Radiography	- Bitewing radiographs are indicated in cases where there is doubt about the clinical integrity of an occlusal surface on clinical examination - If no dentin involvement is seen on radiographic examination, the tooth may be sealed and kept under clinical and radiographic review

19.3 ENAMEL ETCHING

Teeth to be sealed are first etched by phosphoric acid. The purposes of etching are:

- To provide a porous surface into which a resin can readily flow, set, and be retained;
- To provide a high energy surface for good wetting by the resin;

The aim is to achieve a surface free of moisture and other contaminants. The technique is outlined in Table 19.2.

Table 19.2. Technique for fissure sealing

Technique	Rationale
Clean tooth with a non-fluoride prophylaxis paste or pumice/water slurry	Contaminants may adversely affect the etching procedure. Fluoride incorporated in the enamel makes it more acid resistant
Wash with oil-free water, dry and isolate	Produces a clean dry surface
Apply H_3PO_4 etchant gel for 15-20 s with a dabbing (not rubbing) motion	Rubbing may damage the delicate microscopic network in the etched enamel
Limit etchant to at-risk area	Resin flows quickly over all etched surfaces and excess resin may require removal due to occlusal interferences, with potential for damage to underlying enamel
Rinse with water for 15 s	Complete removal of etching debris and residual acid
Dry	Moisture gives a lower energy (less wettable) surface
Check etched surface – it should have a chalky dull opaque appearance	Only visual assessment will recognize a correctly etched surface
If etching is inadequate, re-apply etchant	Must have a porous surface for micromechanical retention
If inadvertent contamination (e.g. by saliva) occurs, repeat etching procedure	Must have a reactive surface
Apply resin into all occlusal pits and fissures	
Confine sealant to etched surface only	
Visible light cure sealant if indicated	
Remove unpolymerized surface layer of resin	Oxygen inhibits free radical addition polymerization

19.4 SEALANT MATERIALS

19.4.1 Resin-based sealants

Early sealant materials were based upon ultra-violet light activated resins, but current systems may be chemically cured or visible light cured. Currently, the most commonly used resin is bis-GMA or Bowen's resin (Figure 11.13) although other dimethacrylates (for example, a urethane dimethacrylate, Figure 11.14) may be used. This is a viscous resin and other monomers are therefore added, such as triethyleneglycol dimethacrylate (TEGDMA; Figure 11.12), to produce a material that flows over the etched surface. Light cured materials have the benefit over chemically cured materials in that they do not require mixing and will therefore not contain air bubbles that may be incorporated during the mixing procedure. The operator is also in control of the time of set and the polymerization time is likely to be less than that for chemically curing materials. Some sealant materials contain inorganic filler particles (such as silica) in order to improve the wear resistance of the material. This also makes the fissure sealants more readily visible on the tooth surface, and, some sealant materials have specially added tints for this purpose. Advantages of colored sealants include:

- The extent of sealant application may be seen more clearly;
- Defects such as an air bubble are more easily visualized;
- Defective margins are more easily seen and repaired;
- Parents and patient can see the treatment which has been carried out;
- Sealant retention is more easily documented, either in a clinical trial or in the dental office.

A potential disadvantage of colored sealants is that they may mask the presence of occlusal caries.

Some manufacturers include fluoride-containing fillers in their formulations, but evidence indicating the effect of this addition on caries is scant.

19.4.2 Success of resin-based fissure sealants

Results of studies on the longevity of fissure sealants are very encouraging, with retention rates of at least 50% being reported at 10 years; caries reduction closely parallels the retention rate. Success is dependent upon careful clinical technique, with the operator ensuring that the tooth being treated is isolated from moisture contamination (often an exacting procedure in a young patient). It is also important that the entire etched surface is covered and that the fissures are penetrated by sealant. The clinician must also check that excess material does not flow interproximally and that the sealant does not interfere with normal occlusal relationships. As with any other form of treatment, it is essential that sealants be checked at regular intervals so that sealant may be added to any areas where material has been lost. Sealant longevity is dependent upon the position of the tooth in the mouth, the skill of the operator, the age of the child and the degree of eruption of the tooth. An increased success rate is achieved for:

- Teeth nearer the anterior of the mouth;
- Operators of higher skill;
- Older children;
- More fully erupted teeth.

The dental profession has been slow to adopt sealants, but there is evidence that they are increasingly being used as a routine part of preventive practice.

19.4.3 Other sealant materials

Thinly-mixed glass-ionomer materials (Chapter 26) have been suggested as being suitable for fissure sealing, although there is relatively limited evidence as to the effectiveness of this technique. Some results have demonstrated up to 80% retention of glass-ionomer fissure sealants after 2 years, while others have reported a total or substantial loss of sealants after 6 months. Glass-ionomer cements have been recommended to be used on fissures of more than 100 μm in width.

A 'compomer' based sealant (Section 27.10) has recently been introduced, but no long-term clinical data are yet available.

19.5 THE SEALANT RESTORATION

An extension of the sealant procedure may involve the use of resin composite (Chapter 27) or glass-ionomer (Chapter 26) materials in the restoration of a small-access occlusal cavity, with the application of a resin-based fissure sealant to the remaining fissures. Such a restoration has been termed a preventive resin restoration or sealant restoration, or, in cases where glass-ionomer materials are used, a preventive glass-ionomer restoration. These techniques are indicated if radiographic examination of the tooth indicates that the extent of carious attack is limited to the outer third of dentin.

Caries is removed with a small round bur or by other ultraconservative cavity preparation methods. The enamel and dentin and the remaining fissures are etched, a dentin and enamel bonding agent applied, the cavity restored with resin composite and the sealant applied and cured. For a preventive glass-ionomer restoration, glass-ionomer is applied to the cavity, and when set, the enamel margins of the cavity and the fissures are etched as appropriate, the tooth rinsed and dried and the sealant applied and cured. The occlusion should be checked and adjusted as necessary; sealant should be re-applied to any areas of glass-ionomer which have been exposed during adjustment.

19.6 SUMMARY

Fissure sealants are recognized as a useful preventive treatment in the susceptible patient, but should be combined with other preventive measures such as dietary advice, oral hygiene instruction and fluoride treatment. Appropriate case selection is important in the cost analysis. Diligent placement technique is essential.

FURTHER READING

Feigal R J (1998). Sealants and preventive restorations: review of effectiveness and clinical changes for improvement. *Pediatric Dentistry* **20**: 85-92.

Kidd, E A M, Joyston-Bechal S (1994). Update on fissure sealants. *Dental Update* **21**: 323-326.

Moore C E, Jackson G S (1988). Pit and fissure sealants: One more time. *Journal of the Canadian Dental Association* **54**: 728-730.

Ripa L W (1993). Sealants revisited: an update of the effectiveness of pit-and-fissure sealants. *Caries Research* **27**(supplement 1): 77-82.

Chapter 20

Fluoride-containing Materials

Summary: A wide variety of fluoride-containing materials is available for application by the dental healthcare worker or patient and these have demonstrable properties in relation to caries control. A number of restorative materials also contain fluoride, either inherently present in the material as a result of its manufacturing process, or added deliberately by the manufacturer. The effect of these materials on caries control requires further investigation in clinical practice.

20.1 INTRODUCTION: FLUORIDATION OF WATER SUPPLIES

A first possible connection between the prevalence of dental caries and diet was made in 1892. It was suggested that a cause of the increase in dental caries at that time might be a change in the type of bread eaten, given the change to white flour from flour which contained the fluorine-containing wheat husk. Nine years later, McKay, in Colorado Springs, noticed that the teeth of many of his patients were affected by a stain which he called 'mottled enamel.' For 30 years, McKay continued his search for the etiological factor of mottling, and in 1931, Trendly Dean was appointed to carry out research on mottled enamel. By 1936, he had concluded that there was a relationship between the severity of mottled enamel, the fluoride concentration in the water supply and caries incidence. He also concluded "the possibility of controlling dental caries through the domestic water supply warrants thorough study." Further studies indicated that the maximum benefit in terms of reduction in caries incidence occurred at 1-2 ppm fluoride, with minimum risk of mottling up to levels of 1.5 ppm. This work led to the decision to fluoridate water supplies in the USA at the level of 1 ppm. Subsequent work, worldwide, has confirmed these findings, with caries reductions in deciduous teeth of between 20% and 80% being recorded, and for permanent teeth between 20% and 90%. Fluoride in drinking water appears to have a greater caries-inhibitory effect on approximal or smooth surfaces than on pit or fissure caries, and the rate of progression of caries is slower in a fluoride area than in an area where the water supply is not fluoridated. Also, fluoride appears to have a life-long caries preventive effect. The safety of fluoridation of water supplies has been reviewed on a number of occasions and has been found to be safe, and does not induce cancer or increase mortality due to cancer.

20.2 MECHANISMS OF FLUORIDE ACTION

The interaction between fluoride and enamel is complex, and, generally, it is thought that one of two reactions takes place so that either fluoroapatite or calcium fluoride are formed:

$$Ca_{10}(PO_4)_6(OH)_2 + 2F^- \longrightarrow Ca_{10}(PO_4)_6F_2 + 2OH^- \quad \ldots(1)$$

$$Ca_{10}(PO_4)_6(OH)_2 + 20F^- \longrightarrow 10CaF_2 + 6PO_4^{3-} + 2OH^- \quad \ldots(2)$$

These reactions improve the stability of the enamel apatite lattice through substitution of hydroxyl groups by fluoride; the effect is to render the enamel less soluble in dilute organic acids such as may be present in plaque which has been exposed to dietary sugars. Although the incorporation of fluoride into tooth substance during formation may be the ideal means by which teeth are provided with an increased resistance to caries throughout life, topical application of fluoride to the tooth surface may also produce caries inhibition.

20.3 APPLICATION OF FLUORIDE

20.3.1 Dietary constituents

There are situations in which fluoridation of the water supply may be impractical or politically unacceptable and there are communities that do not have piped water supplies. In such situations, fluoride dietary supplements may be provided in the form of fluoride tablets or drops. These supplements demand the co-operation of the patient (or caregiver) for a long period of time. They are therefore considered not to be generally suitable as a public health measure and should therefore only be directed towards those children who require them and who live in areas with suboptimal fluoride levels in the drinking water. Tablets have been considered to be more effective than drops, as tablets may dissolve slowly in the mouth, thereby providing an additional topical effect. The recommended optimum dosage varies according to the age of the patient but is generally considered to be 0.50 mg F^- per day for the under-four years age group and 1.00 mg in the 4 to 16 age group (Table 20.1). These supplements should be used to complement regular twice-daily use of 1000 ppm fluoride toothpaste. Ideally, toothbrushing and the taking of fluoride drops or tablets should occur at different times. However, to reduce the risk of enamel opacities, children under the age of 6 years and at low risk of developing dental caries should use a toothpaste containing no more than 600 ppm of fluoride. Children at higher risk of caries should use a standard (1000 ppm) or higher (1450 ppm) toothpaste, and accept that there may be a small risk of developing enamel opacities due to fluoride consumption slightly in excess of ideal.

Table 20.1. Recommended fluoride supplements where water fluoride concentration is less than 0.3 ppm fluoride[‡,§]

Age	Dose per day
0 – 6 months	Nil
6 months – 2 years	0.25 mg F^- (0.55 mg NaF)
2 – 4 years	0.50 mg F^- (1.1 mg NaF)
> 4 years	1.00 mg F^- (2.2 mg NaF)

Domestic salt is another possible vehicle for ensuring adequate consumption of fluoride for caries control but the caries preventive effect of fluoridated salt has been difficult to measure due to the other preventive programs in place.

20.3.2 Topical fluoride

A number of vehicles are available by which fluoride may be applied to tooth surfaces, including aqueous solutions, gels and dentifrices. Some may be applied by the dental healthcare worker, others by the patient. In general,

‡ These recommendations will be reviewed at 2000 and at appropriate intervals as new evidence becomes available or when community measures such as salt or water fluoridation are introduced.

§ Dental Practitioners' Formulary 1996-1998.

the solutions applied by health care workers are of high fluoride concentration and are applied at infrequent intervals (for example, once or twice per annum) while those used by the patient tend to be of low fluoride concentration and used often (e.g. every day).

1. Fluoride solutions applied by the dental healthcare worker. These solutions are principally aqueous solutions of sodium or stannous fluoride, or acidulated phosphate systems. Early workers used 0.1% sodium fluoride solutions, but aqueous stannous fluoride was later shown to be more effective at reducing caries. These are often used as 2% solutions, despite research that indicated that a 1% solution was just as effective. Their principal disadvantages are their chemical instability, which necessitates the mixing of a fresh solution for each application and the potential for brown staining of the margins of restorations.

More recently, it has been demonstrated that fluoride uptake by enamel was higher at lower pH levels. Accordingly, in 1963, a 1.23% fluoride solution acidified by acid sodium phosphate was used and shown to increase the uptake of fluoride in enamel. These solutions, containing 1.23% available fluoride in a 0.1M phosphoric acid at pH 2.8, are known as acidulated phosphate fluoride (APF), and have been shown to cause caries reductions of up to 50% when applied at six-month or annual intervals. Difficulties associated with the application of these solutions include control of the solution, nausea if swallowed and excessive salivation of the patient during application. By the addition of methyl or hydroxyethyl cellulose, APF solutions have become available as gels, with the advantage that they are much more easily controlled in the mouth, especially if a close-fitting special tray is used. Less material is therefore used, with an associated reduction in cost, and as the material is thixotropic, it is more likely to flow into approximal areas. Reductions in caries incidence of up to 40% have been reported. Fluoride-containing gels may be considered to be effective in patients with high caries risk, but their cost-effectiveness in cases of low or moderate caries risk has been questioned.

2. Concentrated fluoride materials. A number of fluoride-containing varnishes have been developed, based on the concept that a high-concentration fluoride, in contact with tooth substance for a longer time would produce a high uptake of fluoride. They have been considered to be the quickest and easiest of all topical fluoride materials to apply. Most fluoride agents of this type have a fluoride ion concentration of between 10,000 and 23,000 ppm which causes reaction (2) in Section 20.2 to predominate, forming crystals of calcium fluoride, while the other reaction, although more beneficial to the enamel, proceeds at a much slower rate.

One such varnish is a suspension of sodium fluoride in an alcoholic varnish, providing 2.26% fluoride. Others use polyurethane varnish or polyurethane-based adhesive coatings. Tests have shown demonstrable fluoride uptake by enamel following fluoride varnish application and that it may be at least as effective as fluoride-containing solutions and gels in caries reduction. A recently introduced product contains 6% NaF and 6% CaF_2 in a synthetic resin suspension.

3. Fluoride applied by the patient. The patient may apply fluoride by the use of fluoride-containing dentifrices and mouthwashes. These are described in Chapter 21.

20.4 FLUORIDE PROPHYLACTIC PASTES

Investigations have demonstrated that small amounts of surface enamel may be removed during prophylaxis using commercially available prophylactic pastes containing the frequently used abrasives, such as pumice, silica, zirconium silicate and alumina. This loss of surface enamel is undesirable since it contains the highest levels of fluoride. It is for this reason that fluoride compounds have been added to prophylactic pastes. Earliest pastes contained 1% NaF, later pastes contained 9-10% stannous fluoride with lava pumice or insoluble metaphosphate as abrasive. Some reduction in caries incidence has been claimed using these pastes but, in general, the results have not been as significant as those demonstrated by other methods of fluoride application.

20.5 COMBINATION OF FLUORIDE THERAPY

Preventive therapies by way of prescriptions of fluoride-containing materials may be prescribed for patients in addition to dietary advice on the reduction or elimination of sucrose-containing foods and drinks from the diet. It would appear that there is no benefit in prescribing more than one systemic fluoride measure at any one time although combinations of various topical fluoride methods and the combination of topically and systemically administered fluoride may be beneficial in reducing caries. However, while fluoridation of public water supplies at the optimum level may confer no risk to the population, there *are* risks of dental fluorosis if children ingest excessive amounts of fluoridated toothpaste, especially if they are already receiving fluoride through the public water supply or by dietary supplements. It is therefore recommended that the toothbrushing of children under the age of six years should be supervised to prevent excessive ingestion, that a pea-sized amount of toothpaste should be used and that mouthrinsing with fluoride materials should not be contemplated in children below five years.

20.6 BENEFITS AND RISKS

From the above, it is apparent that there may be substantial benefits in terms of caries reduction from the application or use of a wide variety of fluoride-containing materials. However, there is an attendant risk of acute or chronic toxicity. Acute toxicity may follow the ingestion of a large dose of fluoride, with the amount ingested in relation to the body weight of the individual being of greatest significance. The probable toxic dose is thought to be around 5 mg/kg body weight, so for a 5 year-old child, a toxic dose would be approximately 100 mg F. Since a standard tube of fluoride toothpaste contains 125 g of toothpaste, a quarter of a tube of toothpaste containing 1500 ppm could be a toxic dose. Acute toxicity presents as nausea, muscle spasm, convulsions and cardiovascular and respiratory depression. Initial emergency treatment should be aimed at inducing vomiting if this has not already occurred, slowing absorption by administering 1% calcium chloride which binds the fluoride, although milk, a rich source of calcium, could be substituted. The patient should referred urgently to hospital.

The outcome of chronic toxicity is dental fluorosis, thought to be caused by a disturbance of the late maturation phase of enamel mineralization. Dental fluorosis is manifested as thin white lines in the enamel, but may present as more severe brown discoloration, opaque white patches and pitting. A dose of 0.1 mgF/kg body weight is considered to be necessary to cause fluorosis. When the whole of a toothbrush is covered with toothpaste, approx.1-1.5 g of paste are applied. It is therefore apparent that the toxic potential for a toxic effect is related to the amount of toothpaste ingested, and this is variable. Risks are higher with mouthrinses, which are therefore not recommended for children under six years of age. The margin of safety with tablets is narrow, especially if combined with treatment by other sources of fluoride.

20.7 FLUORIDE IN RESTORATIVE DENTAL MATERIALS

Some tooth filling materials contain fluoride as an essential component in their formulation, such as silicate cements (no longer in use as anterior restorative materials) and glass-ionomers (Chapter 26). Attempts have been made to incorporate fluoride-releasing agents to other materials such as resin composites and amalgam .

20.7.1 Silicate and glass-ionomer cements

Silicate cements have been in use since 1871 but are now only of historical importance since their widespread use decreased in the early 1970s with the advent of alternative tooth-colored direct restorative materials. However, it was realized that, despite the high solubility of the material, especially in dilute organic acids such as are found in plaque, the incidence of secondary caries around restorations of silicate cement was low. This finding was considered to be due to the high levels of fluoride released by the material as it dissolved in the oral fluids. Sections of sound enamel directly exposed to the silicate cement were found to contain high levels of fluoride while those areas separated from the silicate by even a thin layer of dentin contained much lower levels of fluoride. Given the similarities between the glasses used for silicate cements and those subsequently used in glass-ionomer cements, it may have been anticipated that glass-ionomer cements would possess similar cariostatic properties to silicate cements. However, caries reduction is a function not only of the amount of fluoride incorporated in the enamel surrounding the restorations, but, possibly more importantly, of the amount of fluoride in solution adjacent to the restoration or tooth surface. It is also a function of the time for which these levels are maintained, given that low levels of fluoride in solution may reduce the rate of enamel demineralization. Indeed, trace amounts of fluoride in solution are equally effective in decreasing demineralization or enhancing remineralization as compared with structural fluoride. Levels of fluoride in plaque are also of relevance in cariostasis, given that the fluoride may inhibit plaque metabolism and acid production, and also by acting as a storage site for fluoride which, in turn, may inhibit demineralization and promote remineralization. Release of fluoride from dental materials may therefore be deemed to exert a beneficial, cariostatic effect, especially if the fluoride is made available in solution around and adjacent to the restoration.

Restorations in glass-ionomer materials are widely recognized to release fluoride, with the amount of fluoride release being dependent on factors such as time of mixing (with shorter mixing times producing greater release of fluoride), powder-to-liquid ratio, method of manipulation (hand mix or mechanical mix) and the material itself. Fluoride release from glass-ionomer cements occurs as a result of the setting reaction of the material (this is described in detail in Chapter 26), with the initial rate of fluoride release being high but dropping steadily throughout the life of the restoration. Figure 20.1 shows typical data for the cumulative fluoride release.

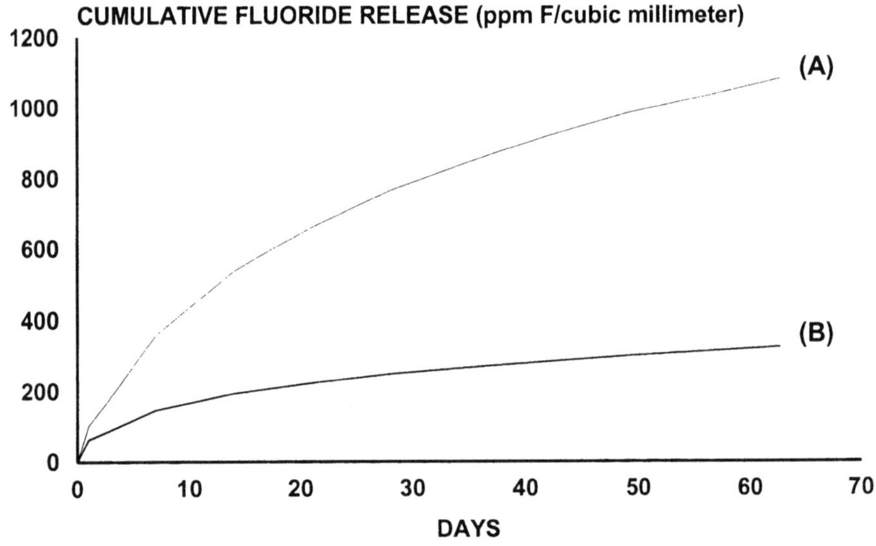

Figure 20.1. Cumulative fluoride release of (A) glass-ionomer cement, (B) resin-modified glass-ionomer cement, ppm/mm^3 of material, in distilled water.

Glass-ionomer restorations take up fluoride and subsequently release it, i.e. they may be 'recharged' with fluoride if fluoride-containing materials are applied to the restoration surface. This may be of importance in maintaining the long-term therapeutic concentrations of fluoride in solution at the material-enamel interface. The effects of glass-ionomers in the clinical situation are likely to be different from those in the laboratory, given that glass-ionomer restorations *in vivo* are continually flushed with saliva that may reduce the effect of the fluoride release. However, glass-ionomer materials have been shown to possess antibacterial properties *in vitro* but this appears to be insufficient for the inhibition of the growth of plaque *in vivo*. Plaque adjacent to glass-ionomer restorations contains greater amounts of fluoride than plaque not adjacent to restorations. There is no general agreement on the extent to which the antimicrobial effect of glass-ionomer contributes to caries prevention, if at all. In this respect, it has recently been suggested that glass-ionomer materials may not exert as great a cariostatic effect as originally anticipated.

20.7.2 Fluoride-containing resin composites

Resin composite materials are discussed in Chapter 27. A number of different approaches to the development of fluoride-releasing composites have been made. Firstly, water-soluble fluoride salts may be added to the polymer matrix-forming material, with the soluble fluoride then dissolving in the water that diffuses into the material. This approach is not ideal as the fluoride salt washes out of the material, leaving a porous structure with an associated decrease in the physical properties of the material. Matrix-bound fluoride in the form of acrylic-amine-HF salts have also been considered, and although these would appear to be an ideal means of producing a fluoride-releasing system, they suffer from disadvantages such as poor stability and discoloration which have prevented their use in restorative materials. However, these materials have been successfully used in adhesive composites for orthodontic brackets and fluoride-releasing sealants. The majority of composites for which fluoride release is claimed contain fluoride-releasing filler systems. These materials appear to maintain adequate physical and mechanical properties despite their release of fluoride. Two principal types have emerged, (i) leachable glass fillers and (ii) the sparingly soluble compounds such as YbF_3, which releases fluoride when water diffuses into the material:

$$YbF_3 + 3OH^- \longrightarrow Yb(OH)_3 + 3F^-$$

In vivo fluoride release may be substantially less than *in vitro* data and the clinical significance of fluoride release from composite materials has still to be determined.

20.7.3 Fluoride-containing amalgam

Stannous fluoride, yielding 0.5% F, has been added to amalgam (Chapter 24) in an attempt to impart cariostatic properties, but the results are equivocal.

20.7.4 Efficacy of fluoride in dental restorations

As a result of many laboratory studies, it is possible to quantify the amount and duration of fluoride release. However the extent to which this fluoride causes a reduction in secondary caries is not fully known until properly designed clinical trials have been completed. Recent hopes that glass-ionomer cements possess cariostatic properties are largely based on information that is anecdotal or indirect.

FURTHER READING

Naylor M N, Murray J J (1989). Fluorides and dental caries. *The Prevention of Dental Disease* (editor: Murray J J) 2nd edition. Oxford University Press, Oxford. pp 115-199.

van Rijkom H M, Truin G J, van't Hof M A (1998). A meta-analysis of clinical studies on the caries-inhibiting effect of fluoride gel treatment. *Caries Research* **32**: 83-92.

Murray J J, Rugg-Gunn A J, Jenkins G N (1991). *Fluorides in Caries Prevention*, 3rd edition. Butterworth-Heinemann, Oxford.

Murray J J. Winter G B, Hurst C P (1977). Duraphat fluoride varnish. A 2-year clinical trial in 5-year-old children. *British Dental Journal* **143**: 11-17.

ten Cate J M (1990). In vitro studies on the effects of fluoride on de- and remineralisation. *Journal of Dental Research* **69** (Special Issue): 614-619.

Arends J, Dijkman G E H M, Dijkman A G (1995). Review of fluoride release and secondary caries reduction by fluoridating composites. *Advances in Dental Research* **9**: 367-376.

Mjør I A (1996). Glass-ionomer cement restorations and secondary caries: A preliminary report. *Quintessence International* **27**: 171-174.

Ellwood R P, Blinkhorn A S, Davies R M (1998) Fluoride: How to maximise the benefits and minimise the risks. *Dental Update*. 25: 365-368, 370-372.

Chapter 21

Dentifrices and Mouthwashes

Summary: Dentifrices and mouthwashes are widely used to promote oral health. In this chapter the functions of the main constituents of these products are discussed.

21.1 DENTIFRICES

A *dentifrice* may be defined as a substance used with a toothbrush to clean the accessible surfaces of teeth and to deliver active components to the mouth to prevent dental and periodontal disease.

21.1.1 Historical development

Dentifrices have been available for many thousands of years, but scientific development began with the production of materials containing ammonia or urea, with pH > 7, in attempts to reduce caries by neutralizing acids. In the 1950s fluoride-containing materials became available, and these have been, and are, significant in reducing caries. These were the first 'therapeutic' dentifrices.

Fluoride-containing dentifrices are now so commonly used that it is only with difficulty that non-fluoride toothpastes can be purchased. They have been shown to reduce caries and are believed to have been largely instrumental in the reduction in caries seen in many western countries since their introduction. Early work demonstrated that sodium fluoride was inactivated by common abrasive systems in toothpaste, calcium carbonate and calcium phosphate. Considerable effort was therefore made to finding fluoride and abrasive systems that were compatible. Among those developed were stannous fluoride/calcium pyrophosphate formulations, but these had the disadvantage of causing a brown/black stain and were subsequently withdrawn. This was replaced by a dentifrice containing sodium fluoride with a silicon dioxide abrasive system, but at the present time, dentifrices, in general, contain sodium monofluorophosphate which is compatible with commonly used chalk-based abrasive systems. Currently available products contain concentrations from 0.4 mg to 1.5 mg fluoride per gram of paste (*circa* 1000 ppm), and lower fluoride concentrations are available for children, for whom abuse through over-ingestion may cause enamel opacities in developing teeth. Children considered to be at low risk of caries or those who are taking fluoride supplements should use low-fluoride formulations containing no more than 600 ppm of fluoride.

21.1.2 Requirements

There are a number of requirements for the ideal dentifrice:
1. Biocompatibility. There must be no harmful effects to the oral tissues, nor should the material be toxic if it is swallowed.
2. Abrasivity. The dentifrice must be sufficiently abrasive to clean teeth, without removing tooth substance.
3. Ability to prevent oral disease. Ideally the material should prevent caries and have antiplaque and anticalculus action. The potential to desensitize teeth is also of value.
4. Patient acceptability. The material must ideally have a pleasant taste and odor and be able to effectively counter halitosis.

21.1.3 Constituents

Modern dentifrices are complex formulations, including both therapeutic and non-active ingredients. Tables 21.1 and 21.2 outline some of the more important therapeutic and non-therapeutic constituents that are or have been used.

21.1.4 Future developments

Research is being carried out to develop a formulation that will perform functions such as caries and plaque inhibition and have antibacterial and desensitizing agents, which will all be fully compatible with each other.

Table 21.1. Therapeutic constituents of dentifrices

Function	Constituent	Comments
Anticaries agent (fluorides)	Sodium fluoride Sodium monofluorophosphate	0.2-0.3% (1000-1500 ppm F) 0.76-1.14% (1000-1500 ppm F)
Anticaries agent (non-fluoride)	These include: phosphates, calcium salts, some metals	Some phosphates can inhibit caries. Calcium carbonate can have a dual action – an abrasive as well as a neutralizing agent
Anticalculus agents	Disodium or tetrasodium pyrophosphate; tetrapotassium pyrophosphate; zinc citrate or chloride	Act as crystal growth inhibitors
Desensitizing agents	Sodium or potassium salts; strontium chloride	Heavy metal salts can occlude the dentinal tubules

Table 21.2. Non-active constituents of dentifrices

Function	Constituent	Comments
Abrasives	Calcium carbonate, silica, dicalcium phosphate	To remove plaque and stains; degree of abrasivity is important.
Detergent	Surface active agent, e.g. sodium lauryl sulfate	Aids in wetting the surfaces of teeth
Humectant	Glycerol	Retains moisture to prevent hardening of the paste
Binder	A colloid	Prevents separation of solids and liquids
Flavor	E.g. spearmint, peppermint, Menthol	Improves patient acceptability
Preservatives	E.g. benzoates	Prevent bacterial growth

21.2 MOUTHWASHES

A mouthwash can be used for a number of purposes:

- To remove or destroy bacteria;
- To act as an astringent;
- To deodorize;
- To have a therapeutic effect by relieving infection or preventing dental caries.

The following types of constituents have been employed as antibacterial agents:

- Phenolic compounds;

- Quaternary ammonium compounds;
- Essential oils, such as oil of peppermint and oil of wintergreen.

Zinc chloride, zinc acetate and aluminum potassium sulfate are examples of astringent ingredients.

Other ingredients include ethanol, dyes, sweetening agents and surface active agents.

Water is the chief constituent of mouthwashes. Some products are supplied as concentrates, to be used after dilution.

The use of fluoride mouthrinses has been shown to be a useful adjunct to a caries preventive regimen. Neutral sodium fluoride is the most commonly tested compound, and because of its ease of formulation, low cost, ease of storage, lack of taste and low risk of staining, it is the mouthwash of choice. Concentrations of between 20 and 100 ppm fluoride are effective. These solutions are normally used for 1 to 2 minutes daily, with 5 ml of solution being sufficient for young children, 7 ml for 10-15 year-olds, with older children and adults requiring 10 ml.

FURTHER READING

Preston A J (1998). A review of dentifrices. *Dental Update* **25**:159-163.

Chapter 22

Plaque-resistant Tooth Coatings

Summary: The emerging field of tooth coatings for the prevention of plaque is reviewed. Control of dental plaque is of great importance in the prevention of caries and periodontal disease.

22.1 DENTAL PLAQUE

As already noted, dental plaque is comprised mostly of bacteria that adhere to the tooth surface as a film (Section 8.5.2). It belongs to the large field of biofilm research, which includes pellicle and dental stain. Dental plaque is very important in dentistry and it is the common etiologic factor that leads to the two primary dental diseases, caries and periodontal disease. Control of dental plaque therefore is an important preventive measure.

The most common method of controlling plaque is by mechanical means, such as toothbrushing or dental floss. However these are home care procedures and as such they are not professionally supervised. So there is always a question about patient compliance. Further, not all patients are competent in the use of toothbrush or floss in inaccessible areas in the dentition, and plaque may grow unchecked and precipitate dental disease. Chemotherapeutic agents such as chlorhexidine are effective anti-plaque agents. However on prolonged usage, they may interfere more broadly with the oral microflora, and they have a tendency to stain the teeth which is a strong disincentive to extensive use. Further consideration of chemotherapeutic agents belongs to the subject of Oral Therapeutics.

22.2 DENTAL PLAQUE CONTROL BY MODIFICATION OF THE TOOTH SURFACE

A chemically clean enamel surface has a relatively high surface energy that makes it a reactive site for the attachment of salivary films called pellicle. Pellicle forms quite rapidly, usually within an hour. The primary step in dental plaque development requires the adherence of bacteria to the pellicular surface of enamel. A high-energy surface is more reactive than a low energy one, so it appears that an alternative approach to plaque control would involve chemically modifying the surface to produce a much lower energy level. This idea has been suggested in the literature and it has given rise to a new class of materials, called *plaque-resistant materials*. Clinical studies have found less plaque growth on low energy surfaces. Even after the substrate is coated with salivary pellicle, the plaque resistant property can be transferred through the adsorbed protein films and still remain effective.

22.3 PRODUCING A LOW ENERGY TOOTH SURFACE

In an earlier chapter the concept of hydrophobic and hydrophilic nature have been introduced (Section 18.2.2). However both of these properties may exist in the same molecule. Such a molecule is called *amphiphilic*, since it has both properties. Amphiphilic molecules have unusual properties, the most important of which is the ability to form films spontaneously on surfaces. If the surface is hydrophilic then the film will form with the hydrophobic surface facing outward (Figure 22.1). These films are said to be self-orienting. Such a hydrophobic outer surface has a low energy level and has a low attraction for molecules less hydrophobic than itself. Further, such molecules that do adhere are easily removed. The most common amphiphilic molecules are soaps, which have an obvious cleaning function. However common soaps are not retained very long on the surface, and their effect is very short term. If the beneficial effect of self-orienting films in reducing plaque adherence is to be realized, they must be retained on the tooth surface for considerable period of time.

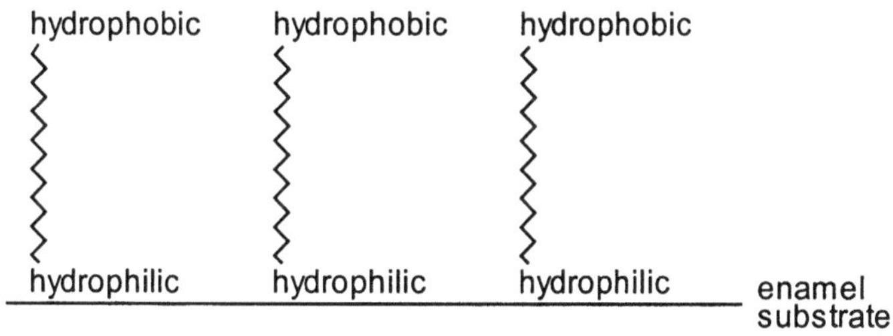

Figure 22.1. Diagram of a self-orienting film formed from amphiphilic molecules, with the hydrophobic part facing outward.

22.4 SPECIFIC TOOTH SURFACE MODIFYING MATERIALS

The idea of plaque-resistant materials is an emerging field and there are only a few examples of workable systems. But it seems likely that with time these materials will grow in importance.

Octapinol is a substituted amino alcohol which when daily-treated on the tooth surface, showed plaque prevention over a seven day period *in vitro* in an artificial mouth system that included saliva. *In vivo* experiments in beagle dogs over one year demonstrated that regular application of octapinol significantly reduced plaque accumulation. There are no further reports on the use of this material and it may be regarded as a 'proof of concept' material. From a practical point of view daily application is difficult to achieve, except for those molecules which can be applied in a dentifrice.

Polydimethylsiloxane (silicone oil) is the most studied tooth-surface altering material. It adsorbs onto the tooth surface and forms a hydrophobic film due to the low surface energy as outlined above. Enamel surface treated for 1 minute with silicone oil and placed intraorally at different time periods up to 3 hours showed the delayed formation of acquired pellicle as observed by scanning electron microscope. An experimental toothpaste containing silicone oil/triclosan was shown to improve gingival health in a clinical study. It should be pointed out that in this example the silicone oil film is being used as a carrier to localize the antibacterial triclosan onto the surface of the tooth. So the approach can be regarded as a combination of the plaque resistant and the antimicrobial methods. Silicone oil does not adhere strongly to enamel thus the effect in delayed pellicle formation seemed to disappear during a 3 hour follow up-period.

Substantive polymeric coating (SPC) is an approach different from the silicone method. SPC is a graft polymer of polysiloxane and methacrylate groups that form a self-orienting film on the tooth surface. The material subsequently polymerizes on the tooth surface, which gives it greater retention on the tooth. This approach has just been reported in the literature and appears to hold out considerable promise as the first practicable system for use in the dentist's office.

22.5 CONCLUSION

The use of plaque resistant materials belongs to the area of preventive dentistry. With the exception of pit and fissure sealants, and some chemotherapeutic agents, dentistry has very few preventive-specific materials. This new group, if it can be reduced to practice, should stimulate the practice of preventive techniques as part of the overall program of dental care.

FURTHER READING

Rølla G, Ellingsen J E, Gaare D (1994). Polydimethylsiloxane as a tooth surface-bound carrier of triclosan: A new concept in chemical plaque inhibition. *Advances in Dental Research* **8**:272-277.

VII

DIRECT RESTORATIVE MATERIALS

Chapter 23

Direct Restorative Materials: Classification and Overview

Summary: This chapter defines the various dental applications of directly placed restorative materials and classifies materials according to their setting reactions.

23.1 INTRODUCTION

Many materials that are used in dental treatment are placed directly into the mouth in the unset state, with solidification taking place *in situ*. There are numerous dental applications for such materials, including:
- Pit and fissure sealants, as discussed in Chapter 19;
- Permanent tooth restorative materials;
- Provisional (temporary) tooth restorative materials;
- Materials used in association with restorative materials; this group includes bases, liners, varnishes and bonding agents;
- Luting agents for the cementation of laboratory fabricated metallic castings and ceramic and resin composite veneers and restorations;
- Orthodontic cementing media;
- Pulp capping materials;
- Materials used in endodontics.

23.2 DEFINITIONS

Some of the terms referred to above require definition:

1. A *restorative material* is intended to restore both form and function to a tooth.

2. The term *cement* often causes confusion because it is used both as a noun and a verb. Two definitions can be given for the dental usage of the word as a noun:
- One definition is to restrict the term to the acid-base reaction materials, where an acidic (proton donor) liquid that reacts with a basic or amphoteric (proton acceptor) powder to give a set material (see Section 23.4);
- In general, a cement is a non-metallic material that is mixed to a plastic consistency, followed by setting; this can include materials that set by a polymerization reaction.

3. A *cavity base* is a cement that is placed within the cavity preparation, often with the intention of protecting the pulp from thermal changes, from harmful chemicals or from electrical stimuli.
4. A *liner* is applied in a thin layer to the walls and floor of a cavity preparation. Liners can include varnish materials (see below) or calcium hydroxide preparations.
5. A *varnish* is a solution of a resin in a volatile solvent that evaporates *in situ*, leaving a thin coat of resin.
6. A *bonding agent* or *bonding system* is used to secure adhesion of a restorative material to enamel and/or dentin.
7. A *luting agent* is a cement applied to give retention to veneers, inlays, crowns, bridges and orthodontic appliances.

It should be noted that in these definitions there is always the potential for overlap – that is, between cement and luting agent, and between liner and base. Also, there can be a choice of several materials for any one application, and many materials are used for a number of applications.

23.3 OVERVIEW OF SETTING REACTIONS

One useful way of classifying this very diverse group of materials is according to their chemical composition and setting mechanisms, as outlined in Table 23.1.

Table 23.1. Setting mechanisms of directly placed dental materials

Mechanism	Example	Chapter
1. Acid-base reaction	Dental cements based on zinc oxide: - Zinc oxide-eugenol and related materials - Zinc phosphate - Zinc polycarboxylate	25

Mechanism	Example	Chapter
1. Acid-base reaction (continued)	Dental cements based on fluoroaluminosilicate glasses: - Silicate cement (obsolete) - Glass-ionomer cement	26
	Some calcium hydroxide materials	25
2. Polymerization reaction	Pit and fissure sealants	19
	Resin composite restoratives	27
	Polyacid-modified resin composites ('compomers')	27
	Resin-based cementing agents and adhesives	28, 44
	Some calcium hydroxide materials	25
3. Combination of acid-base and polymerization reaction	Resin-modified glass-ionomers	26
4. Amalgamation reaction	Dental amalgam	24
5. Evaporation of a solvent	Varnish	
6. No setting reaction	Gutta percha	29

23.4 CLASSIFICATION OF ACID-BASE REACTION CEMENTS

There are five principal types of acid-base reaction cements, four of which are currently in use. These are based on two powder types, which are basic or amphoteric:

- Zinc oxide, the reactions of which have been described in Section 15.5;
- Fluoroaluminosilicate (FAS) glass - see Section 15.6.

Three proton-donor liquid types are possible:

- Eugenol and analogous compounds;
- Aqueous phosphoric acid solutions;
- Aqueous solutions of poly(acrylic acid).

Of the six theoretically possible powder/liquid combinations, five produce setting materials. This is illustrated in Figure 23.1, where the rectangles represent powder types and the circles represent liquid types. A cement is represented by the intersection of a rectangle and a circle. Of the five possible materials, one is no longer in use - namely silicate cements. In the past these were used for anterior tooth restorations, but resin composites and other materials have now superceded them.

Details of acid-base reaction cements are given in Chapters 25 and 26. It should be noted that Figure 23.1 is a simplification because:

- Only major components are considered here. Dental cements often contain other components to modify their properties;

– There are a number of cements derived from the major types that are not included in this diagram.

In Figure 23.1 it can be seen that glass-ionomer cements are included. There are now resin-modified glass-ionomers, which are designed to set both by an acid-base mechanism and by polymerization.

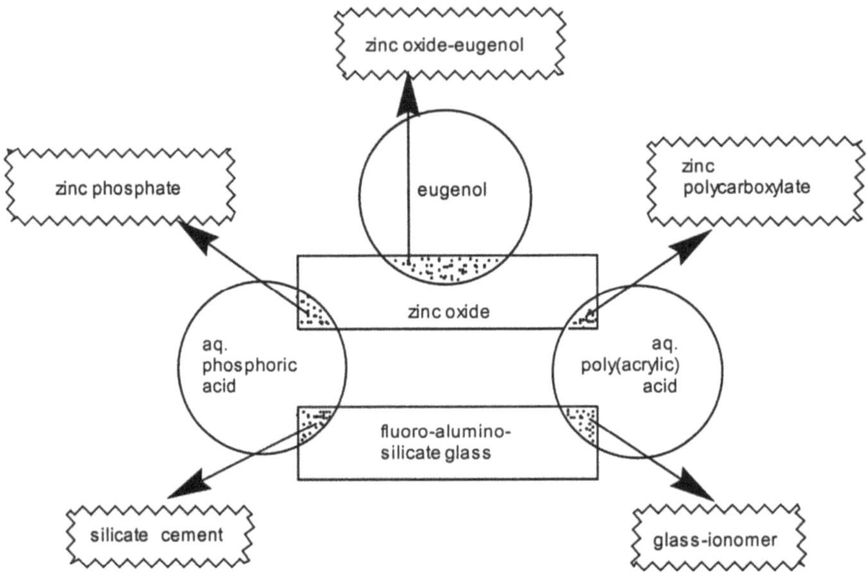

Figure 23.1. Illustration of the five principal types of dental acid-base reaction cements.

23.5 CLASSIFICATION OF POLYMERIZING MATERIALS

There are many dental materials that set by free radical addition polymerization, which reaction may be either activated by visible light or by tertiary amines. These include pit and fissure sealants (Chapter 19), resin composite filling materials (Chapter 27) and resin based cements and adhesives (Chapters 28 and 44).

In the last few years some materials have become available which are derived from resin composites. They set only by polymerization but also contain some of the constituents of glass-ionomers. They are termed 'polyacid-modified resin composites' or 'compomers,' the latter word being derived from *COMP*osite ion*OMER*. Their properties are given in Section 27.10.

23.6 OVERALL CLASSIFICATION: THE 'CONTINUUM' OF MATERIALS

The above classes of material are used both for dental restorations and as luting agents. It is now recognized that there is a 'continuum' of composition for these materials, and this is illustrated in Figure 23.2

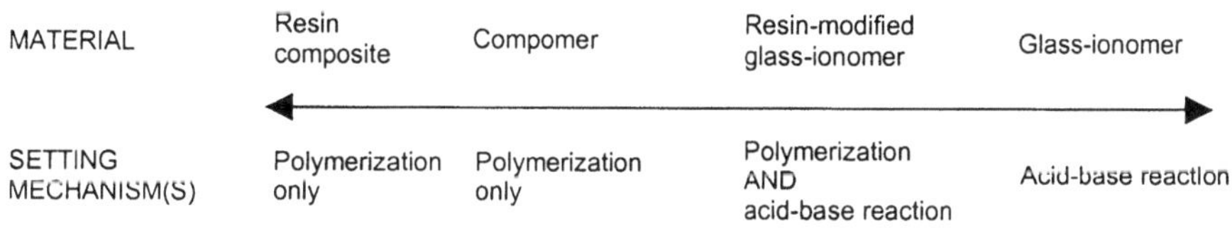

Figure 23.2. The 'continuum' of materials.

FURTHER READING

These materials are further discussed as follows:

- Chapter 19: pit and fissure sealants;
- Chapter 24: dental amalgam;
- Chapters 25 and 26: acid-base reaction cements, including resin-modified glass-ionomers;
- Chapter 27: resin composites and compomers;
- Chapter 28: dentin bonding systems;
- Chapter 29: materials in endodontics.

In chapters 43 and 44, these materials are assessed, and their general comparative properties noted. Guidelines are also given on the principles and practice of material selection.

Chapter 24

Dental Amalgam and Related Materials

Summary: The composition and properties of contemporary amalgam materials are given, together with the important practical points in their manipulation, including mercury hygiene. Methods of achieving retention of amalgam are reviewed.

24.1 INTRODUCTION

An *amalgam* is an alloy of mercury with another metallic material. Mercury is a liquid at room temperature; its freezing point is –39°C. It can readily undergo amalgamation reactions with metals such as silver, tin and copper to give a set material.

Dental amalgam has been a widely used filling material for posterior teeth, although its use is beginning to decline, because of concerns about the use of mercury, and the increasing desire from patients for tooth-colored restorations in posterior teeth. Mercury is mixed with an alloy powder to give a plastic material that is packed into the prepared cavity. This sets to form a hard and strong material.

Alloys for use with mercury for dental applications are often referred to as dental amalgam alloys. Strictly speaking this is a misnomer; they are not amalgam alloys, but alloys from which an amalgam can be prepared.

24.2 COMPOSITION

Alloys for the preparation of dental amalgam may be broadly classified into two types:

- Alloys with ≤ 6% copper, used until the 1970s;
- 'High copper' or 'copper enriched' alloys, typically 12-30% Cu.

24.2.1 Older formulations (≤ 6% Cu)

Until the 1970s, alloys for the preparation of dental amalgam contained less than 6% copper - the chemical formulation of these materials has changed little over the years. Typical composition ranges for these materials are presented in Table 24.1. An important difference between alloys containing zinc and those that are zinc-free is discussed in Section 24.6.8. Some alloys contain or have contained up to 2 to 3% mercury - such alloys amalgamate more rapidly.

Table 24.1. Composition of older formulations of alloy (≤ 6% Cu)

Element	Weight percent	Element	Weight percent
Silver	67-74	Copper	0-6
Tin	25-27	Zinc	0-2

The principal difference between different alloys is their particle size and shape. Lathe cut alloys (Section 24.3) may be coarse or fine grain; the latter are to be preferred (Section 24.8). Alloys are particle size blended – that is there is a distribution of sizes to give greater packing efficiency of the particles. As an alternative to lathe cut materials, spherical particle alloys are available. Some alloys contain a blend of lathe cut and spherical particles.

24.2.2 'Copper enriched' or 'high copper' alloys

These have been available since the 1970s, and have largely superceded the lower copper materials.

Copper enriched alloys are of the following types:

1. Blended alloys. These are sometimes referred to as 'dispersion modified' alloys. They are admixtures of two parts by weight of conventional composition lathe cut particles plus one part by weight of spheres of a silver-copper eutectic alloy (70% Ag + 30% Cu, approximately - see Figure 13.9) The approximate overall composition is given in Table 24.2.

Table 24.2. Overall composition of blended 'copper enriched' alloys

Element	Weight percent	Element	Weight percent
Silver	69	Copper	13
Tin	17	Zinc	1

2. Single composition alloys: a number of different types are available, as detailed in Table 24.3.

Table 24.3. Types of single composition 'copper enriched' alloys

Type	Composition
Ternary alloys in spherical form	Either: 60% Ag, 25% Sn, 15% Cu
	Or: 40% Ag, 30% Sn, 30% Cu
Ternary alloys in spheroidal form	As above
Quaternary alloys in spheroidal form	59% Ag, 13% Cu, 24% Sn, 4% In

24.3 MANUFACTURE OF ALLOY

Conventional alloys are prepared by fusing together the pure metals to form an ingot that is then homogenized and cut into filings. Homogenization helps to ensure that each filing has similar composition and properties. The size and shape of the particles of cut alloy are of great importance (Section 24.8).

A freshly cut alloy reacts very rapidly with mercury. This may be explained partly by the dislocations and imperfections in the alloy lattice, which can increase its chemical reactivity. If the alloy filings are stored at room temperature for a few months the reactivity gradually decreases — such alloys are said to have been aged. The same results can be achieved much more rapidly by boiling the filings in water for 30 minutes. This rapid method of aging the filings is usually carried out by the manufacturer, to give a product of stable properties.

Spherical particles are prepared by an atomization process in which the molten alloy is sprayed into an inert atmosphere, when the droplets of alloy solidify as spheres. Spherical particles are easier than irregular shaped particles to grade with respect to their particle size. A blend of sizes from 10 to 37 μm has been suggested.

24.4 MANIPULATION

24.4.1 Mercury hygiene

It is important to realize that exposure to mercury vapor is a hazard for dental personnel. Good attention to detail is of paramount importance. Table 24.4 summarizes the main points in mercury hygiene.

Table 24.4. Practical points in mercury hygiene

Factor	Practical points
Personnel	Personnel should be familiar with the hazards of mercury, the importance of good mercury hygiene practices and the symptoms of mercury exposure. Periodic monitoring for mercury exposure should be carried out
Working environment	Good ventilation; frequent replacement of air filters; periodic monitoring of mercury in dental offices; work surfaces impervious to mercury and with restraining edges, to confine mercury in the event of spillage
Handling	Single-use precapsulated alloys are preferred; reusable capsules should be checked for mercury leakage during trituration; A no-touch technique of handling should be used; a mercury spill kit should be available for use if necessary
Placement	Ultrasonic condensers are contraindicated (they are no longer available in most countries)
Removal	Old amalgam restorations should be removed with copious cooling, preferably under rubber dam – heating amalgam will release mercury
Amalgam scrap	Scrap amalgam should be stored in sealed bottles and covered by a sulfide solution; appropriate filters must be attached to water drainage systems to prevent mercury contamination of the public water system

24.4.2 Proportioning and trituration

The alloy/mercury ratio is important. In the set amalgam it is desirable to have less than 50% mercury (Section 24.6.4). Most amalgams are supplied in closed capsules that contain the appropriate amounts of alloy and mercury. Prior to use, a capsule is 'activated' to break the sealed portion of the capsule that contains the mercury. The activated capsule is mixed on a mechanical amalgamator, for the time specified by the manufacturer for the material. Older materials were proportioned by weight or volume, and often mixed in a mortar and pestle. These methods have been superceded, since it is desirable to minimize the exposure of dental personnel to mercury vapor.

The choice of trituration time is important, and will depend both on the type of alloy and the speed of the mixer. Time will typically be from 5 to 12 seconds. In particular copper enriched alloys may require precise control of trituration conditions. Some such products require high energy mixing to break up the oxide coating that forms on copper-rich particles.

24.4.3 Condensation

For full details of this, and other clinical procedures, a textbook on operative dental surgery should be consulted. The mixed material is packed into the cavity in increments in such a way that:

- Each portion is properly adapted by a condenser of suitable size;
- A load of up to 4 to 5 kg is applied to each increment;
- As the mix is condensed, some mercury-rich material rises to the surface. Some of this can be removed, to reduce the final mercury content, and improve the mechanical properties (Section 22.6.4). The remainder will assist bonding with the next increment, to avoid the production of a weak laminated restoration.

A material should be condensed as soon as possible after mixing. If it is left too long, and has begun to set:

- Proper adaptation to the cavity will be impossible;
- Elimination of excess mercury will be difficult;
- Bonding between increments will be poor;
- Lower strength values will result.

Mechanical condensers are also available, which apply vibration to pack the amalgam. These are contra-indicated, as they can increase the amount of mercury vapor in the dental operatory.

Amalgams prepared from spherical alloys need less packing pressure than those prepared from lathe cut alloys. However, condensation can be more difficult for spherical alloys, as the condenser point tends to pass right through the material instead of developing pressure. Generally spheroidal particle amalgams condense with more resistance than spherical materials.

24.4.4 Trimming and carving

When the cavity is overfilled, the top mercury-rich layer can be trimmed away and the filling carved to the correct contours. The amalgam prepared from a coarser grain alloy may be more difficult to carve, as the instrument may pull out large pieces of alloy from the surface. Spherical alloys are used where ease of carving is desired.

24.4.5 Polishing

Conventional amalgams are polished not less than 24 hours after insertion - that is, when the material has gained considerable strength. Since amalgams from copper enriched alloys gain strength rapidly (Table 24.6), some manufacturers suggest that they can be polished shortly after insertion.

24.5 SETTING REACTIONS AND STRUCTURE

24.5.1 Nature of the alloy

Silver and tin can form an intermetallic compound, of formula Ag_3Sn. This is called the gamma (γ) phase of the silver-tin system. It contains 73.15% silver and 26.85% tin. An alloy for dental use should have silver and tin in proportions close to this, though copper may replace a small amount of the silver. The silver contributes to the resistance to tarnish of the amalgam. It reacts very readily with mercury, and makes amalgamation of the alloy easier. If too much tin is present, contraction occurs on setting of the amalgam and the strength and hardness of the set material are reduced.

Copper may replace silver to some extent; it increases the hardness and strength of the amalgam. Zinc, if present, acts as a scavenger for oxygen in the fusion of the alloy, to facilitate alloy manufacture.

24.5.2 Setting mechanism and structure (older formulations, ≤ 6% Cu)

The reaction between dental amalgam alloys and mercury is very complex. Considered here are a few facts related to the reaction between the intermetallic silver-tin compound (Ag_3Sn) – the γ phase – and mercury. During and after mixing the γ phase dissolves in the mercury. Reaction occurs to give formation and crystal growth of at least two phases:

- The intermetallic compound Ag_2Hg_3, with a body-centered cubic structure, called the γ_1 phase;
- A tin-mercury intermetallic compound ($Sn_{7-8}Hg$) with a hexagonal structure called the γ_2 phase.

These reactions may be written as:

$$Ag_3Sn + Hg \longrightarrow Ag_2Hg_3 + Sn_{7\text{-}8}Hg + Ag_3Sn \text{ (unreacted)}$$

or:

$$\gamma + Hg \longrightarrow \gamma_1 + \gamma_2 + \gamma \text{ (unreacted)}$$

The structure of the set material is heterogeneous, consisting of a core of unreacted γ and a matrix of the γ_1 and γ_2 compounds, the latter of which forms a continuous network. After setting, further reactions may occur by diffusion processes.

24.5.3 Setting mechanism and structure ('copper enriched' alloys)

The main feature of these materials is that the set structure is essentially free of the γ_2 component.

1. Blended alloys. The reaction is essentially that between a mixture of Ag_3Sn plus Ag-Cu spheres and Hg, and takes place in two stages. The first stage is the reaction between Ag_3Sn and Hg as outlined previously for the reaction of lower copper-containing alloys. The Ag-Cu does not participate at this stage. This is followed by a reaction between the γ_2 component and Ag-Cu spheres, leading to the production of a copper-tin compound, and more γ_1 phase, thus:

$$Sn_{7\text{-}8}Hg + Ag\text{-}Cu \longrightarrow Cu_6Sn_5 + Ag_2Hg_3$$

or:

$$\gamma_2 \quad + Ag\text{-}Cu \longrightarrow Cu_6Sn_5 + \quad \gamma_1$$

The Cu_6Sn_5 is present as a 'halo' surrounding the Ag-Cu particles. The final set material consists of a core of Ag_3Sn and Ag-Cu surrounded by a halo of Cu_6Sn_5, and a matrix of γ_1 phase.

2. Single composition-alloys. The structure of the materials is similar to that given above, except that the Cu_6Sn_5 is present in the γ_1 matrix rather than as a halo.

It should be noted that other constituents are present in some amalgams. For example, experiments have shown that alloys in which about 10% of gold is substituted for some of the silver also produce amalgams free of the γ_2 phase.

Figure 24.1 shows SEM pictures of two amalgam prepared from different types of 'copper enriched' alloys.

The absence of the γ_2 phase in contemporary materials has great significance in terms of:

- Corrosion properties (Section 24.6.2);
- Strength (Section 24.6.4);
- Creep properties (Section 24.6.5);
- Durability of the margins of amalgam restorations (Section 24.6.6).

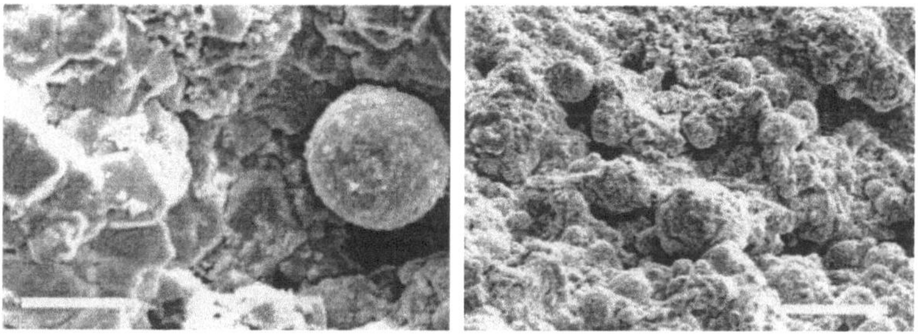

Figure 24.1. Structure of amalgams prepared from 'copper-enriched' alloys; Left, blended alloy, showing Cu-Ag sphere (horizontal line = 10 μm); Right, single composition spherical alloy (horizontal line – 50 μm).

24.6 PROPERTIES

24.6.1 Toxicity

The wisdom of using a restorative material containing mercury has often been questioned, and is currently a matter of debate. The potential danger of any form of mercury is related both to the form in which the mercury is present and to the quantity and frequency of exposure.

Table 24.5 lists the forms of mercury, with comments on these.

Table 24.5. Forms of mercury

Form of mercury	Comment
Mercury liquid	- High vapor pressure at room temperature - Avoid skin contact, as Hg may be absorbed - A few people show an allergic response to Hg
Mercury vapor	- Very toxic; particular danger for dental staff - Good mercury hygiene in dental clinic is imperative - Small quantities have been found in expired air from patients with amalgam restorations - Patient unlikely to be exposed to Threshold Limit Value of mercury because of dental fillings
Intermetallic compounds	- These are formed in set amalgam - They are comparatively insoluble
Organometallic compounds	- These are very toxic - It has been shown that methyl mercury can form in the presence of oral streptococci - Quantities are small, and there is no evidence of harmful effects

There is no evidence of harmful effect of amalgam, except for patients who are allergic to mercury. Such allergies are not common.

24.6.2 Corrosion reactions

Amalgam can tarnish in the presence of sulfur, to give a layer of sulfides on the surface of the restoration.

In the case of the older lower copper amalgams, the set material is heterogeneous, which can encourage corrosion. Of the three phases present, the γ_2 is the most active electrochemically, being anodic in relation to both the γ and γ_1 phases. As γ_2 corrodes, essentially two products result:

- Ionic tin is produced: in the presence of saliva, corrosion products such as SnO_2 and $Sn(OH)_6Cl$ are formed;
- Hg is produced, which can react with some of the remaining hitherto unreacted γ phase.

For the 'copper enriched' amalgams different behavior is observed, since essentially no γ_2 is present in the set material. Cu_6Sn_5 is the phase most prone to corrosion. However, the corrosion currents associated with these systems are considerably less than that with conventional amalgam. Thus the volume of corrosion products is less than with conventional amalgam. No mercury is produced as a result of the corrosion of γ_2-free amalgams.

Some practical considerations are important in relation to corrosion. Corrosion resistance is greatly improved if the amalgam is polished. This process removes pits and voids on the surface, which aid concentration cell corrosion (Section 14.3.2). If amalgam comes in contact with a gold restoration, an electrolytic cell may be set up leading to corrosion of the amalgam and incorporation of mercury on the gold restoration. Corrosion of conventional amalgam can have a significant effect on long term mechanical properties. It has been shown, for example, that tensile strength is reduced by 30% when the network of γ_2 has corroded.

24.6.3 Marginal leakage

The initial marginal leakage of an amalgam restoration according to *in vitro* tests reduces with time, because of sealing of the micro-fissures by products of corrosion breakdown. However, since there is little corrosion with contemporary high-copper amalgams, the use of amalgam bonding techniques (Section 24.7.2) has been suggested as a means of minimizing leakage.

24.6.4 Strength

The following factors can lead to the production of a weak amalgam restoration:

- Undertrituration;
- Too high a mercury content;
- Too low condensation pressure;
- Slow rate of packing;
- Corrosion;
- Contamination with blood or saliva during placement.

The rate of development of strength of an amalgam is of importance (Figure 24.2). With amalgams that develop strength slowly, there is danger of early fracture of such a restoration. Generally, spherical and copper enriched amalgams have high early strengths (Table 24.6). Of the phases present in conventional amalgams the γ_2 is the weakest and softest.

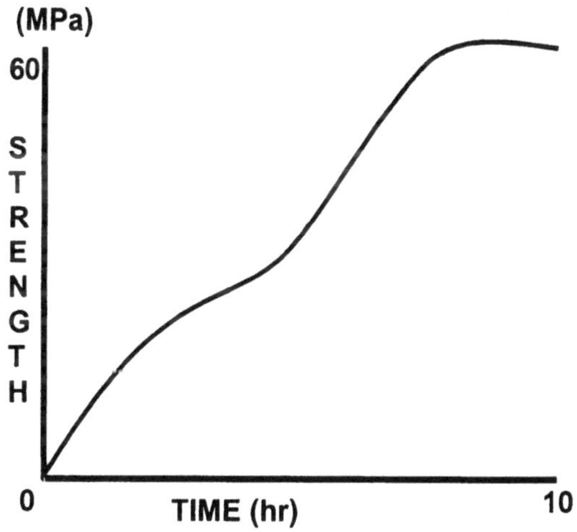

Figure 24.2. The rate of increase of tensile strength of an amalgam with time.

Table 24.6. Typical properties of dental amalgam

Amalgam type	Compressive strength at 1 h (MPa)	Compressive strength – fully set (MPa)	Static creep (%) after 7 days under pressure of 38 MPa
Conventional, Lathe cut	120-170	380-450	2.5-3.5
Conventional, spherical	140-180	380-450	0.3-1.5
Blended alloys	120-220	410-460	0.2-1.7
Single composition ternary alloys	230-320	460-540	0.02-0.3
Quaternary alloys (with indium)	210-240	430-480	0.06-0.1

24.6.5 Creep

In general, set alloys with no γ_2 phase show less creep than conventional materials (Table 24.6).

24.6.6 Marginal failure

'Ditching' of the margins of amalgam is a common occurrence. Clinical trials have shown that new alloy formulations show much less marginal breakdown than conventional materials. Poor technique can cause breakdown – for example, an unsupported ledge of amalgam extending over the enamel may fracture during mastication.

In general, materials with high creep values have been shown to have poorer durability of margins. This does not, however, necessarily prove that there is a cause and effect relationship between the two phenomena.

A theory has been propounded which links marginal breakdown with corrosion characteristics. It has been suggested that the mercury corrosion product (from conventional materials) reacts to form more γ_1 and γ_2 material, with associated expansion, termed 'mercuroscopic expansion.' The expanded material, weakened by corrosion, protrudes away from the supporting tooth structure, and fractures.

24.6.7 Thermal diffusivity

From the data in Table 6.1, it can be seen that dental amalgam is a conductor of heat, whereas the enamel and dentin it replaces is a thermal insulator. Consequently, large amalgam restorations may be lined with a thermal insulating cement to protect the pulp from temperature changes in the mouth caused by hot and cold foods and liquids (Section 43.4.5).

24.6.8 Dimensional changes

Ideally there should be little or no contraction on setting of a dental amalgam, otherwise a gap between filling and cavity walls may result, enhancing the possibility of further decay. Too great an expansion should also be avoided, as this will cause the filling to protrude from the cavity.

In laboratory experiments, where free expansion is measured, it has been shown that a greater expansion on setting will results if:

- A higher alloy/mercury ratio is used;
- There is a shorter trituration time;
- Lower pressure during condensation is used;
- The alloy has a larger particle size;
- If there is contamination by water before setting in zinc-containing materials. This will result in an electrolytic reaction between zinc (the anode) and the other metals which are cathodic (see Table 14.1) and the water as an electrolyte. Hydrogen is evolved as a result of this reaction. The pressure of the evolved hydrogen may cause the amalgam to flow. This causes an expansion, which may not appear within the first 24 hours, but may become evident some days after insertion of the restoration.

24.7 RETENTION OF AMALGAM

24.7.1 Pins

Pins are used to enhance the retention of restorations for which there is insufficient tooth substance to provide a retentive cavity or in cases where achievement of retention would necessitate the removal of sound tooth substance. Their use is generally obviated by the use of materials that either adhere to or can be bonded to tooth substance.

The use of pins for retaining restorations was first described in 1887. The use of threaded stainless steel orthodontic wire was described in 1958, but is little used today. In this technique, a hole is drilled with a twist drill of slightly greater diameter than the wire, and the threaded wire, of either 0.5 mm or 0.7 mm diameter, is cemented into the hole using zinc phosphate cement. Two other types are available. Friction lock pins use the elasticity of dentin for their retention. A hole is made using a twist drill 0.03 mm smaller in diameter than the pin of 0.55 mm diameter, which is then forced into the cavity.

The majority of pin systems currently in use comprise a twist drill and self-threading stainless steel or gold-plated stainless steel pins. The twist drill is 0.03 mm smaller than the pins which vary according to type from 0.5 mm to 0.7 mm in diameter and are usually 0.5 cm in height. After cutting the pin hole, the pin then cuts its thread into the dentin and the elasticity of the dentin and the thread retain the pin in position. When the pin reaches the bottom of the hole, it shears away from the top which has retained it in the handpiece.

Contrary to the original belief, pins do not strengthen restorations. The pins act as lines of weakness within an amalgam restoration. Amalgam does not bond to the pin material. Pins may cause cracking of the surrounding dentin and may generate stresses within the dentin. The potential for iatrogenic damage is high, either by creating an exposure of the pulp or a perforation of the periodontal membrane. It may be that pin use will decrease as a result of these problems and with the recent development of adhesive techniques and materials.

24.7.2 Bonding agents

Amalgam restorations traditionally have been retained by mechanical features such as undercuts, slots and keys. However, it has been demonstrated that it is possible to bond amalgam restorations to the cavity wall and/or base by the use of adhesive resins. These are discussed in detail in Chapter 28.

The clinical technique involves the use of an autopolymerized dentin bonding system placed in accordance with the manufacturers' instructions followed by condensing the amalgam into the cavity before the autocuring bonding system is polymerized.

Despite the fact that amalgam bonding systems are being used more widely, there is little or no *in vivo* or *in vitro* information to demonstrate the effectiveness of the bond under the dynamic loading conditions which may occur in clinical use. However, it is increasingly being realized that if the dentin underlying an amalgam restoration is 'sealed' with a bonding system, post-operative sensitivity is reduced, given that that it has been considered that sensitivity results from microleakage.

24.8 THE SELECTION OF AN AMALGAM ALLOY

A number of questions must be asked in selecting an amalgam alloy.
1. Should a lower copper or 'copper enriched' alloy be used? High copper alloys appear to be superior in many of their properties. Their better strength is probably not very important; correctly manipulated conventional materials are sufficiently strong. The better marginal integrity of high copper amalgams is important. The conventional materials are still used in some countries, particularly because of their lower cost.
2. Which type of conventional alloy? Finer grain alloys are to be preferred in terms of ease of carving; however, amalgams produced from extremely fine particles have a greater γ_2 content.

There appears to be little advantage in using spherical alloys of the conventional type, except in terms of ease of carving.

Zinc-free alloys are preferred in situations where moisture control is difficult.
3. Which type of copper enriched alloy? The dispersion-modified alloys have produced excellent results in clinical trials. Alloys containing spheroidal particles may be easier to manipulate than those that are all spherical.

24.9 ALTERNATIVES TO AMALGAM

In attempts to avoid the use of mercury, liquid gallium alloys have been available (containing gallium, indium, tin and silver) which can react with a silver-tin-copper alloy to give a set material. These products are contraindicated, because clinical research has shown that the materials expand, causing fracture of both tooth and restoration.

An experimental approach to eliminating the use of mercury is the cold-welding of surface-treated silver particles to form a cohesive mass.

FURTHER READING

Chapter 43 gives guidelines for the selection of materials for the restoration of teeth, and compares amalgam with alternative restorative materials. Section 43.4.5 discusses choice of materials to be used in conjunction with amalgam.

American Dental Association Council on Scientific Affairs (1998). Dental amalgam: update on safety concerns. *Journal of the American Dental Association* **129**: 494-503.

Anderson M H, McCoy R B (1993). Dental amalgam. The state of the art and science. *Dental Clinics of North America* **37**: 419-431.

Craig R G (1986). Biocompatibility of mercury derivatives. *Dental Materials* **2**: 91-96.

Dunne S M, Gainsford I D, Wilson N H F (1997). Current materials and techniques for direct restorations in posterior teeth. Part 1: Silver amalgam. *International Dental Journal* **47:** 123-136.

Marshall S J, Marshall G W Jr (1992). Dental amalgam: the materials. *Advances in Dental Rresearch* **6**: 94-99.

Mitchell R J, Okabe T (1996). Setting reactions in dental amalgam. Part 1. Phases and microstructures between one hour and one week. *CriticalReviews in Oral Biology and Medicine* **7**:12-22.

Okabe T, Mitchell R J (1996). Setting reactions in dental amalgam. Part 2. The kinetics of amalgamation. *CriticalReviews in Oral Biology and Medicine* **7**:23-35.

Chapter 25

Acid-Base Reaction Cements: (1) Zinc Oxide-Based Materials and Calcium Hydroxide

Summary: The chemical reactions of zinc oxide have been reviewed in Section 15.5; in this Chapter a number diverse cements containing zinc oxide are discussed. Cements containing calcium hydroxide are also included.

25.1 INTRODUCTION

In Chapter 23 an overview of the setting mechanisms of directly placed dental materials has been presented. This includes a large group of materials collectively known as 'acid-base reaction' cements. These cements have been classified into five principal types, of which four are in current dental use. This chapter considers the materials based on the reactions of zinc oxide (Section 15.5). In addition another group of materials is discussed — those containing calcium hydroxide — although not all of them have an acid-base setting reaction mechanism.

25.2 GENERAL FEATURES OF ACID-BASE REACTION CEMENTS

Though chemically diverse, there are a number of similarities between all acid-base reaction cements:

- They are usually supplied as powder-liquid formulations;
- The liquids are acidic (proton donors);
- The powders are basic or amphoteric (proton acceptors);
- Setting is by an acid-base reaction;
- The powder is present in substantial stoichiometric excess, so only partly reacts with the liquid;

- The set material is thus heterogeneous, consisting of unreacted powder particles (the core) surrounded by a matrix of reaction products.

25.3 ZINC PHOSPHATE AND RELATED MATERIALS

25.3.1 Composition

The powder contains zinc oxide as the principal constituent. Magnesium oxide may be present, up to about 10%. Very small quantities of other oxides, or metallic salts (e.g. fluorides) may be present.

The liquid is an aqueous solution of phosphoric acid, containing about 30% to 40% water, that is, the solution maybe as much as 60% H_3PO_4. Zinc and/or aluminum phosphates are also present, formed by dissolving zinc oxide and/or aluminum hydroxide in the liquid.

25.3.2 Manipulation

Cement consistency is important. The thicker the mix, the stronger is the set material. Thus for a cavity lining, a thick mix should be used. For cementation purposes a thinner mix is required, to permit the cement to flow as the restoration is being seated.

In terms of proportioning it is not customary to measure the powder and liquid but every effort should be made to obtain consistent proportioning for the required consistency. Too thin a mix should be avoided, because, in addition to affecting the strength, a thin mix has a lower pH and the set material is more soluble.

Mixing is carried out on a cool glass slab, adding the powder to the liquid in small increments to prolong the working time, and completing the procedure within 1 to 1½ minutes.

The liquid should be kept in a stoppered bottle; loss of water from the liquid will lower its pH and slow down the setting. Liquid that has become cloudy because of loss of water should be discarded.

The powder is of similar composition to those of other cements (for example, zinc oxide-eugenol cements, see below), but each powder should only be used with the liquid supplied for it, to ensure the correct setting time and other properties.

Increase in temperature accelerates the rate of reaction of the cement. Thus the cement sets faster at mouth temperature than at room temperature.

When used for luting the cement should be applied to the inlay (or crown, or bridge) before it is applied to the prepared cavity. If the opposite procedure were done, the cement in the tooth may begin to set before the restoration is seated.

25.3.3 Setting reaction

Surfaces of the particles of zinc oxide react with phosphoric acid, to give an insoluble phosphate. Magnesium oxide, if present, will react similarly. The final set material is heterogeneous, consisting in general of a core of unreacted zinc oxide particles in a matrix of zinc phosphate.

During setting heat is given out since the reaction is exothermic. Some shrinkage also occurs.

25.3.4 Setting time

This depends on the composition and formulation of the materials, as well as on a number of manipulative variables.

The powder is generally prepared commercially by heating the ingredients to above 1000°C, causing granulation, by a sintering process. Subsequently the solid is ground to a very fine powder. The rate of reaction of the powder with the liquid depends on the temperature to which it was heated; a higher temperature reduces the reactivity of the powder. It also depends on the particle size after grinding - a finer material reacts more quickly, since a greater surface area is exposed to the liquid.

The buffering agents added to the liquid slow down the rate of reaction and improve the working time of the cement.

Manipulative variables also influence setting time. The following four factors will give acceleration of the setting reaction:

- A high powder/liquid ratio;
- Fast rate of addition of powder to liquid;
- The presence of moisture;
- Higher temperature.

25.3.5 Properties

1. Biological properties. The pH of the freshly mixed cement may be between 1.6 and 3.6. The pH rises during setting, and approaches neutrality within one to two days. A thinner mix has a lower pH and takes longer to reach neutrality. Adverse pulpal reactions may occur because of a lack of

bond between the material and dentin. Protecting the pulp with zinc oxide-eugenol, calcium hydroxide or a dentin bonding system can minimize these reactions.

Zinc phosphate cement has low thermal diffusivity (Table 6.1), so can protect the pulp from heat changes if used in sufficient thickness.

2. Interfacial properties. These cements do not form chemical bonds with enamel or dentin. The retention of cemented restorations depends on the mechanical interlocking of the set material with the surface roughness of the cavity and restoration.

3. Chemical properties. The solubility of a set zinc phosphate cement depends on the powder/liquid ratio. A thinner mix gives a more soluble material. The solubility of the cement in distilled water is very low, but is higher in solutions of lower pH. The solubility of the cement as measured by a lactic acid erosion test is high.

4. Mechanical properties. These cements are stronger than zinc oxide-eugenol materials and they have adequate compressive and tensile strengths for use as bases under restorations of dental amalgam or as luting materials.

5. Optical properties. The set cement is opaque, owing to the large quantity of unreacted zinc oxide in the set material. As a consequence zinc phosphate cement is not recommended for luting translucent restorations.

6. Practical considerations. In terms of rheological properties, the mixed unset cement appears to be near-Newtonian in behavior (Figure 25.1) with a viscosity of approximately 120 Pa.s. Viscosity-time curves do not show a horizontal plateau corresponding to a working time (Figure 25.2).

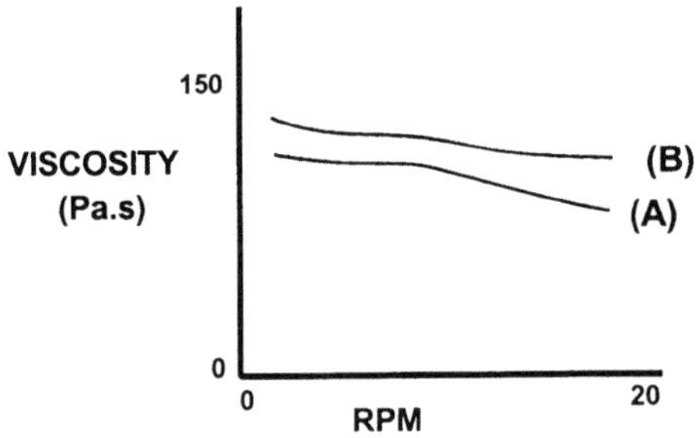

Figure 25.1. Viscosity at 25°C of mixed cements as a function of rate of testing.(A) zinc phosphate, (B) zinc polycarboxylate. After Vermilyea S, Powers J M, Craig R G (1977). Rotational viscometry of a zinc phosphate and a zinc polyacrylate cement. *Journal of Dental Research* **56**:762-767.

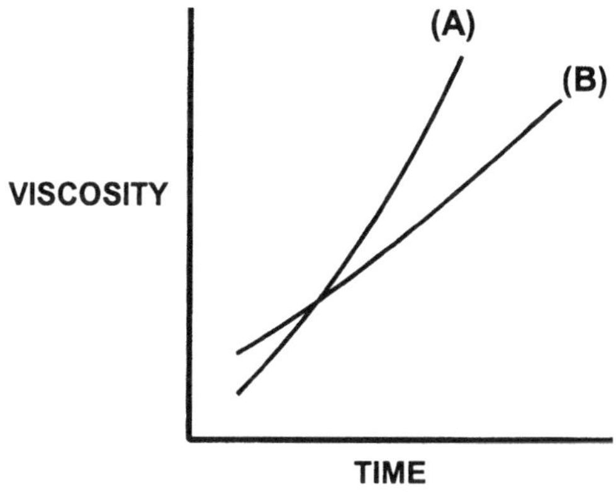

Figure 25.2. Increase in viscosity with time of (A) zinc phosphate (B) zinc polycarboxylate cement. After Vermilyea S, Powers J M, Craig R G (1977). Rotational viscometry of a zinc phosphate and a zinc polyacrylate cement. *Journal of Dental Research* **56**:762-767.

Low film thickness is an important consideration for luting cements. For most materials this is less than 40 μm and can be as low as 15 μm. Clearly this property depends on, among other things, the particle size of the powder, as supplied, and the extent to which this is changed during setting.

25.3.6 Related materials

Copper cements are similar to phosphate cements, except that the powder contains a copper compound in addition to zinc oxide. If copper(I) oxide (cuprous oxide) is used, the cement is red, while copper(II) oxide (cupric oxide) gives a black material. Black copper cements are considered to be bactericidal, and were used at one time to prolong the life of deciduous teeth, if all the carious tooth substance could not be removed.

25.4 ZINC OXIDE-EUGENOL (ZOE) AND RELATED MATERIALS

25.4.1 Composition

The powder consists of zinc oxide with magnesium oxide being present in small quantities. Zinc acetate (or other salts), in quantities up to 1%, are used as accelerators for the setting reaction.

The liquid is comprised of eugenol, the major constituent of oil of cloves. Olive oil, up to 15% may also be present. Sometimes acetic acid, to act as an accelerator is included.

25.4.2 Manipulation

ZOE cements are mixed by adding the powder in small increments to the liquid, until a thick consistency is obtained. A powder/liquid ratio of between 4/1 and 6/1 by weight will give a material of the required properties; with experience, a suitable consistency can be recognized without weighing the materials. As a rule, a thin glass slab and stainless steel spatula are used.

25.4.3 Setting reaction

On mixing the powder and liquid a chemical reaction takes place to form zinc eugenolate. Absorption of the eugenol by the zinc oxide may also occur.

Other factors to be noted are that the setting reaction between pure zinc oxide and pure eugenol will not occur in the absence of water. Thus, a mixture of zinc oxide and eugenol, without added accelerators, can be kept in a desiccator for several days without undergoing much change. Also the set materials contains both some unreacted zinc oxide and eugenol.

25.4.4 Setting time

This depends on many factors related to the formulation and usage of the material. It depends on the method of preparation of the powder and its particle size — a finer powder will have a greater surface area exposed to the eugenol, so can react more quickly. Accelerating additives are usually present to give a clinically acceptable working and setting time.

The powder/liquid ratio is important, as a thicker mix gives a faster setting material. Also exposure to moisture on mixing or the addition of water will accelerate the reaction. Increase in temperature also causes faster setting.

25.4.5 Properties

1. Biological properties. Eugenol itself has been considered to be an irritant chemical, but when mixed into a cement the effect on the pulp is minimal.

Because of their low thermal diffusivity, these cements can insulate the pulp from oral temperature changes. They can also protect the pulp from the phosphoric acid of phosphate cements. ZOE cements are bacteriostatic.
2. Interfacial properties. These cements do not adhere to enamel and dentin and as a result, leakage may occur if the cement is exposed at a cavity margin.
3. Chemical properties. The solubility of the set cement in water is high - by far the highest of all dental cements - mainly due to the elution of eugenol. This is a contraindication for their use as permanent luting agents.
4. Mechanical properties. These are the weakest of all the cements (except calcium hydroxide, Section 25.6).
5. Optical properties. The set cement is opaque.

25.4.6 Modified ZOE materials

1. Resin bonded cements. Zinc oxide-eugenol cements are available which contain either:
- Hydrogenated rosin comprising about 10% of the powder; or,
- Polystyrene dissolved in eugenol, to give a 10% solution.

The function of these additives is to increase the strength of the cement.
2. EBA cements. The letters EBA are an abbreviation of *ortho*-ethoxybenzoic acid (formula in Figure 15.2). The formulation of cements containing EBA is given in Table 25.1.

Table 25.1. Composition of EBA cements

Powder	% by weight	Liquid	% by volume
Zinc oxide	60-74	Eugenol	37.5
Fused quartz or alumina	20-34	*o*-ethoxybenzoic acid	62.5
Hydrogenated rosin	6		

In comparing these cements with the unmodified accelerated ZOE materials, there are three factors of note:
- A higher powder/liquid ratio can be used for the EBA materials (7/1 or greater); this thick mix behaves thixotropically during crown cementation;
- The mechanical properties of EBA cements are better than unmodified ZOE products.
- Biocompatibility is good, making these cements one of the materials of choice for root-end fillings (Chapter 29).

3. Special zinc oxide-eugenol products. Some zinc oxide-eugenol materials contain antibiotics such as tetracyclines, and steroids as anti-inflammatory

agents. Their principal use is in reduction of pulpal pain and as an initial root canal dressing. Another product also contains barium sulfate, which is radiopaque.

25.5 ZINC POLYCARBOXYLATE CEMENTS

25.5.1 Composition

These cements are based on the reaction of zinc oxide (small quantities of magnesium oxide may also be present) with poly(acrylic acid). The polymer may be supplied as a viscous aqueous solution of concentration 30-40%, or as a dry powder, blended with the zinc oxide. In the latter case, the blended powders are mixed with water to activate the cement.

25.5.2 Manipulation

Since poly(acrylic acid) solutions are more viscous than the liquids of other cements, this affects the ease of mixing of the material.

If the cement is being used to secure adhesion to enamel and dentin, it is important that the tooth surface should be clean and saliva-free. The cement should be applied to the tooth as soon as possible after mixing, otherwise poor adhesion may result. If a cement mix begins to 'cobweb' on manipulation, it should be discarded. There is a continuous increase in cement viscosity during manipulation of the material (Figure 25.2).

Polycarboxylate cement will adhere to instruments, particularly those made of stainless steel. Thus mixing implements should be cleaned immediately after mixing.

25.5.3 Setting reaction

This involves the formation of a salt, zinc polyacrylate (Section 15.5). Like other acid-base cements, the set material is a cored structure containing a considerable quantity of unreacted zinc oxide.

25.5.4 Setting time

This depends on the composition and method of manufacture of the powder and liquid. A faster setting time is achieved at higher temperatures.

25.5.5 Properties

1. Biological properties. These cements have very little irritant effect on the pulp.
2. Interfacial properties. These cements adhere to enamel and dentin, and proposed mechanisms for this are discussed in Section 26.6.
3. Chemical properties. These cements are more soluble than zinc phosphate materials. Some products may also absorb water, which can cause the material to become soft and gel-like.
4. Mechanical properties. Zinc polycarboxylate cements are almost as strong as phosphate materials in compression, and stronger in tension.
5. Other physical properties. These cements are good thermal insulators.
6. Optical properties. In common with all zinc oxide-containing cements, the set cement is very opaque, because of the large quantity of unreacted zinc oxide that is present.
7. Rheological properties of the mixed material are broadly similar to those of zinc phosphate cements (Figures 25.1 and 25.2).

25.6 CALCIUM HYDROXIDE FORMULATIONS

25.6.1 Composition

The simplest products of this type contain only an aqueous suspension of calcium hydroxide. However, such materials are not sufficiently strong to withstand the forces transmitted during packing a filling material such as amalgam.

Other products contain in addition either aqueous methyl cellulose or a resin dissolved in a volatile solvent such as chloroform; these materials are more cohesive and stronger that the above.

One product is a light-cured resin containing calcium hydroxide.

A number of calcium hydroxide cements contain a phenolic compound such as a disalicylate which can form a chelate with calcium hydroxide, which is present in stoichiometric excess. These materials are supplied as two pastes:

- One paste contains typically 50% calcium hydroxide and zinc oxide, as reactants, zinc stearate as accelerator and a liquid to act as a carrier. This liquid may be ethyl toluene sulfonamide or a paraffin oil;
- The other paste has a disalicylate as reactant - e.g. butylene glycol disalicylate, together with fillers and compounds to confer radiopacity.

25.6.2 Properties

1. Biological properties. Calcium hydroxide can neutralize the free phosphoric acid of a phosphate cement; a thickness of about 0.25 mm is sufficient to serve as an effective barrier against the passage of acids. The pH of these materials is around 11 - 12; this degree of alkalinity is inimical to the survival of microorganisms found in carious dentin. Because of their low thermal diffusivity, these cements can insulate the pulp from oral temperature changes.
2. Interfacial properties. These cements do not adhere to enamel and dentin and as a result, leakage may occur if the cement is exposed at a cavity margin.
3. Chemical properties. The solubility in water is high for some of the two paste materials. It has been reported that, when used as a cavity liner, some versions of the material may 'disappear' as a result.
4. Mechanical properties of the two paste materials: Compressive strength after 24 hours is 6-10 MPa and tensile strength 1-2 MPa - this is much weaker than the other cements discussed in this chapter.

25.6.3 Applications

Calcium hydroxide cements can be used under cements containing phosphoric acid, to protect the pulp from chemical damage. They have often used as a lining material under polymer-ceramic composite restorations. They can be used for pulp capping, as they can stimulate the formation of secondary dentin. However, this latter application is controversial at this time (Section 43.4.6).

FURTHER READING

Section 43.4.6 discusses materials for pulp capping. Chapter 44 gives guidelines for the choice of cements for luting.

Øilo G (1991). Luting cements: a review and comparison. *International Dental Journal.* **41**: 81-88.

Milosevic A (1991). Calcium hydroxide in restorative dentistry. *Journal of Dentistry.* **19**: 3-13.

Chapter 26

Acid-Base Reaction Cements: (2) Glass-Ionomer and Related Materials

Summary: This chapter considers glass-ionomers and a number of materials derived from them. These cements are adhesive to tooth tissue and are translucent, and are finding applications as luting agents and tooth restorative materials.

26.1 GLASS-IONOMER (POLYALKENOATE) CEMENT

26.1.1 Composition and nature of components

These cements contain an ion-leachable glass — a fluoroaluminosilicate (FAS) glass (Section 15.6) that can react with a water-soluble polymeric acid to yield a cement. As originally formulated, the glass was a calcium aluminosilicate containing fluoride. A typical glass is prepared from some six components (Table 26.1) which are fused together at 1000-1300°C, followed by quenching and grinding.

Table 26.1. Typical components of a glass-ionomer cement powder**

Constituent	Weight %	Constituent	Weight %
SiO_2	30.1	CaF_2	34.5
Al_2O_3	19.9	NaF	3.7
AlF_3	2.6	$AlPO_4$	10.0

In the structure of the glass, aluminum enters the silica network - see Figure 15.3. The ratio of Al_2O_3 to SiO_2 is critical for the correct reactivity. Glasses are not necessarily homogeneous; phase separation can occur. Fluoride is an important component because:

** Wilson A D, McLean J W (1988). *Glass-Ionomer Cement.* Quintessence, Chicago. p.22.

- Fluoride contributes to the therapeutic value of the cement (Chapter 20);
- It assists the manufacture of the glass by lowering fusion temperature;
- It enhances working characteristics and mechanical properties of the cement;
- Under certain conditions fluoride can give a more translucent glass.

Radiopaque glasses are used in some materials; in these, barium or strontium may replace calcium. Another variant is for the manufacturer to give glass powders an acid treatment, which reduces the surface concentration of calcium, giving a cement of greater working time (see setting mechanism below).

For the water-soluble polymer component, originally poly(acrylic acid) was used. Many current materials use a copolymer of acrylic acid with itaconic or maleic acid (Figure 26.1). In general this will be referred to as a poly(alkenoic acid), hence the cements are sometimes known as 'polyalkenoates.' Instead of a viscous aqueous solution, the polymer is often supplied as a dry powder blended with the glass. Such products are mixed with water or tartaric acid solution. Some are supplied in encapsulated form for mechanical mixing.

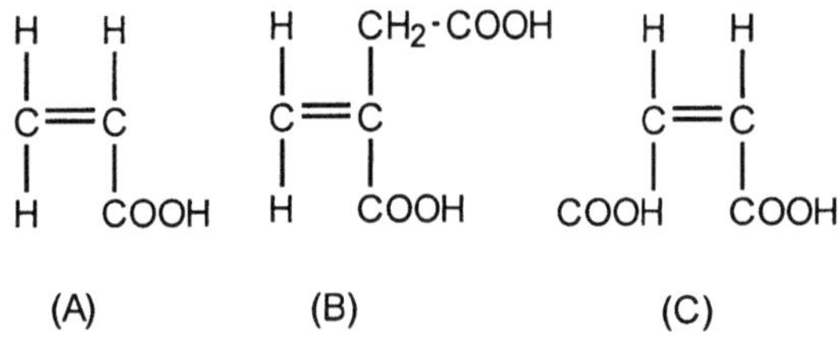

Figure 26.1. Formulae of (A) acrylic acid (B) itaconic acid (C) maleic acid.

Other constituents include tartaric acid, which is important because it can usefully increase the setting rate. Tannic acid is sometimes incorporated because it can adhere to collagen.

26.1.2 Setting reaction

On mixing the basic glass with the aqueous poly(alkenoic acid), an acid-base reaction ensues. The outer layers of the glass particles are decomposed, giving release of Ca^{2+}, Al^{3+} and F^- ions (Fig 26.2). The cations migrate into the aqueous phase, and cross-link the polyalkenoate chains, causing hardening of the material. Over a long period further hardening occurs, as more cations bind to the polyalkenoate chains.

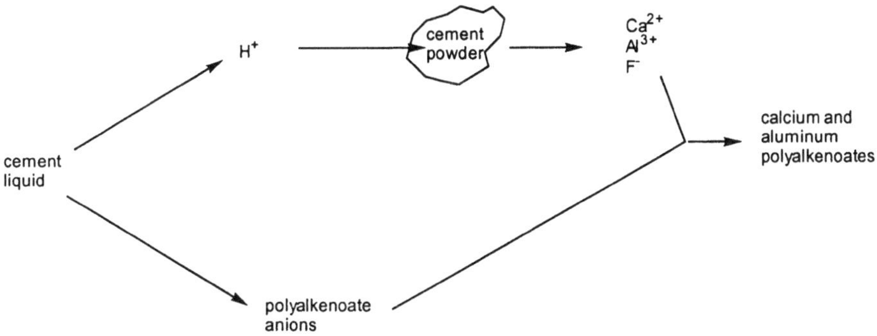

Figure 26.2. Reactions in glass-ionomer cements.

26.1.3 Setting time

This depends on both the composition of the material and the manner in which it is manipulated. In relation to formulation, composition and reactivity and particle size of glass powder are important, as well as the presence of additives such as tartaric acid which increases the speed of set.

In relation to manipulation, the proportioning of constituents and temperature of mixing are important.

26.1.4 Structure of set material

The set cement is heterogeneous containing a core of unreacted glass particles (Figure 26.3). Only about 20%-30% of the glass reacts. The core particles are sheathed by a siliceous hydrogel. These are bound together by the matrix of reaction products. Water is an essential component in the materials; this is of two types: loosely bound water, capable of being removed by desiccation and tightly bound water, which cannot be easily removed. Fluoride is also present.

The strength of the set material is the result of a combination of ionic cross-links, hydrogen bridges and entanglements of the polyalkenoate chains.

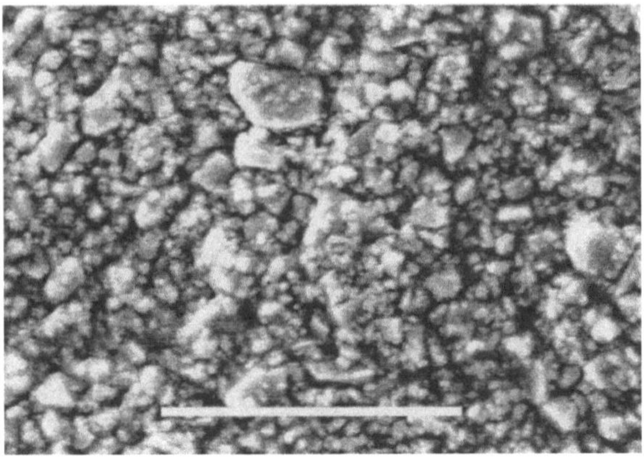

Figure 26.3. Heterogeneous structure of a set glass-ionomer cement (the horizontal bar represents 50 μm).

26.1.5 Properties

1. Biological properties. Glass-ionomers have been reported to cause some inflammatory response, which resolves within a month. The cement has little effect on the gingival tissues. Some luting cements have been reported to cause post-operative sensitivity. This appears to be worse for thinner mixes of cement. This can be largely avoided by not desiccating the tooth prior to cementation. Anticariogenic properties may result from the release of fluoride by these cements.
2. Adhesive properties. These cements adhere to enamel and dentin, and to base metal casting alloys. Suggested mechanisms for bonding to tooth tissue and practical points in obtaining adhesion are discussed in Sections 26.6 and 26.7.
3. Chemical properties. In terms of resistance to oral fluids, glass-ionomer cements, when fully hardened, are more durable than other types of cement. This has been confirmed both by *in vivo* tests and by acid erosion experiments. However, as the set cement may take up to 24 hours to mature, it is generally recommended that freshly set cement must be protected from exposure to moisture.
4. Mechanical properties. In terms of compressive strength, glass-ionomers are superior to all those prepared from a zinc oxide powder. However, the materials are brittle with low tensile strength, so cannot be used for high stress-bearing tooth restorations.

5. Esthetics. Although some early polyalkenoate cements were disappointing in terms of translucency, many modern materials offer reasonable esthetics.
6. In common with all cements, these materials have low thermal diffusivity.

26.1.6 Classification and applications

Conventional glass-ionomer cements may be classified into three groups:
1. Type I, luting cements. These are fine grain materials with low film thickness when set.
2. Type II, restorative materials. Examples of applications include:
- Abrasion and erosion cavities;
- Restoring deciduous teeth;
- Restoration of Class III and Class V carious lesions;
- Tunnel restorations;
- Combined with resin composite in a laminate or 'sandwich' technique (Section 27.7);
- Repairing defective margins in restorations.
3. Type III, lining materials. Applications include:
- Cavity lining in situations where fluoride release is considered to be of value;
- As a base under an amalgam or resin composite restoration.

It must be noted that because of their brittle nature, glass polyalkenoate cements are contra-indicated for:
- Load-bearing restorations in permanent teeth;
- Class IV restorations;
- Core (foundation) restorations;
- Situations where optimum esthetics are required.

26.1.7 Manipulation

It is important that the cement should be mixed at the correct powder/liquid ratio, particularly for Type II cements. Many materials are supplied with pre-proportioned constituents in capsules, designed for mechanical mixing. Rapid mixing is required. Moisture isolation of the tooth is desirable. A dentin surface conditioner – usually a 25% aqueous solution of poly(acrylic acid) – is supplied with some materials to enhance bonding. Pulpal protection by a calcium hydroxide cement is important if the underlying dentin is less than about 0.5 mm thick. Protection of the freshly set cement from moisture by application of a varnish or unfilled resin is important. Table 26.2 outlines the main points in the procedure for placement of glass-ionomer restorations.

Table 26.2. Placement of glass-ionomer restorations

Technique	Rationale
Choose shade of material before cavity preparation	After isolation, the isolated tooth may dry and change color
Check that cavity is free from caries	Residual caries may prejudice longevity of completed restoration
Isolate tooth	The performance of the material is prejudiced by contamination
Condition tooth – for example with 25% aqueous poly(acrylic acid) solution	Improves adhesive bond strength
Mix material to correct consistency and place in cavity	Optimum mechanical properties and minimal solubility depend on a thick mix of material
Adapt glass-ionomer to margins with a placement instrument	Adaptation is essential to chemical interaction between cement and tooth substance
Use a matrix where possible	Improves surface finish
Do not disturb material after it loses its glossy surface	Crazing of the surface may result from prolonged manipulation
Leave matrix in place until setting is complete	The matrix protects the restoration from drying out in addition to producing contour
Remove excess with a blade and finish the restoration with discs or stones lubricated with petroleum jelly	The petroleum jelly helps to prevent dehydration during finishing
Apply layer of unfilled light-activated resin and cure	Glass-ionomers must be protected from moisture during the maturation phase
Check that the layer of resin has not produced a ledge at or beyond the cavity margin	A ledge could attract plaque

Note that for resin-modified glass-ionomers (discussed below), conditioning may or may not be advocated by the manufacturer. These products require visible light curing following placement.

26.2 CERMETS AND RELATED MATERIALS

In cermet (*CER*amo*MET*al) cements an ion-leachable glass and fine silver powder, are heated to over 1000°C to form an amorphous mass which is ground to make a powder which is mixed with a poly(alkenoic acid) to form a set cement.

The general properties of such materials are:

- Biocompatibility is similar to conventional glass-ionomers;
- Fluoride release, however, is less than for conventional glass-ionomers;
- Slightly improved physical properties and wear resistance when compared to conventional glass-ionomers;
- Adhesion to enamel and dentin;
- Poor esthetics.

Suggested applications for cermets include:

- Use as core build-up (foundation) materials (see Chapter 39);
- Filling materials for posterior teeth where the occlusal forces are minimal.

An alternative material is available in which the powder is simply an admixture of FAS glass and dental amalgam alloy powder (Ag_3Sn). Apart from its radiopacity, the physical properties of this material are little different from conventional glass-ionomer.

26.3 RESIN-MODIFIED GLASS-IONOMER CEMENTS

Resin-modified glass-ionomers (RMGI) were developed to overcome some of the problems of traditional glass-ionomers, including their short working time, long setting time and brittleness. In addition to an FAS glass and poly(alkenoic acid), simple resin-modified materials also contain a monomer such as 2-hydroxyethyl methacrylate (HEMA) or Bis-GMA, (Figure 11.13) together with a photoinitiator such as camphorquinone (Figure 27.7) in materials designed to be visible light cured. These products set by two mechanisms:

- Polymerization of the monomer; this may be by visible light cure or chemical cure. One material (see below) utilizes both of these methods of activation;
- The acid-base glass-ionomer reaction. It is therefore apparent that these materials will always set in the absence of light, because of the conventional acid-base reaction. But note that optimum properties are only achieved if the polymerization reaction also takes place.

Some products contain more complex polymer systems in addition to HEMA. For example, a poly(alkenoic acid) modified with pendant methacrylate groups, in addition to HEMA, is present in some products

(Figure 26.4). This molecule is capable of polymerizing and also reacting with the glass.

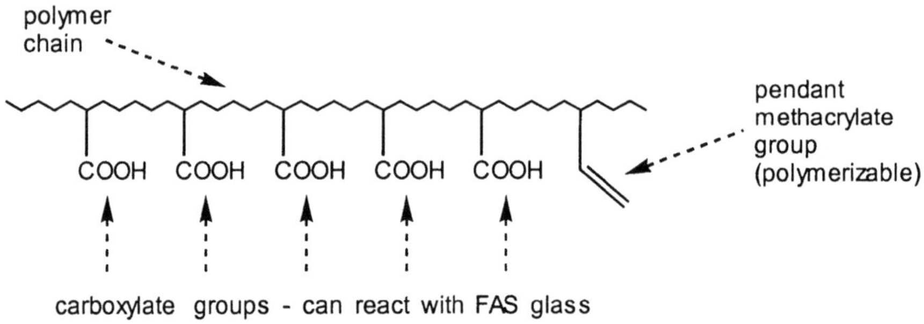

Figure 26.4. Representation of a modified poly(alkenoic acid) with pendant methacrylate groups.

A further variant is that some products claim to have a 'tri-cure' mechanism. That is, they are designed to set by three mechanisms (Figure 26.5):

- The acid-base reaction;
- Visible light curing of methacrylate groups;
- Chemically activated polymerization of methacrylate groups.

A number of advantages are claimed for this system. In addition to the benefits of visible light curing, it also provides an extended working time with rapid setting, and the development of good mechanical properties even in areas that are inaccessible to the curing light.

The general properties of resin-modified glass-ionomers are:

- Biocompatibility similar to conventional glass-ionomers;
- Fluoride release similar to or better than conventional glass-ionomers;
- Adhesion to enamel and dentin;
- Improved physical properties, especially with regard to tensile strength;
- Wear resistance similar to conventional glass-ionomers;
- Satisfactory esthetics.

Suggested applications include:

- Use as core build-up materials;
- Restoration of Class III and Class V cavities;
- Restoration of posterior teeth where the occlusal forces are minimal;
- Luting materials for orthodontic brackets;
- Cavity linings and bases.

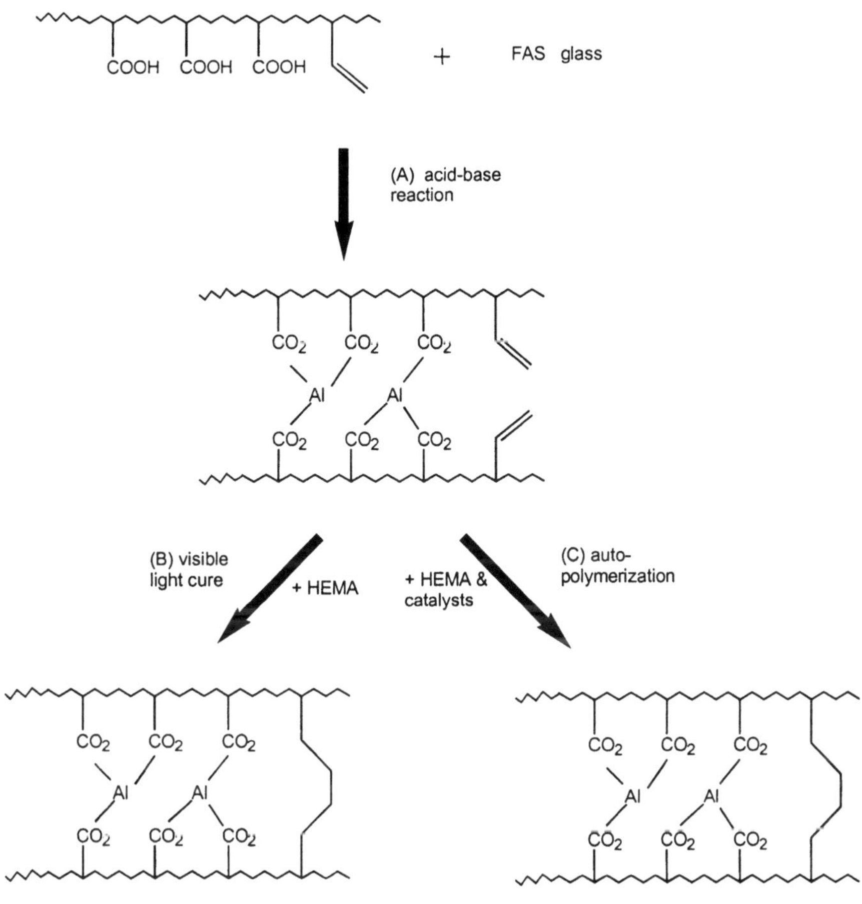

Figure 26.5. 'Tri-cure' mechanism of a resin-modified glass-ionomer.

26.4 RESIN-MODIFIED GLASS-IONOMER LUTING MATERIALS

The materials described above are available as restorative and base materials, differing mainly in glass composition and resin type. RMGIs are also available as luting materials, which are not cured by visible light, but set by a combination of the conventional glass-ionomer acid-base reaction and the polymerization of a chemically activated resin. Advantages of these materials include:

- Fluoride release;
- Adhesion to tooth substance;
- Low solubility in oral fluids;
- Ease of handling and easy post-cementation clean-up;
- Adequate mixing and working time combined with fast set.

The principal disadvantage appears to be a setting expansion of some of these materials, particularly under conditions of high humidity. This has been reported to have caused fracture of all-porcelain crowns. No other sequelae to this setting expansion, such as pulp pressure symptoms, have been reported.

26.5 HIGHER VISCOSITY GLASS-IONOMER CEMENTS

Higher viscosity glass-ionomer cements (also termed 'condensable' glass-ionomers) were developed in the early 1990s, principally in response to the Atraumatic Restorative Treatment technique. This is a minimal instrumentation technique designed for less industrialized communities. These materials are more easily handled than conventional glass-ionomers and have been considered, by virtue of their high viscosity, to be capable of being condensed into a tooth cavity in a manner similar to amalgam. The increased viscosity is a result of finer particle grain size distribution and the addition of poly(acrylic acid) to the powder of some materials. The majority of these materials are metal-free, but one product contains a silver-tin-copper alloy.

This group of materials has similar properties to conventional glass-ionomers in terms of biocompatibility, fluoride release, adhesion to enamel and dentin and esthetics. Physical properties – specifically tensile strength and abrasion and wear resistance – are better than conventional glass-ionomers.

26.6 ADHESION MECHANISMS FOR POLY-CARBOXYLATES AND GLASS-IONOMERS

It is widely accepted that bonding to enamel and dentin occurs by some type of ionic mechanism, although the precise mechanism is not understood yet. Chelation of the calcium of hydroxyapatite has been suggested. This is thought to be unlikely, because it would involve the formation of an 8-membered ring. Based on infrared spectroscopic evidence the formation of strong ionic bonds between polyacrylate (polyalkenoate) ions and surface calcium ions of apatite in enamel and dentin was proposed. It was then suggested that initial adhesion was by the formation of strong hydrogen bonds, which, over a period of time, are replaced by ionic bonds.

More recently, it has been postulated that polyacrylate ions enter the molecular structure of hydroxyapatite, so displacing and replacing surface phosphate ions - see Figure 26.6.

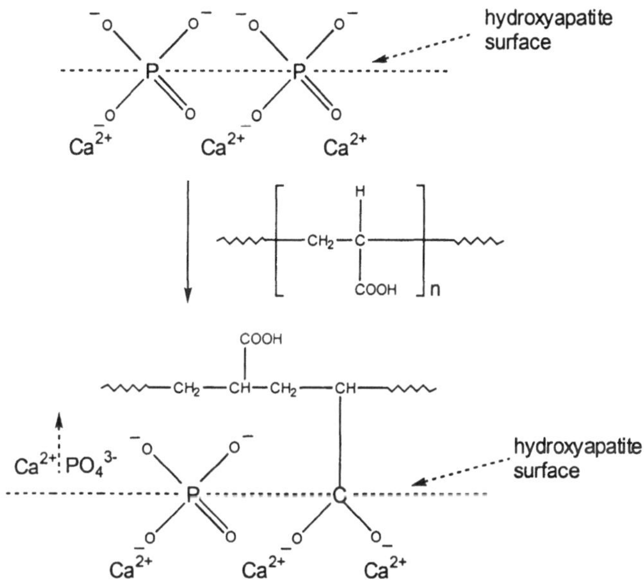

Figure 26.6. A proposed mechanism of bonding of glass-ionomers to hydroxyapatite. After Wilson A D, Prosser H J, Powis D M (1983). Mechanism of adhesion of polyelectrolyte cements to hydroxyapatite. *Journal of Dental Research* **62**: 590-592.

One area of interest is this – do these materials bond to collagen? It is believed that this is not the case. Note that the bond to enamel is better than the bond to dentin.

26.7 PRACTICAL POINTS IN OBTAINING ADHESION

Good bonding requires careful attention to detail. Etching is not helpful, since the adhesion is chemical rather than micromechanical in nature. Indeed, it has been claimed that bond strength decreases as surface roughness increases. It is evident that the cement must be applied to a clean surface, for interaction between polyalkenoate ions and calcium ions to occur. A great variety of conditioning agents for dentin has been recommended, including 10% citric acid and a 25% aqueous solution of poly(acrylic acid). Some resin-modified glass-ionomers are supplied with a special primer which contains a poly(alkenoic acid) co-polymer, HEMA and photoinitiators.

FURTHER READING

In Chapter 39, glass-ionomer cements and related materials are critiqued as core build-up materials. Chapter 43 deals with the choice of materials for the restoration of teeth. Chapter 44 considers the choice of cements for luting.

Frankerberger R F, Sindel J, Kramer N (1997). Viscous glass-ionomer cements: A new alternative to amalgam in the primary dentition. *Quintessence International* **28**: 667-676.

McLean J W, Prosser H J, Wilson A D (1985). The use of glass ionomer cements in bonding composite resins to dentine. *British Dental Journal* **158**: 410-414.

Mount G J (1990). Polyacrylic cements in dentistry. *American Journal of Dentistry* **3**: 79-84.

Mount G J (1995). Some physical and biological properties of glass ionomer cement. *International Dental Journal* **45**: 135-140.

Naasan M A, Watson T F (1998). Conventional glass ionomers as posterior restorations. A status report for the American Journal of Dentistry. *American Journal of Dentistry* **11**: 36-45.

Sidhu S K, Watson T F (1995). Resin-modified glass ionomer materials. A status report for the American Journal of Dentistry. *American Journal of Dentistry.* **8**: 59-67.

Wilson A D, Kent B E (1972). A new translucent cement for dentistry. The glass ionomer cement. *British Dental Journal* **132**: 133-135.

Wilson A D, McLean J W (1988). *Glass-Ionomer Cement.* Quintessence, Chicago.

Chapter 27

Resin Composites and Compomers

Summary: Resin composites and materials derived from them are widely used as directly placed tooth colored restorative materials. The available materials differ considerably in composition and properties. This chapter discusses the composition, properties, manipulation and applications of these materials.

27.1 INTRODUCTION AND HISTORICAL PERSPECTIVE

Combinations of polymers and ceramics are now widely used in restorative dentistry. Chapter 11 gives the background to polymers, including the mechanism of free radical addition polymerization, which is of particular relevance. The theory of composite materials is discussed in Chapter 16.

Silicates are now rarely used as anterior restorative materials because of problems such as high solubility and a high incidence of pulp death. As a result, polymeric filling materials were developed, with the earliest being based on chemically activated acrylics, the chemistry of which is discussed in Section 11.3. These acrylic filling materials had far from ideal requirements because of high water absorption, high coefficient of thermal expansion, discoloration, high shrinkage on polymerization, high incidence of secondary caries and low strength.

To overcome some of the above problems, ceramic-filled polymers were developed. Some early materials were based on acrylic resin, but in the early 1960s dimethacrylate polymers were proposed. Since then considerable development has taken place in filler technology. Modern composite materials are ceramic-filled dimethacrylates. Such materials have been widely used for restoration of cavities in anterior teeth and are now finding application for restorations in posterior teeth in load-bearing situations.

27.2 CONSTITUENTS OF COMPOSITES

The components of modern composites may be listed as:
- Principal (higher molecular weight) monomers;
- Diluent (lower molecular weight) monomers;
- Inorganic fillers;
- Silane coupling agents;
- Polymerization inhibitors;
- Initiator/activator components;
- Ultra violet stabilizers.

27.2.1 Principal (higher molecular weight) monomers

Many composites are based on an aromatic dimethacrylate system, the monomer being the reaction product of bisphenol-A and glycidyl methacrylate, often called Bis-GMA or Bowen's resin (formula in Figure 11.13). This highly viscous monomer can undergo free radical addition polymerization to give a rigid cross-linked polymer. A small number of products use alternative monomers that are described as urethane dimethacrylates (Figure 11.14). The properties of composites based on these monomers are generally similar to those of materials containing Bowen's resin. There appears to be good compatibility between products using Bowen's resin and urethane dimethacrylate – that is, a bonding resin based on Bowen's resin will bond satisfactorily to a composite based on urethane dimethacrylate. However this does not imply that the components of bonding systems, such as primers and resins, are necessarily interchangeable (see Chapter 28).

27.2.2 Diluent (lower molecular weight) monomers

Other monomers are included in composite formulations to reduce the viscosity of the material to enable proper blending with the inorganic constituents, and to facilitate clinical manipulation. These monomers are also difunctional, having two reactive methacrylate groups per molecule. Two examples are ethylene glycol dimethacrylate and triethylene glycol dimethacrylate (Figure 11.12). Greater quantities of diluent monomer give composite materials of lower viscosity, but also with greater shrinkage on polymerization.

27.2.3 Inorganic fillers

1. Types of fillers. A wide variety of fillers has been used. Early composites contained glass fibers and beads, synthetic calcium phosphates and fused silica. The filler particle in early materials, termed *macrofilled composites*, were generally between 5 – 10 µm, producing restorations with surfaces that were difficult to polish and which therefore stained readily. Wear resistance was poor, as the filler particles were readily lost from the material.

Manufacturers developed *microfilled composites* during the 1970s. These products contain colloidal silica filler of particle size about 0.04 µm, resulting in a material that is easily polished (Figure 27.1).

Current materials may contain lithium aluminosilicates, crystalline quartz, or barium aluminoborate silica glasses. This latter material has the following formulation (weight %): SiO_2, 50; BaO, 33; B_2O_3, 9 and Al_2O_3, 8. Many composites contain a combination of a barium glass and another filler. Many current materials are termed *hybrid composites* because the filler is composed of a variety of particle sizes, the majority being typically 1 – 1.5 µm, but with the spaces between the larger particles being filled with particles which may be as small as those in the microfilled materials (Figure 27.1).

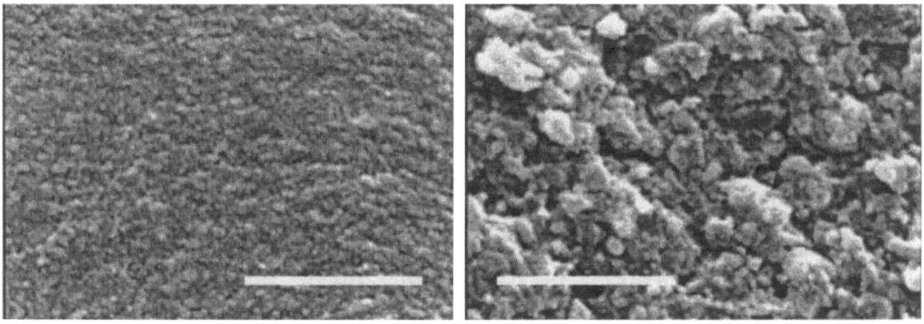

Figure 27.1. SEM of resin composites; left: microfilled composite; right: hybrid composite. The horizontal bars represent 10 µm.

A strontium glass was incorporated in one product; it was claimed that this softer material rendered the composite easier to polish.

One material uses only one, as opposed to two or more types of filler. This is a synthetic mineral of zirconia/silica, fabricated in such a way as to produce particles with rounded edges. Particle size is in the range 0.01 µm (smaller than in the microfilled materials) to 3.5 μm, with a mean of 0.6 μm (Figure 27.2). There is a 'continuum' of filler particle sizes.

A number of composite materials also contain a fluoride-containing filler (Section 20.7.2).

A number of recently introduced materials have used alternative filler technologies in an attempt to produce a 'condensable' material that handles in a manner similar to amalgam (Section 27.9.2). The following four approaches to filler technology are being used:

- Fibers, 40-60 μm long, 6-10 μm diameter, 70% volume of filler (Figure 27.2);
- Trimodal particle size distribution; filler particles designed to interlock during the packing procedure;
- 66 % total volume of three fillers, one of which is porous and becomes impregnated by resin;
- A non-slumping filler.

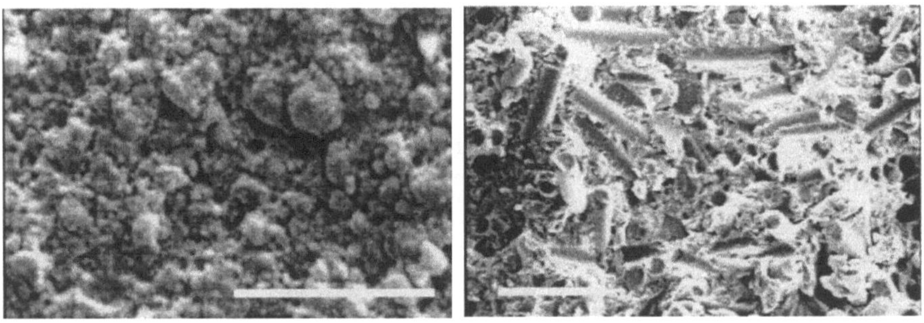

Figure 27.2. SEM of resin composites; left: with zirconia/silica filler - horizontal bar = 10 μm; right: with fibrous filler - horizontal bar = 100 μm.

2. Quantity of filler. Composites with the larger size particles contain typically 78% (by weight) of filler. Some recent products for posterior restorations contain up to 87% filler. Some recently introduced 'flowable' composites contain about 60% filler (Section 27.9.1). However, microfilled composites contain less inorganic filler. It is technically difficult to add larger quantities of microfine silica to a fluid monomer, since it acts as a thickening agent and confers thixotropy. It is usual for a microfine filler to be prepared in a matrix of cured resin, which is then ground, and incorporated in a difunctional monomer. Present day microfilled composites contain from 25% to 63% SiO_2 (by weight).

3. Effects of fillers on properties. The incorporation of inorganic fillers has the following effects on a polymer:

- Improvement in mechanical properties such as compressive strength, modulus of elasticity and hardness;
- Reduction in coefficient of thermal expansion;
- Contribution to the esthetics; glass particles are able to modify the optical appearance of the composite, so as to match the color of the surrounding tooth material;
- Reduction in the contraction on setting;
- Less heat evolved in polymerization because a smaller quantity of resin is used;
- The composite is radiopaque if the filler contains Ba, Sr, or Zr.

4. Classification of materials. – See Table 27.1. Available products can be classified according to filler type, but it has also been suggested that they be classified according to particle size, given that the filler content and filler size have been shown to directly determine the physical and mechanical properties of composite materials. Accordingly *ultrafine* materials have a mean particle size in the range 0.5 to 4.0 μm and *fine* materials with particles in the range 4.0 – 10.0 μm.

Table 27.1. Classification of resin composite materials

Type	Typical filler content	Particle size (μm)	General comments
Macrofilled	78 weight % 55 volume %	1-35	Difficult to polish; surface becomes rougher in service due to abrasion of resin matrix; surface may attract plaque
Microfilled	35-63 weight %	0.04	Easy to obtain and maintain smooth surface. Poorer mechanical properties. Some products have poor wear resistance
Hybrid filled (Figure 27.3)	> 80 weight %	0.5-2 and 0.04	Improved polishability compared to macrofilled; better wear resistance than microfilled
Continuum filled (Figure 27.4)	86.8 weight %	0.01-3 mean 0.9	Contains a synthetic zirconia/silica filler
Flowable	< 60 weight %	-	Used by addition of small increments to achieve restorative contour
Packable ('condensable')	≥86 weight %	-	Intended to be packed in a manner similar to dental amalgam

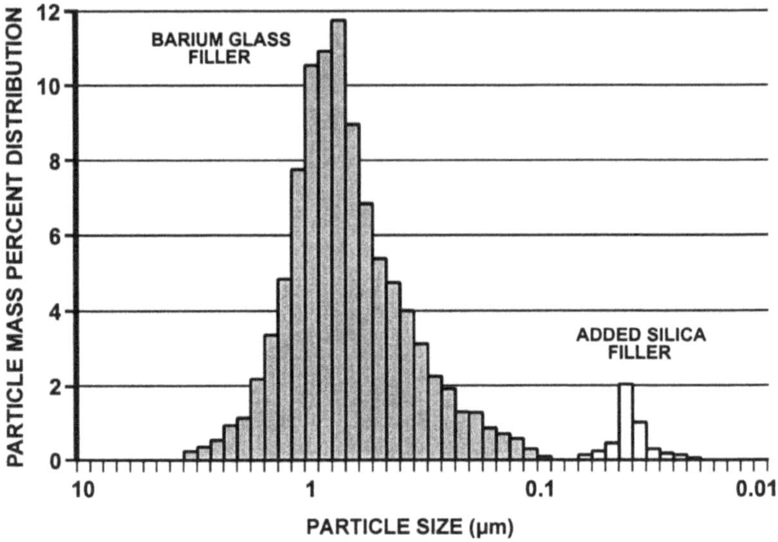

Figure 27.3. Filler particle size distribution for a hybrid composite.

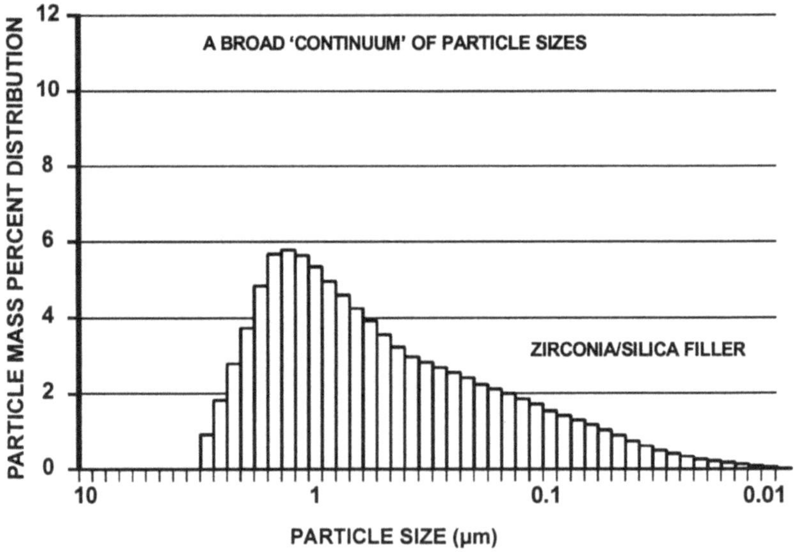

Figure 27.4. Filler particle size distribution for the 'continuum' filled resin composite.

27.2.4 Silane coupling agents

It is important, if reinforcement of the polymer by the filler is to occur, that the two constituents should be bonded together. To achieve this, the filler is usually treated with a vinyl silane compound (Figure 27.5).

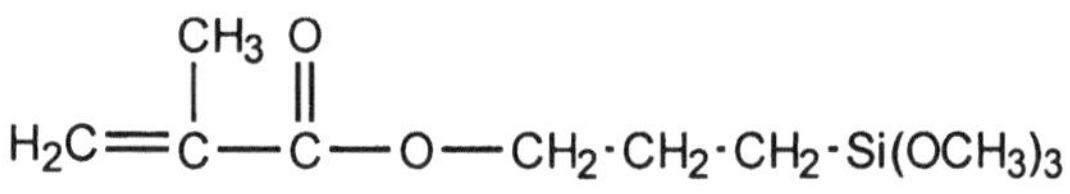

Figure 27.5. Vinyl silane compound (γ-methacryoxypropyl trimethoxysilane).

27.2.5 Polymerization inhibitors

Since dimethacrylate monomers will polymerize on storage, an inhibitor is necessary. Hydroquinone has been widely used, but was responsible for causing discoloration of the material. The monomethyl ether of hydroquinone is now used (Figure 27.6). Only a few parts per million of this compound are required.

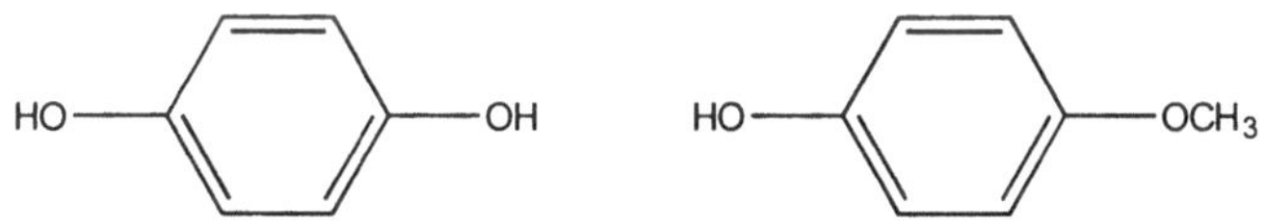

(A) (B)

Figure 27.6. (A) Hydroquinone (1,4-dihydroxybenzene); (B) Monomethyl ether of hydroquinone.

27.2.6 Initiator/activator systems

Composites may be classified according to method of curing – that is – chemical activation or visible light cure.

1. Chemical activation. Benzoyl peroxide initiator and tertiary amine activators, or sulfinic acid type initiators may be employed. Of the tertiary amines, N, N-dimethyl-*p*-toluidine was used as activator, but now N, N-dihydroxyethyl-*p*-toluidine is now most widely used (Figure 11.7).

2. Visible light activation. Visible light cure (VLC) composites have been developed which contain an α-diketone such as camphorquinone and an amine. On application of visible light of wavelength 460-485 nm, free

radicals are generated (Figure 27.7). Visible light cured materials are now very widely used.

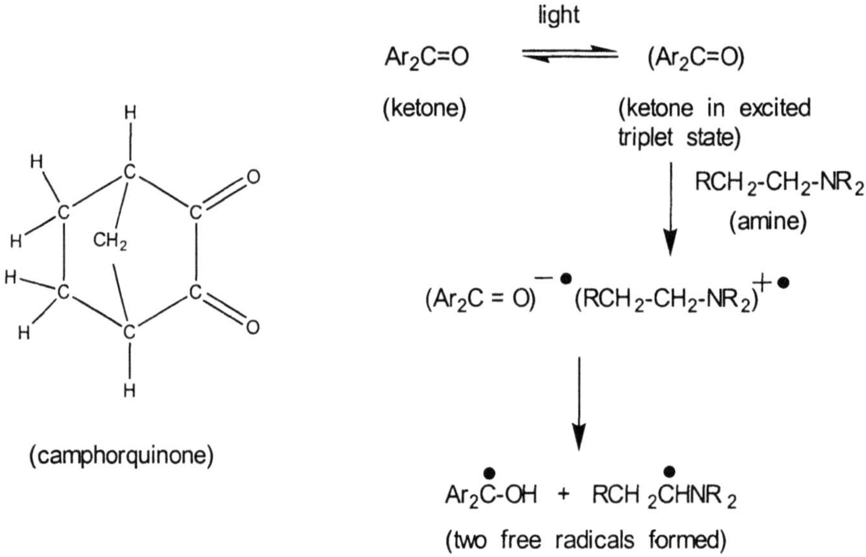

Figure 27.7. Left: camphorquinone; Right: system for visible-light activation of polymerization.

27.2.7 Ultra violet stabilizers

To prevent discoloration of composites in service, compounds are incorporated which absorb electromagnetic radiation. Clinical evidence suggests that this improves color stability. (Example 2-hydroxy-4-methoxybenzophenone - Figure 27.8.).

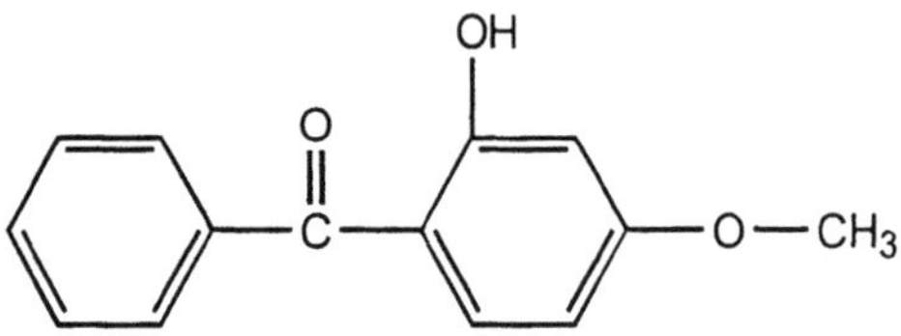

Figure 27.8. 2-hydroxy-4-methoxybenzophenone.

27.3 LIGHT SOURCES

The available lights for curing composites may be classified as in Table 27.2. The light output will have a spectral distribution similar to that in Figure 7.2B.

Table 27.2. Classification of visible light curing sources

Mode of transmission of light	General comments
Fiber optic system	Fiber optic system needs to be handled with care to avoid fracture of the glass rods
Fluid-filled hose	Avoids above problem, but fluid may deteriorate over a period of time
Pistol grip	These lights are generally more compact and lightweight than the above

The light curing unit will comprise the following:

- A quartz-halogen bulb of adequate light output (e.g. 420 mW/cm^2);
- A transformer and control circuitry;
- Appropriate light filters;
- A switch and timing device;
- A curing tip: This may vary from around 4 mm to 7 mm in diameter. Larger tips are ideal for curing larger restorations, provided that the light intensity is sufficient. Light tips should be autoclavable.
- Ideally the unit should incorporate a light meter or means of measuring the light output at the tip, so that the operator may check the output regularly.

An important requirement is that light-curing units should not be adversely affected by disinfecting solutions.

Recently introduced high intensity lights derived from plasma technology have been reported to cure resin composite restorations in times of less than 5 seconds. However, the effects of this rapid cure on stresses associated with polymerization shrinkage are not fully quantified. Furthermore, it has been reported that there is substantial heat present at the light tip which may damage soft tissues with some systems.

27.4 SELECTION OF MATERIALS

1. Chemical *versus* visible light curing. An advantage of chemical activation is that no elaborate equipment is needed. However, there are many benefits of visible light activation. Command setting means that there

is no increase in viscosity until application of light. Also since VLC materials require no mixing, problems of air incorporation are avoided.
2. Microfine *versus* conventional fillers. Microfilled materials can both take and retain good surface finish. However materials with higher inorganic content have better mechanical properties and lower coefficients of thermal expansion.

27.5 TECHNIQUES OF MANIPULATION

27.5.1 General considerations

1. It has been recommended that enamel margins should be beveled. This permits a gradation of shade from restoration to tooth and a greater bonding area. However in load bearing locations, a thin edge of composite at the beveled area will be liable to fracture. Bevels should therefore not be applied to the occlusal aspects of cavities for composite restorations in posterior teeth.
2. It was previously considered that a base was required to protect exposed dentin. Traditionally this was believed to be necessary to avoid the possibility of irritation from chemical constituents of the restorative procedure and material. However it is now believed that greater danger to the pulp comes from ingress of microorganisms at the restoration-tooth interface. A dentin bonding system (Chapter 28) should therefore be employed to cover all the internal surfaces of the cavity.
3. Since pulp capping with dentin bonding systems is controversial, for cavities with 0.5 mm of the pulp, a base may be indicated. In such situations, the base materials of choice are:

- Glass-ionomer cements (either conventional or resin-modified materials);
- Calcium hydroxide cements, although these materials do not bond to dentin.

Eugenol-containing materials should be avoided, since eugenol can act as a plasticizer for the polymer component of the composite.
4. Bonding to enamel. All enamel surfaces contacted by resin should be etched. However the etchant should be carefully confined to the area immediately around the cavity, as resin will adhere to all etched areas. The consequent need to remove this excess resin could cause damage to sound enamel. The rules of acid etching should be followed carefully (Table 19.2).

5. When a light cured intermediate resin or bonding agent is being used, it should be polymerized prior to application of the restorative material.
6. Cellulose acetate matrix bands should be used to apply pressure to the material and give optimum surface finish.
7. Contamination by blood or saliva should be avoided.

27.5.2 Chemically activated materials

The two pastes should be mixed thoroughly in the correct proportion (usually equal volumes). During mixing of some products, tints can be added to enhance color matching between composite and tooth. Contamination of one paste by the other should be avoided. As far as possible, incorporation of air during mixing should be avoided, as this will have an adverse effect on physical properties. The mixed material should be placed in the cavity without delay.

27.5.3 Visible light cure (VLC) materials

In general, most commercially available light sources will polymerize most light-cured materials to a depth of 3 mm, though some systems are more efficient than others.

Under-curing may result:

- If the light is not sufficiently close to the surface of the material being polymerized;
- If the light is of insufficient intensity;
- If the light is attenuated by passage through a restoration or tooth substance;
- If the light source is of the incorrect wavelength.

Under-curing results in a material with a hard outer 'skin' and soft material at the base of the cavity. Darker shades of material absorb more light, so require longer curing to achieve the same depth of cure as lighter shades. Over-curing is not harmful, so it is advisable to err on the side of longer curing times rather than shorter. Note that in some instances the material may begin to polymerize if exposed to strong ambient lighting in a dental operatory.

It has recently been considered that the rapid curing of a composite restoration by a light of high intensity has the potential to set up stresses within the composite and at the interface between composite and tooth substance, thus militating against good adhesion. Proponents of this concept advise on of the following procedures:

- Use of a light source the intensity of which builds up to its maximum value over a period of 30 seconds or longer;
- Curing of the restoration through tooth substance, for example, through a cusp;
- Bringing the light down to the restoration gradually over a period of 30 seconds or longer.

However other practitioners emphasize the chairside convenience of high speed curing.

27.5.4 Finishing procedures

If surface finishing is required, this is probably best achieved by:

- Contouring the material with a fine (15 μm) diamond bur or 8 to 12 fluted tungsten carbide bur;
- Polishing with a composite finishing system comprising for example, abrasive discs, impregnated rubber points and 50 μm aluminum oxide paste.

Surface glazes are supplied with some materials; these are essentially unfilled polymers. Though a glaze can give a smooth surface initially, it is unlikely that its esthetic benefit will be long lasting. However the benefits of glazing are that microscopic voids on the surface are filled, and the surface of the restoration is further cured, with potential benefits in terms of hardness and wear resistance.

Tables 27.3 and 27.4 summarize the rationale for the most important practical points in the placement of light-activated composites in anterior and posterior teeth.

27.6 APPLICATIONS

1. Restorations of anterior teeth. Composites are now the most widely used materials for this application. Although microfine-filled materials are recognized as being the most esthetic composites, they may not be sufficiently durable for larger restorations.

Table 27.3. Placement of light activated resin in anterior teeth

Technique	Rationale
Choose shade of material before cavity preparation	After rubber dam placement isolated tooth may dry and change color
Check that cavity is free of caries	Residual caries may prejudice longevity of completed restoration
Bevel labial aspect of cavity margin	May improve esthetics, and may increase area for bonding
Apply dentin and enamel bonding agents in accordance with manufacturer's instructions	Failure to adequately bond restoration may prejudice result
Insert composite increments ≤ 2.5 mm	Thicker layers may not cure fully, especially darker shades of material
Cure the composite by gradually bringing the light towards the restoration	Fast initial curing may set up stresses within the restoration
Cure in excess of manufacturer's recommended time	VLC composites cannot be overcured
Finish restoration (Section 27.5.4) taking care that enamel margins are not damaged	
Place a layer of glaze/unfilled resin and light cure	Will fill microscopic voids and may improve initial esthetics

Table 27.4. Placement of light activated resin composite in posterior teeth

Technique	Rationale
Choose shade	A slight mismatch may be desirable so that enamel and composite may be differentiated during finishing
Check occlusion prior to cavity preparation	Ideally occlusion should not be directly on cavity margins
Prepare cavity; ensure that it is caries free	As for anterior restorations
Do not bevel occlusal margins	Thin flashes on margins of composite will fracture
Apply dentin and enamel bonding agents Alternatively the deepest portion of the cavity may be filled with glass-ionomer or a flowable composite	As for anterior restorations
Use a matrix that can be pushed out to form a tight contact	Composite cannot be condensed like amalgam
Place a thin layer of material at the gingival margin and light cure	This layer is furthest from the light, therefore the most difficult to cure
Place composite in increments; each increment should touch only one wall of the cavity	Incremental cure gives a better overall cure
Cure in excess of manufacturer's stated time	As for anterior restorations
Surface finishing	As for anterior restorations

2. Restorations of posterior teeth. There is great current interest in the application of composites as alternatives to dental amalgam. They can be recommended for use where esthetic considerations are of importance. For long lasting restorations it is essential that the operator is aware of the optimum methods of placement and factors influencing success, in particular that these materials perform best in small-to-medium sized cavities. Restorations of composite are much more technique-sensitive and time consuming to place than restorations of amalgam.
3. Composites have been recommended as core build up (foundation) material for crowns. Chemically cured materials may be particularly appropriate in this respect, as they do not require incremental build-up.
4. Other applications include:
- Luting of resin-bonded bridge systems (Chapter 44);
- Inlay materials (Chapter 37);
- Polymeric crown and bridge materials (Chapter 38);
- Laminate veneer systems are available to improve the esthetics of stained and discolored teeth. A thin polymeric or ceramic veneer is cemented to acid etched enamel by a resin.

27.7 ASSESSMENT OF COMPOSITES

1. Biological considerations. When composites are used in conjunction with a dentin bonding system the risk of pulpal irritation is negligible. Plaque can accumulate on a poorly polished composite surface, though this is less of a problem with small particle hybrid or microfilled composites.
2. Bonding. Composites are not adhesive to enamel and dentin, so bonding systems must be employed. In contemporary systems the enamel and dentin are treated simultaneously using a total-etch technique.
3. Chemical properties. The solubility of composites is very low. The polymer component absorbs some water that may make the material swell; this may partially counteract polymerization shrinkage. This is more apparent with the less heavily filled microfilled materials than with hybrid-filled composites.
4. Mechanical properties. These are generally good, though microfilled materials are generally less rigid than hybrid composites. Chemically cured composites may be less rigid than visible light cured materials because of the presence of air that was incorporated during mixing.
5. Esthetic considerations. Modern composite materials are color stable, may have similar translucency to enamel and may provide good long-term

esthetics. A wide variety of shades and translucencies is available with many systems.

6. Thermal properties. Composites have less thermal expansion than unfilled resins (Table 6.2). They also have low thermal diffusivity (Table 6.1).

7. Dimensional change on setting. Monomers which are in current use in dental composites shrink on polymerization by between 1% and 3% by volume.

The forces from polymerization shrinkage:

- May be sufficient to compromise bonding to dentin;
- May cause stresses to develop within the restoration if a bonding system with good adhesion has been employed (Chapter 28).

These stresses are detrimental to a restoration given that they become concentrated either internally at the interface of filler particles and the resin matrix or externally at the interface between restoration and tooth. If the stress exceeds the adhesive or cohesive strength of the substrates involved, separation will occur. Stresses are greatest in cavities with a high ratio of bonded to unbonded surface area – the so-called *configuration factor*. The clinician must therefore counter the potential for formation of these stresses. A number of possible strategies are available:

- Use of a material that flows, especially as it develops rigidity – some chemically cured and some flowable materials (Section 27.9.1) fulfill this criterion;
- Use of a material of lower modulus to fill part of the cavity – the base layer of the restoration may be built up in glass-ionomer (the laminate or sandwich technique), a flowable composite or a compomer;
- Use of a bonding system which is inherently more flexible or which is capable of being placed in a thick layer that acts as a stress absorber;
- Slow curing of the resin;
- Curing the resin in small increments each of which touches only one wall of the cavity. This is desirable for better curing of the material and hence the material has better properties. However, recent finite element analysis research has questioned the effectiveness of the incremental curing technique in reducing stresses;
- Fill as much of the cavity as possible with pre-cured composite or ceramic inserts.

8. Surface finish. With some composites it is difficult to obtain a smooth surface finish by abrading and polishing techniques. Also, abrasive wear in service roughens the material, because the polymer phase wears more

rapidly than the harder ceramic material. However, materials with microfine fillers can take and retain a smooth surface finish.

9. Radiopacity. This is essential if the composite is to be used in a posterior tooth. Most materials are more radiopaque than tooth substance.

10. Rheological properties. Unmixed composite pastes are usually Bingham bodies (Figure 27.9). Chemically activated composites show a continued increase in viscosity from the conclusion of mixing (Figure 27.10).

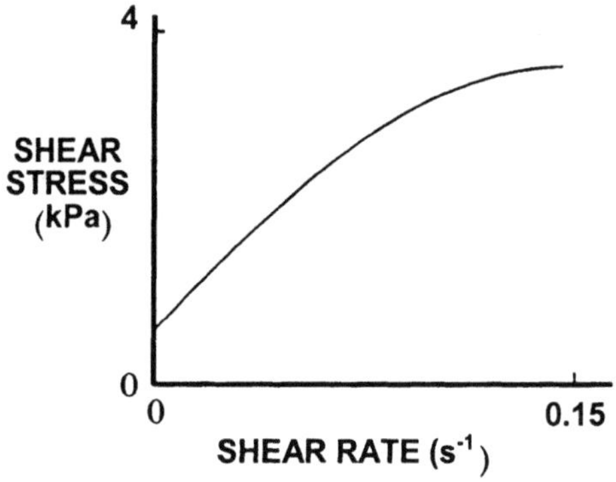

Figure 27.9. Rheological characteristics of a composite paste (compare with Figure 5.3). After Braden M (1977). Rheology of composite filling material pastes. *Journal of Dental Research*. **56**: 627-630.

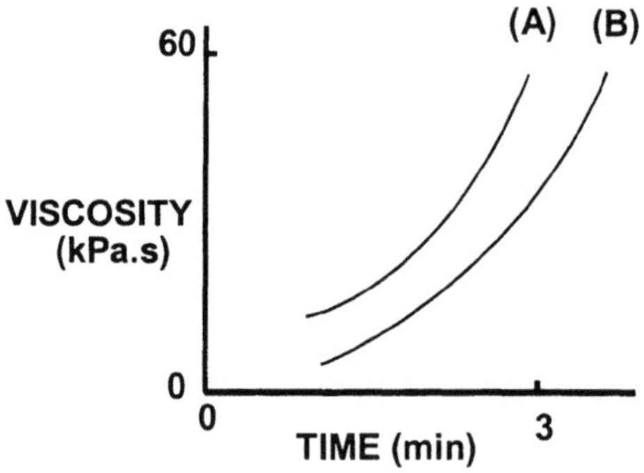

Figure 27.10. Apparent viscosity at shear rate of 13 s^{-1} versus time, for setting composites (A) marcofilled (B) microfilled material. After Watts D C, Combe E C, Greener E H (1980). Capillary rheology of two composite resin systems. *Journal of Oral Rehabilitation*. **7**: 475-480.

27.8 RESIN-BASED LUTING MATERIALS

Resin composite luting materials were developed in the early 1970s for use with the earliest type of adhesive bridge (the so-called *Rochette bridge*). These cements were essentially less heavily filled chemically cured composites, with a filler loading of about 65% by weight. Since their introduction, there has been substantial technical development, producing materials that make a major contribution to contemporary dentistry.

The available materials may be classified according to their method of curing, which may be by visible light, or by chemical curing or by a combination of the two (dual cure).

27.8.1 Visible light and dual cure materials

Light cure resin composite luting materials polymerize by a similar mechanism to the restorative materials. Dual cure products also contain a system for chemical activation of polymerization, which ensures that the material will polymerize even if it does not receive sufficient light of the appropriate wavelength. This can be of value in the deepest areas of a cavity beneath an inlay or crown.

Light cured materials are used mainly for the placement of porcelain veneers while dual cure materials are used for placement of composite or ceramic inlays and dentin-bonded all-ceramic crowns.

Where cements are used for luting translucent restorations or veneers, it is imperative that account is taken of the shade of the cement because this will contribute to the overall shade of the restoration. Some manufacturers offer try-in pastes of similar shades to the luting materials. These are water-based non-setting materials. For dual cure cements, supplied as two paste systems, one of the pastes alone may be used for determining shade, provided that the material does not start to polymerize under the influence of operatory lighting.

27.8.2 Chemically cured materials

Chemically cured materials are used for placement of resin retained bridges, any metal restoration for which a resin cement is indicated and for placement of bonded amalgams.

A number of chemically cured luting materials have been considered particularly appropriate for bonding to metal – either the metal retainers of resin-bonded bridges or in bonding amalgam restorations to tooth substance. These include materials based on the resin monomer 4-META (4-methacryloxyethyl trimellitic anhydride – formula in Figure 28.3). 10% 4-META material with 90% methacrylate has shown good shear bond strengths to non-precious metal and enamel and dentin. A version of this material has been developed for amalgam bonding, and a critique of it is given in Section 24.7.2.

Another material, which is a dimethacrylate in which phosphate ester groups are incorporated in a Bis-GMA resin has also shown bond strengths of approximately 30 MPa to sandblasted nickel-chromium alloy. This, and the 4-META material, form the basis by which resin-bonded bridge retainers may be bonded to tooth substance. However, it is always desirable that resin-bonded bridge retainers have some inherent retention and resistance form, as this will help protect the bond between metal and tooth from twisting and torquing forces, notwithstanding the forces which may pull the restoration directly from the tooth.

Resin-based luting materials possess many ideal properties, including low solubility in oral fluids, good compressive and tensile strengths, low film thickness and good color stability. However, if any areas of luting material are exposed to occlusal loading at the margins of ceramic and composite inlays, porcelain veneers and dentin-bonded crowns, the wear resistance of the luting material is generally poorer than that of the restoration. This potential deficiency may be minimized by careful observation of the occlusion pre-operatively and designing the restoration outline to minimize occlusal loading at the cavity margins. Resin-based materials that do not possess any inherent bond to enamel and dentin may be used in conjunction with enamel etching and a dentin bonding system.

Resin-based luting materials suffer, along with all resin-based materials, from oxygen (or air)-inhibition, i.e. the presence of oxygen prevents the polymerization of the surface layer of the material. As these materials are less heavily filled than resin-based restorative materials, the effect will be more evident with luting materials. It is therefore desirable to cover the exposed luting material with an air-inhibition gel, often a glycerine- or polypropylene-based material. The use of such gels may improve marginal adaptation by preventing removal of the uncured surface layer of material when the restoration margins are being finished and polished.

27.9 OTHER RESIN COMPOSITE VARIANTS

A number of newly introduced variants on the 'conventional' composites described above have achieved clinical acceptance, although there is little information on their effectiveness. It would therefore appear that their acceptance has been because their users favor their handling characteristics. Among these materials are, flowable composites, high viscosity composites and ceramic-polymer (ceromer) materials.

27.9.1 Flowable composites

The majority of these are light cured, radiopaque materials that are dispensed directly on to the tooth surface. They are broadly similar to resin cements, with filler loading and particle size less than hybrid composites, resulting in a material of low viscosity. Filler content is generally less than 50% by volume, so polymerization shrinkage will be greater than for hybrid materials. The lower modulus of elasticity may allow the material to flex and flow under the conditions thought to occur in Class V cavities and the flow of the material may also be useful in absorbing stresses caused by polymerization shrinkage as discussed above. Flowable composites are available in a range of shades and a number of formulations are claimed to contain fluoride.

These materials are generally used with a technique by which small amounts of material are applied incrementally to build the restoration contour – as opposed to overfilling and finishing techniques used for conventional composites. Hand instruments are used minimally.

Claimed advantages of these materials are that they are fast and easy, that excellent access can be achieved using the syringe tips in which they are often supplied. However questions remain concerning their wear resistance and durability under conditions of occlusal loading. Suggested uses include restoration of Class V cavities, amalgam repair, pit and fissure sealant, glaze for composite Class I restorations and as a base for Class I, II and III laminate restorations.

27.9.2 Condensable composites

In an attempt to overcome some of the difficulties with placement of posterior composite restorations, a number of manufacturers have developed 'condensable' resins, for which amalgam-like packability is claimed, with the potential to achieve better contact points more easily

(Section 27.2.3). The better control of placement may also assist in achieving correct occlusal form. However, the increased viscosity may also increase the potential for formation of voids. There are no long-term clinical data for these materials.

27.9.3 Ceramic-polymer ('ceromer') materials

The majority of these are laboratory materials for the construction of crowns (Section 37.5) but one has been adapted for direct-placement restorations. This material has a molecular structure that is more highly cross-linked than Bis-GMA and the material is more elastic than conventional composites. Esthetic properties are good, wear resistance appears to be acceptable and there is little potential for wear of the opposing dentition. No data are available on long-term durability of these materials.

27.10 POLYACID-MODIFIED RESIN COMPOSITES (COMPOMERS)

Figure 23.2 shows the 'continuum' of tooth colored restorative materials. Polyacid-modified resin composites (commonly known as compomers) can be considered to be composite resins with the addition of some glass-ionomer components such as an acid-decomposable glass and the bonding of poly(acrylic acid) molecules to the resin monomer which forms the matrix. These glass ionomer characteristics are, however, insufficient to promote the acid-base reaction typical of glass-ionomer materials. Thus compomers do not set in the dark; visible light activation of polymerization is required.

Compomers were introduced in the early 1990s and are formulated as anhydrous one-component materials, commonly presented in capsules that are shrink-wrapped to prevent contamination of the unused product by moisture. An original aim of the manufacturers of earliest compomers was to produce a material which bonded to tooth substance without the need for acid etching: in this respect, they have largely been successful since retention rates of compomer restorations placed in class III and class V cavities without etching have been good. Most recently, it has been suggested that microleakage is reduced when enamel margins are etched prior to restoration placement.

27.10.1 Composition

The first commercially available compomer was composed of the materials shown in Table 27.5.

Table 27.5. Composition of the first commercially available compomer[††]

Compomer	Primer/adhesive
Urethane dimethacrylate resin	PENTA (Figure 27.11)
TCB resin (a bi-ester of 2-hydroxyethyl methacrylate and butane tetracarboxylic acid)	Triethylene glycol dimethacrylate
	Elastomeric resin
Strontium fluorosilicate glass, 2.5 μm mean particle size, approx. 70% by weight.	Initiators
	Stabilizers
Initiators	Acetone
Stabilizers	

The TCB resin contains two acidic polycarboxylate groups and two polymerizable methacrylate groups. Setting occurs by visible light activated polymerization. Water is absorbed to a maximum of 3% (w/w) by the polymerized matrix over a period of months. This diffuses through the restoration and an acid-base reaction takes place between the strontium fluorosilicate glass filler and the polycarboxylate groups of the monomer. This acid-base reaction causes further cross-linking of the matrix and release of a small amount of fluoride, this being generally in the range of 10% of that released by true glass-ionomers.

This compomer was supplied with a self-etching acetone-based primer containing PENTA (dipentaerythritol penta-acrylate phosphoric acid ester – Figure 27.11), TEGDMA (triethylene glycol dimethacrylate – Figure 11.12) and an elastomeric resin. PENTA produces an ionic bond to the inorganic part of the tooth, while TEGDMA and the elastomeric resin wet and penetrate the dentin surface. It may be considered that the elastomeric resin provides some flexibility to the bonding mechanism and that this helps to prevent dislodgment of the restorations when tooth flexure occurs (see Section 27.7, paragraph 7).

A number of other compomer systems are broadly similar to that described above. However, a recently introduced material contains a fluoroaluminosilicate glass of 3 μm mean particle size. It also contains chemicals in its adhesive solution, which are more akin to a glass-ionomer material, such as a methacrylated polycarboxylic acid.

[††] Manufacturer's information

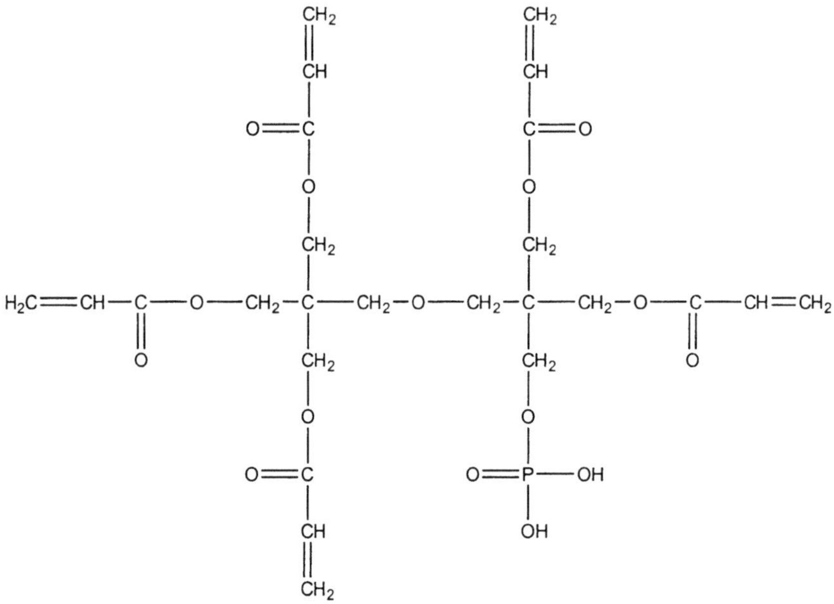

Figure 27.11. PENTA (dipentaerythritol penta-acrylate phosphoric acid ester).

27.10.2 Properties

1. Biological considerations. There is little evidence of adverse pulpal reactions when the bonding systems are employed. Microleakage is reduced when the enamel margins are acid-etched. Fluoride release commences some months after placement of restorations, and is generally in the order of 10% of that released by glass-ionomer materials.
2. Bonding. Compomers are not adhesive to enamel and dentin, so an intermediate bonding system must be employed. Bond strength measurements produce figures that are not as high as with dentin bonding systems, but retention of restorations in non-retentive non-load bearing cavities does not appear to be a problem.
3. Chemical properties. The solubility of compomers is low. The polymer component absorbs some water which permits some long-term acid-base reaction and initiates some degree of fluoride release.
4. Mechanical properties. These are generally inferior to resin composite materials but superior to glass-ionomer materials. Surface hardness is

approximately 50%, compressive strength 70% and flexural strength 80% of typical composite materials.
5. Esthetic considerations. Compomer materials may produce restorations of good esthetics. A wide variety of shades is available with many systems but there is little variation in translucency.
6. Thermal properties. The thermal expansion/contraction of compomers is low. Compomers are good thermal insulators.
7. Dimensional change on setting. Compomers contract slightly on setting but may expand up to 3% due to water uptake following placement.

27.10.3 Critique

Compomers are simple to use and are easy to handle. They are stronger, more esthetic and less soluble than glass-ionomer materials. They may be placed without acid etching and three-year clinical trial data are positive. Wear resistance is less good than resin composite and fluoride release is substantially less than glass-ionomers.

27.11 FUTURE TRENDS

Considerable development is being carried out in the development of resin composites, both in terms of improved filler technology and novel polymerizing systems.

Research has been undertaken in the use of nanofillers, which are smaller than microfillers. The size of these filler particles is below the wavelength of visible light. These nanofillers do not scatter or absorb visible light and therefore provide a means of achieving radiopacity without interfering with the esthetics of the material. Additionally these very small particles may fill spaces between larger particles and allow filler loadings of up to 95 % by weight. This in turn could result in a material with lower polymerization shrinkage and improved physical properties.

A recently introduced variant on the conventional composite filler concept is a 'Polymeric Rigid Inorganic Material' (PRIMM). In this material, the inorganic filler consists of a continuous network of alumina/silicon dioxide ceramic fibers. These fibers, which are approximately 2 μm in diameter, are fused together at selected sites to produce scaffolding units of up to 200 μm. These are silanated to produce chemical bonding to the resin system in a similar manner to conventional resin composites. The use of PRIMM as a scaffolding agent produces a material that may be handled in a manner similar to amalgam, using a specially designed amalgam carrier which resists the abrasive effects of the alumina fibers. These materials may be cured to depths of 5 mm using conventional light units because of the excellent light conducting properties of the alumina fibers. Furthermore, polymerization shrinkage is reduced because the amount of resin material remaining outside the fiber matrix is minimal. However, no long-term data are available on performance. It has also been suggested that PRIMM could be incorporated into glass-ionomer materials with similar effects as for resin-based materials.

The problems caused by polymerization shrinkage have already been emphasized (Section 27.7). To overcome this, research is being carried out into bicyclic monomers that undergo ring-opening polymerization. Spiro-orthocarbonates can produce composites with no setting contraction, but further development is needed before these materials are ready for clinical use. Similarly, oxybismethacrylates (which are bifunctional monomers) also reduce contraction, but further development is needed.

Another concept is the development of anticaries monomer systems. In one such system chlorhexidine has been added to experimental monomers and antibacterial activity was demonstrated by release of chlorhexidine. Monomers with antibacterial properties such as MDPB (a compound of the antibacterial agent dodecyl pyridinium bromide and a methacrylate group) have also been developed and have been shown to inhibit growth of *Streptococcus Mutans* at its surface, with no adverse effects on mechanical properties. Addition of fluoride to resin matrices has also been used as a possible antibacterial measure. However all of these concepts require extensive development and clinical testing before they can be considered for general use.

FURTHER READING

Further discussion of resin composites is given in relation to indirectly placed restorations (Chapter 37) and core build-up materials (Chapter 39). Guidelines on the selection of materials for tooth restorations and for luting cements are presented in Chapters 43 and 44. Appendix II lists and classifies some current resin composites.

Bayne S C, Heymann H O, Swift E J (1994). Update on dental composite restorations. *Journal of the American Dental Association* **125**: 687-701.

El-Mowafy O M, Lewis D W, Benmergui C, Levinton C (1994). Meta-analysis on long-term clinical performance of posterior composite restorations. *Journal of Dentistry* **22**: 33-43.
Willems G, Lambrehts P, Braem M, Vanherle G. (1993). Composite resins in the 21st century. *Quintessence International* **24**: 641-658.
Eick J D, Robinson S J, Byerley T J, Chappelow C C (1993). Adhesives and non-shrinking dental resins of the future. *Quintessence International* **24**: 632-640.
Davidson C L, Seyma-Davidson S (1998). Handling of mechanical stresses in composite restorations. *Dental Update* **25**: 31-35.
Leinfelder K L (1997). New developments in resin restorative systems. *Journal of the American Dental Association* **128**: 573-581.
van Dijken J W V (1996). 3-year clinical evaluation of a compomer, a resin-modified glass ionomer and a resin composite in Class III restorations. *American Journal of Dentistry* **9**: 195-198.
Peutzfeldt A (1997). Resin composites in dentistry: the monomer systems. *European Journal of Oral Science* **105**: 97-116.

Chapter 28

Dentin Bonding Systems

Summary: This chapter traces the significant developments that have occurred in dentin bonding technology. The mechanism of action of dentin bonding systems is discussed, and important points in practical procedures are stressed. Materials are critiqued in terms of clinical performance.

28.1 INTRODUCTION

The production of a stable bond to dentin is a central requirement for the success of resin-based restorative systems, but is also essential for the success of restorations placed in minimal, non-invasive cavity preparations which preserve tooth substance.

The ability to bond reliably and successfully to enamel has been an integral part of restorative dentistry since the early 1960s, but bonding to dentin has proved to be more difficult for a number of reasons:

1. Biocompatibility considerations. These are important because dentin is a vital substrate with tubules communicating to the pulp.
2. The presence of water. Dentin contains up to 20% water by weight. The dentin surface is moist due to tubule fluid outflow. A dentin bonding system must therefore be able to operate satisfactorily on such a moist surface. Note that many resin systems are water-repelling (hydrophobic).
3. The nature of dentin. Dentin close to the amelodentinal junction is a different substrate to that close to the pulp, given that up to 20% of the dentin surface 1 mm from the pulp is made up of tubules while, close to the ADJ, this figure reduces to about 1%. Moreover, sclerotic dentin presents different problems.
4. The effect of operative procedures on dentin. A 'smear layer' composed of debris, particles of mineralized collagen matrix, bacteria and inorganic tooth particles is present on a cut dentin surface. While it was originally

thought that the smear layer was tenaciously attached, it is now considered that it is poorly adherent to the underlying dentin and ideally must therefore be treated to stabilize it or remove it prior to application of a bonding resin. The majority of current systems remove the smear layer.

5. The ability of the bond to resist stresses. The bond to dentin must be sufficient to withstand the polymerization shrinkage of the resin restoration placed against it.

28.2 THE IDEAL BONDING SYSTEM

Dentin bonding systems are typically composed of a number of separate components or materials. A number of requirements for bonding systems are important.

1. Biocompatibility to dental tissues is essential. Furthermore, there should be no potential for sensitization of patients or operators.
2. Bond properties. The system must provide an immediate, permanent, high bond strength. The bond strength should mature rapidly, given that the bonding system will have to withstand the stresses generated by the polymerization shrinkage of the resin-based material placed shortly after the bonding agent. In addition it must provide a bond strength to dentin similar to that to enamel. Failure to do so may result in debonding of the system at the dentin surface while it remains adherent to enamel, with the potential for leakage, sensitivity and secondary caries. There should be no reduction in bond strength when applied to a moist surface.
3. Microleakage. In terms of interfacial properties, the ideal dentin bonding system should minimize microleakage at the margins of restorations and prevent recurrent caries and marginal staining.
4. Chemical compatibility with a wide range of resins and other restorative materials is necessary.
5. Physical characteristics. Low film thickness (*circa* 10 μm), if the system is to be suitable for use with indirect restorations.
6. Practicability. The system should be easy to use and minimally technique sensitive. Good shelf life is important.

28.3 HISTORICAL DEVELOPMENT

Many workers classify the development of dentin bonding systems in terms of 'generations.' This approach is adopted here, but it should be noted that the latest generation systems are not always necessarily superior in performance to earlier products.

1. First generation systems. Earliest reports of the production of a bond to dentin in laboratory studies were published in 1952 by Kramer and McLean and in 1955 by Buonocore. The early dentin bonding systems which these researchers described were essentially dimethacrylates with attached phosphate groups which sought to use the potential for chemical bonding by ionic bonds to the plentiful calcium in the dentin. However, the reported bond strengths were low (typically 5.7 MPa) and were found to decrease after storage in water (2.7 MPa after 5 months), i.e. they were not hydrolytically stable. By 1962, a system had been developed by Bowen which used surface-active N-phenyl glycine - glycidyl methacrylate (NPG-GMA, Figure 28.1) to enhance the wetting of the dentin surface and thereby improve adhesion.

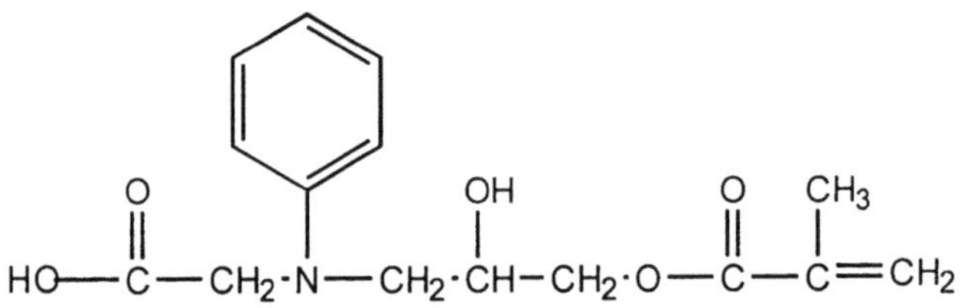

Figure 28.1. NPG-GMA (N-phenyl glycine glycidyl methacrylate).

2. Second generation systems. These consisted of phosphorus-containing esters of Bis-GMA or other unfilled resins. The aim was both to chelate to the calcium in the dentin and to polymerize with the Bis-GMA in the restorative material. These systems were limited by the fact that they only bonded to the smear layer and not to the underlying dentin. Reported bond strengths ranged from 0.7 - 15.3 MPa, typical figures being 2 - 5 MPa. The bond strength was considered to be insufficient to resist the forces caused by polymerization shrinkage of the restorative composite resin.

3. Third generation systems. These materials were introduced in the 1980s, and included chemicals to modify or remove the smear layer and improve the wettability of the dentin surface. Improved hydrophilic resins – often one system would contain a variety of different resins – were also utilized. One system, containing HEMA and glutaraldehyde, was originally thought to bond chemically to collagen that had been treated with EDTA, but it is now generally considered that the method of bonding of this system was as a result of a micromechanical mechanism.

Better retention and marginal integrity were achieved compared to earlier materials, but marginal leakage was not eliminated. The additional stages in manipulation made these materials more complicated and time-consuming than previous materials, but the bond strengths to dentin were generally higher and more reliable in the oral environment. However, bond strengths of these systems were lower than the value generally considered to be that which was required to withstand the stresses generated by the polymerization shrinkage of a resin composite material, generally considered to be between 15 MPa and 20 MPa. The method by which the third generation of dentin bonding agents achieved bonding to dentin was probably by penetration of the smear layer, i.e. many third generation dentin bonding systems used micromechanical means of adhesion rather than the unreliable chemical bonding seen with previous systems.

4. Fourth generation materials. These were introduced in the 1990s and many are still in use at the time of writing. The 'total-etch' technique is often used – that is – enamel and dentin are both etched with, for example, phosphoric acid. This conditioning is followed by application of a primer, followed by a bonding agent. Bond strengths greater than 20 MPa can be achieved and improved resistance to marginal leakage was noted.

5. Fifth generation materials. The aim of these latest materials is to reduce the number of procedural steps required for bonding, for example, by combining primer and bonding agent. However bond strength data indicate that these materials may be very technique sensitive, success being dependent on the moisture content of the conditioned dentin, which should be neither too much nor too little.

The composition, mechanism of action and manipulation of currently available fourth and fifth generation materials are discussed below.

28.4 COMPONENTS OF CONTEMPORARY DENTIN BONDING SYSTEMS

The essential components of a contemporary dentin bonding system are etchants (or conditioners), primers and bonding resins. Each is considered in turn, including the principles by which they operate.

28.4.1 Etchant

An acid etchant which removes the smear layer, opens the dentinal tubules by removing the smear plugs, and decalcifies the uppermost 10-15 μm of the intertubular and peritubular dentin. The majority of currently available systems use 35% phosphoric acid but some systems employ 3% nitric acid, 10% maleic acid or a self-etching primer (see below). When the dentin surface has been etched, only a dense network of collagen remains of 10 to 15 μm depth; this becomes penetrated by the resin components of the bonding system. This etchant component is termed a conditioner by some manufacturers. It should be noted that excessive etching produces deeper decalcification and a thicker collagen network that then may not be totally penetrated by the resin components of the system, resulting in failure under loading and leakage (this type of leakage being known as *nanoleakage*). The manufacturers' suggested etching times should therefore be followed studiously. Sclerosed dentin should be etched for slightly longer than advised.

The use of the same etchant for enamel and dentin - the concept of 'total etch', has the advantage of simplicity and will save time if both enamel and dentin can be etched simultaneously. Etching of dentin initially was met with suspicion by many dental practitioners, but the procedure has been shown not to be detrimental to pulpal tissue provided that the etched dentin surface is adequately 'sealed' by the bonding resin.

28.4.2 Primer

The primer wets and penetrates the collagen network of the decalcified dentin surface, increasing its surface energy. Primers are composed of one or more hydrophilic resin monomers or bifunctional molecules – with a hydrophilic group and a hydrophobic group – such as HEMA (2-hydroxyethyl methacrylate) – Figure 11.5, biphenyldimethacrylate (BPDM) – Figure 28.2 – or 4-META (4-methacryloxyethyl trimellitic anhydride) – Figure 28.3. The hydrophilic group has an affinity for the dentin surface while the hydrophobic methacrylate group has an affinity for resin. Primers are not washed off, once placed, whereas conditioners are normally washed off the dentin surface.

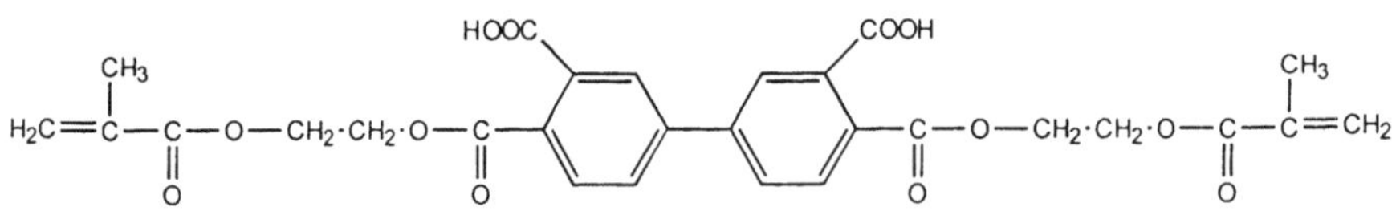

Figure 28.2. A biphenyl dimethacrylate (BPDM) with hydrophilic carboxylate groups and polymerizable methacrylate groups.

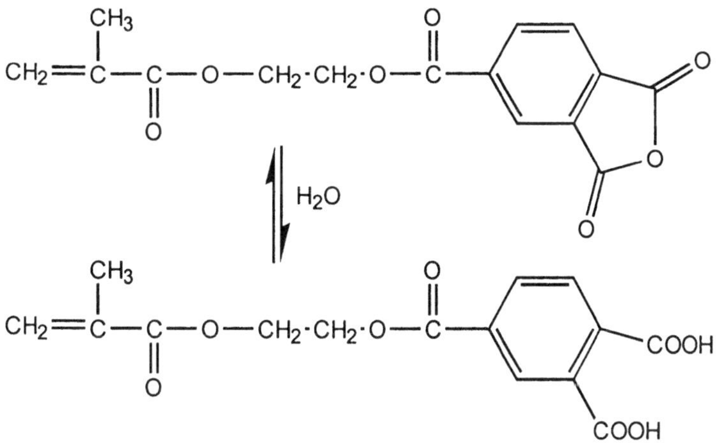

Figure 28.3. 4-methacryloxyethyl trimellitic anhydride (4-META) - top formula - which readily hydrolyzes to form 4-methacryloxyethyl trimellitic acid (4-MET).

28.4.3 Resin

The resin component of the bonding system often consists of a combination of resins such as Bis-GMA. It penetrates the conditioned and primed dentin and copolymerizes with the primer to form an intermingled layer of collagen and resin. This layer is termed the hybrid layer (see below) which is neither resin nor tooth but a hybrid of the two. It is generally considered that the effectiveness of bonding of resin coupling agents is primarily a function of penetration into conditioned dentin.

28.4.4 Reducing the number of components

Some early dentin bonding systems required the operator to carry out up to seven stages during the bonding procedure and it may be considered that the greater the number of stages, or the more technique sensitive the system, the greater the potential for error. Manufacturers have therefore reduced the number of stages; fourth generation systems generally required the application of three solutions - etchant, primer and bonding resin(s). Most recent attempts to reduce the number of stages, to two, has taken manufacturers down one of two routes.

1. Combination of primer and resin - such systems require an etching stage, but commonly are marketed as 'one-bottle' or 'one-stage' bonding systems. However, given the potential for reaction between primer and bonding resin components, the chemistry involved in development of one-stage materials

has been difficult and may result in a reduced shelf life of some such systems.

2. Combination of the etchant and primer, the so-called 'self-etching primers.' Most are phosphate derivatives of hydrophilic monomers, one example being Phenyl-P (Figure 28.4).

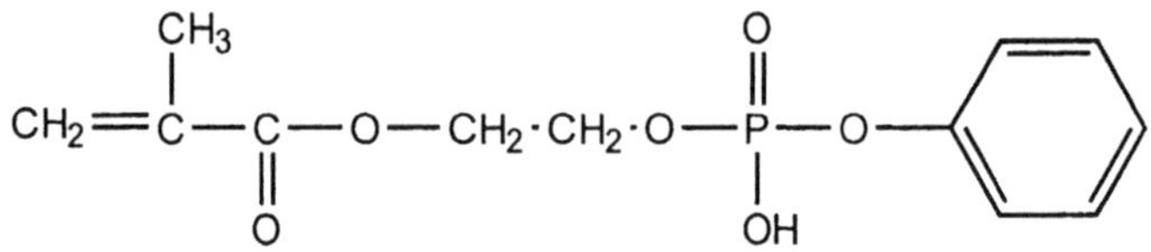

Figure 28.4. Formula of phenyl-P;
2-(methacryloxy)ethyl phenyl hydrogen phosphate.

In one system, the acidic adhesive monomer, Phenyl-P, is present at a concentration of 20%-25%, and at this concentration in the presence of water, the solution is very acidic, with a pH of approximately 1.5. Additionally, the self-etching primer solutions often contain up to 50% HEMA, or other hydrophilic monomers, so that they simultaneously etch and prime the dentin. The self-etching primers must have sufficient acidity to overcome the buffering potential of the dentin, but they must also have sufficient monomer to compete with water when they diffuse through the smear layer. However, the acidity of the primer will be reduced as it penetrate through the smear layer, leaving less acidity to etch the underlying dentin. As the smear layer may not be totally removed by these systems, it has been considered that the partially demineralized smear layer becomes incorporated into a hybrid layer. This may explain why self-etching primers, in general, produce thinner hybrid layers than systems which use etchants such as phosphoric acid.

28.4.5 Etchants *versus* self-etching primers

The etch achieved by the self-etching primers may not be so intense as that achieved by etchants such as phosphoric acid, but this does not appear to be translated into any deficiency of bond strength when self-etching primers are utilized. However, it is necessary to mix the components of some of the self-etching primers and this introduces a further step which takes time.

Contemporary systems increasingly employ a reduced number of bottles as described above, but these 'one-step' systems often require repeated applications of a particular stage, and the total application procedure is therefore not necessarily faster or simpler than earlier 4th generation systems.

28.5 MECHANISM OF ACTION

28.5.1 The hybrid layer

Work carried out using scanning electron microscopy (SEM) in 1982 using the resin 4-META and its 10% citric acid/3% ferric chloride conditioner (10/3) identified, not only a distinct boundary between dentin and resin, but also a diffuse transition zone approximately 5 μm thick between the resin phase and the underlying mineralized dentin. This layer is termed *the hybrid layer,* or *resin-reinforced zone* or *resin-infiltrated layer* and it has been considered to provide a strong union between resins and dentin. Its formation requires the removal of the smear layer and smear plugs, the stabilization of the collagen network which can collapse if desiccated and the application of a suitable monomer mixture which facilitates the diffusion or permeation of resin into the demineralized but stabilized dentin matrix. Although the first hybrid layer was produced following treatment with 10/3 and 4-META, similar layers have been observed with a wide variety of contemporary dentin bonding systems (Figure 28.5). Formation of hybrid layers occurs principally in peritubular dentin.

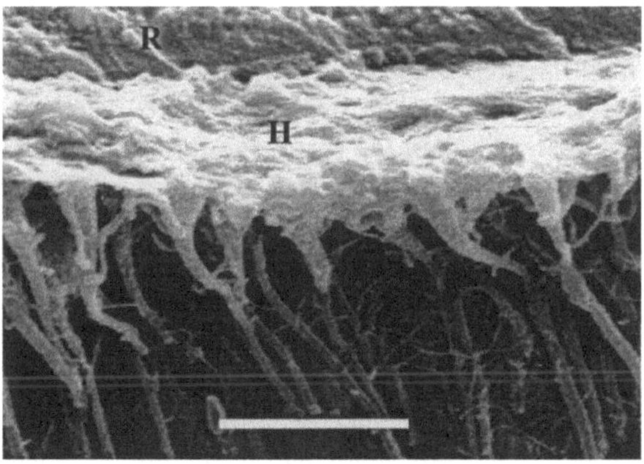

Figure 28.5. Hybrid layer (H) formed between resin composite (R) and dentin. The horizontal bar represents 10 μm.

28.5.2 Intertubular bonding

The hybrid layer produces micromechanical bonding of resin to dentin, but resin tag formation (Figure 28.5) may also contribute to the overall bond strength. Since the dentinal tubules converge towards the pulp, their penetration may generate mechanical retention, as there will be no possible path of withdrawal unless some of the tags fracture. It therefore follows that a stronger resin should produce a stronger bond. Moreover, the bond will be enhanced if the resin actually bonds to the tubule wall or if penetration of lateral channels that join individual dentinal tubules can be achieved. However, this mechanism for bonding can only play a major role where dentinal tubules are present in large numbers, that is, in areas of dentin closer to the pulp.

28.6 BOND STRENGTH MEASUREMENTS *VERSUS* MICROLEAKAGE

Total marginal sealing is one of the ideal characteristics of a restorative system. This is often achieved at enamel margins, but, despite the high bond strengths of contemporary materials, is rarely totally achieved at dentin or cementum margins when using dentin bonding systems. The essential issue is that of bond strength *versus* the forces that might break the bond. Among the factors involved are:

1. Resin-based restoratives shrink up to 3% on polymerization and the forces generated, which are generally considered to be between 15 MPa and 20 MPa, may threaten the bond achieved at the restoration margins or internal surfaces. If a high bond to dentin is not achieved before application of the restorative material, then the shrinkage forces may damage the bond, with consequent microleakage. This may explain the apparent discrepancy between the high bond strength figures achieved by current systems and the fact that microleakage occurs. Bond strength measurements should therefore be carried out early, preferably at 10 minutes or less.
2. Differences in coefficient of thermal expansion between the restorative material and the tooth structure may lead to opening of the margins of the restoration when temperature changes are inflicted on the restoration.
3. Occlusal forces on a tooth may cause flexing of cusps and, if the restoration and its bond to tooth is not able to flex in a similar manner, leakage may occur.

4. Resin-based restorative materials may absorb water and undergo hygroscopic expansion over a period of time, although the degree to which this occurs is dependent upon the type of material and other characteristics. This may help to reduce the potential for marginal gaps.

The clinical manifestations of imperfect marginal seal are marginal staining, sensitivity and ultimately, secondary caries.

28.7 WET BONDING

In the past, water was considered to be a contaminant in any restorative procedure, but especially in bonding procedures because early bonding systems were highly hydrophobic and the presence of water was therefore inappropriate. Water in the dentin bonding mechanism may arise from dentinal tubule fluid, atmospheric water, rinsing procedures and adhesive solutions. Contemporary systems are much less hydrophobic due to the development and increased use of hydrophilic resins such as HEMA. Indeed, it was demonstrated by Kanca in 1992 that increased bond strengths could be obtained when the dentin surface was moist rather than dry. It is difficult to quantify the degree of wetness required, given the different chemical formulae of different systems and their differing modes of action. As a general rule, however, it may be considered that the dentin surface should be left moist and not desiccated. Large amounts of water on the dentin surface may interfere with bonding - the 'overwet phenomenon'.

A number of bonding systems contain acetone or ethyl alcohol as a carrier for the monomers, and these materials are generally able to tolerate increased amounts of water on the dentin surface than other systems which are not acetone-based. When the acetone primer contacts the water on the dentin, the boiling point of the acetone is raised and the boiling point of the water is lowered, a process known as azeotrophism. This causes the evaporation of both the acetone and the water, with the resin being left behind. It has now been established that the collagen network may collapse if desiccated and, in order to achieve penetration of the collagen network by the primer and bonding resin, it is necessary to prevent collapse by keeping the dentin surface moist or by the application of a suitable monomer mixture which facilitates the permeation of resin.

In the past, dentists were taught that all restorative procedures should be carried out in a dry field. The concept of wet bonding has therefore taken some time to gain acceptance. It is important to note that the production of a wet surface does not imply a tolerance for contaminants such as blood, gingival crevicular fluid, saliva or oil. However, given the diversity of the solutions and monomers in the many systems currently available, it is essential that manufacturers' instructions should be followed with each system. Table 28.1 gives general factors in the practical application of dentin bonding systems.

Table 28.3. Practical points in dentin bonding

Technique	Rationale
Isolate tooth	Bonding systems may tolerate some degree of humidity but not contamination with saliva or blood
Remove thin layer of sclerotic dentin	May provide some micromechanical retention and will expose dentin which is more readily bonded to
Provide mechanical retention if this does not involve removal of sound tooth substance	Mechanical retention and resistance form will help the bond resist mechanical stresses applied to the restoration
Apply etchant for recommended period of time	Underetching will give a hybrid layer of less thickness, and while overetching will increase the depth of decalcified dentin, the resin may not completely penetrate this depth and nanoleakage may occur
Wash dentin surface and blot dry; dentin surface should be left moist but not wet	Desiccation will reduce bond strength because of the collapse of the collagen network with the formation of an inadequate hybrid layer
Apply primer and bonding resin; solvents should be allowed to evaporate or gently blown off	Air incorporation within the bonding resin will result in incomplete polymerization of the resin and lower bond strength
Cure bonding resin before application of restorative material	Inadequate curing of the resin must be avoided

28.8 METHODS OF TESTING AND VALIDITY OF TEST METHODS

Dentin bonding systems are normally tested using shear bond strength measurements at 24 hours, and measurements of microleakage at restoration margins. However, the bond will be subjected to more than shear forces, given that tensile and compressive forces may be also applied. Furthermore, bond strength measurements at 24 hours are not appropriate because the bond will be subjected to forces when the restoration is placed and finished and polished. Initial bond strength measurements should therefore be carried out at a maximum of 10 minutes.

28.9 CLINICAL FACTORS IN DENTIN BONDING – PARAMETERS AFFECTING PERFORMANCE

1. It may be considered that materials with the least technique sensitivity will be simpler to use than those with complex application techniques, and, accordingly, it is likely that operators will produce optimum results with a material that is only minimally technique sensitive. However, it is also important for the manufacturers to produce systems that are effective, in both the short term and long term.
2. Bonding to different dentin substrates. In general, retention of resin composite restorations is reduced when bonding is to sclerosed dentin. Patient age appears to be a factor influencing success, possibly related to the above but also perhaps related to the increased tooth flexure in older age. The shape and size of the lesion has also been considered relevant with fewer Class V restorations in resin composite being lost in deep wedge-shaped lesions when compared with shallow, saucer-shaped lesions. Dentin adhesion is better in the maxillary arch than in the mandibular arch, possibly due to less difficulty with moisture control in the maxillary arch.
3. A number of manufacturers have realized that tooth flexure could be a factor in retention/loss of restorations, as demonstrated by the increased number of Class V restorations in resin composite which are lost as compared to more elastic glass-ionomer materials. Some manufacturers have therefore incorporated an elastomeric resin in their bonding systems, while others have incorporated particles in the resin layer, which if present in sufficient thickness, are claimed to produce a stress-absorbing effect. Further, chemical or dual cure systems which require mixing, of necessity, incorporate air bubbles as porosities into the resin layer and accordingly, stresses may be less.

28.10 CLINICAL PERFORMANCE OF DENTIN BONDING SYSTEMS

Criteria for satisfactory clinical performance of a dentin bonding system include:

- The restoration(s) should be retained in place for a significant time;
- The bonding system should prevent ingress of fluids and microorganisms at the restoration margin(s). The implication that there will be no pulpal irritation if the restoration is completed sealed is accepted;

- The survival rate of resin-based restorations is inferior to that of conventional restorations in amalgam or gold. However, Class V cervical lesions are the situation in which dentin bonding systems are most frequently tested clinically, often in non-carious lesions. In such situations, current systems which remove the smear layer, in achieving retention rates in non-retentive Class V cavities typically of over 90% at 3 year recall, have demonstrated improved effectiveness over previous systems in which the smear layer was not removed.

28.11 USES OF DENTIN BONDING SYSTEMS

Adhesive techniques are finding an increasing number of applications in clinical practice, as a result of their increased effectiveness, the potential for less destruction of tooth substance to achieve retention, the increased patient demand for tooth-colored restorations and environmental concerns over mercury-containing restorations. The uses of dentin bonding systems include:

1. Bonding of resin-based restorative materials. The total etch technique may be used with dentin bonding systems in the placement of restorations in resin composite or compomer.

2. Dentin-bonded ceramic restorations. Dentin-bonded all-ceramic crowns (Section 34.8.1) have been shown to be fracture resistant and of good esthetics. Furthermore, they require less tooth preparation than metal-ceramic crowns and use an insoluble luting material. The technique involves the application of a dentin bonding agent of low film thickness to the dentin surface. This then bonds to the ceramic restoration (the fitting surface of which has been etched using hydrofluoric acid to produce a micromechanically retentive surface) by means of a dual-cure resin composite luting material. Similar methodology may be used in the placement of ceramic veneers, and ceramic inlays and onlays. It is necessary to use a dentin bonding system which is of low film thickness as systems which do not fulfil this requirement may pool at internal cavity line angles, and when polymerized, will prevent the restoration from seating.

3. Amalgam bonding. This has been discussed in Section 24.7.2.

4. Reattachment of fractured tooth fragments. As the reliability of dentin bonding procedures improves, so too must the potential for long-term reattachment of fractured anterior tooth fragments. A number of such cases have been described in the dental literature, with the consensus view being that the use of dentin bonding in the attachment procedure provided

improved reliability. Various clinical procedures have been described, but most involve the beveling of the margins of the retained and lost tooth fragments, enamel and dentin bonding and reattachment using just the dentin bonding system, a resin luting system or composite. The use of an adhesive luting system such as 4-META has also been described. Advantages include the reduced time required when compared to a crown procedure, indeed, the potential for an immediate result, and the good shade match of the tooth fragment. The principal disadvantage is the uncertain longevity of the repair.

5. Pulp capping. There has been considerable interest in the potential for dentin bonding agents to be used in the treatment of exposures of the pulp, possibly related to the uncertain success of alternative procedures. The concept is that the exposure site can be totally sealed by the bonding system, and, given that microleakage has been considered to play a major part in pulp death following pulpal exposure, the sealing of the exposure may allow for healing and possible dentin bridge formation. It may be considered that such cases have only a chance of success when the pulp, prior to treatment, is not inflamed or damaged. A number of successfully treated cases have been reported but no long-term studies are available (see Section 43.4.6).

6. Other uses include desensitization of sensitive cervical dentin or cementum, the adhesive luting of bridgework, repair of fractured porcelain and retention of metal frameworks.

28.12 FUTURE PROSPECTS OF DENTIN BONDING

The reliability of dentin bonding has improved substantially during the 1990s, and, as a result, the number of minimally invasive techniques available to the restorative dentist has increased dramatically, to the extent that it is difficult for those who are old enough to remember the era when mechanical retention had to be obtained to retain Class V and other restorations. It can be expected that the effectiveness of adhesive techniques will further improve and that, as a result, all crowns will be placed using an adhesive luting procedure and that reattachment techniques for fractured cusps and teeth will become commonplace, and that all restorations, of whatever material, will be bonded in position.

FURTHER READING

In Appendix III details of the components of some contemporary dentin bonding systems are given.

Nakabayashi N, Nakamura M, Yasuda N (1991). Hybrid layer as a dentin-bonding mechanism. *Journal of Esthetic Dentistry* **3**: 133-138.

Eick J D, Cobb C M, Chappell R P, Spencer P, Robinson S J (1991). The dentinal surface: its influence on dentinal adhesion. Part I. *Quintessence International* **22**: 967-977.

Eick J D, Gwinnett A J, Pashley D H, Robinson S J (1997). Current concepts on adhesion to dentin. *Critical Reviews in Oral Biology and Medicine* **8**: 306-335.

Gwinnett A J (1992). Moist versus dry dentin: its effect on shear bond strength. *American Journal of Dentistry* **5**: 127-129.

Pashley D H, Carvalho R M (1997). Dentine permeability and dentine adhesion. *Journal of Dentistry* **25**: 355-372.

Schulein T M (1988). The smear layer on dentin. A status report for the American Journal of Dentistry. *American Journal of Dentistry* **1**: 264-270.

Chapter 29

Materials in Endodontics

Summary: The composition and properties of materials for root canal filling, root canal perforation repair and retrograde (root end) fillings are discussed.

29.1 INTRODUCTION

There are four situations when materials are required during endodontic therapy:

- Root canal filling materials;
- Root-end filling materials;
- Repair of root canal perforations;
- Temporary restorative materials, as discussed in Section 43.4.7.

29.2 ROOT CANAL FILLING MATERIALS

29.2.1 Definition and classification

A *root filling* is a permanent restoration intended to obturate the root canal system of a tooth. The object of this treatment is to promote long term retention of a healthy root. Materials introduced into the root canal as medicaments are dealt with only briefly.

Root fillings may be classified as in Table 29.1. Most frequently a combination of a core material (Type I) with a sealer cement (Type II) is used.

Table 29.1. Classification of root canal filling materials[‡‡]

Type	Description		Materials
Type I	Core materials (to be used with sealer cements)	1.	Polymer based
		2.	Metallic
Type II	Sealer cements (to be used with core materials)	1.	Non-polymerizing materials
		a.	Powder-liquid formulations
		b.	Paste-paste formulations
		2.	Polymerizing materials
Type III	Materials used without either core materials or sealer cements	1.	Non-polymerizing materials
		a.	Powder-liquid formulations
		b.	Paste-paste formulations
		2.	Polymeric materials

29.2.2 Requirements

There are a number of important requirements for root canal filling systems. A system is considered to include all the materials which, in combination, are used to obturate root canals.

1. Biological properties. The materials should not be irritant to periradicular tissues. They should not provoke an immune response, and not be mutagenic or carcinogenic. They should be bacteriostatic and sterile on insertion.
2. Interfacial properties. The ability to seal root canals laterally as well as apically is important. Adhesion between the root canal filling and canal walls is desirable, given that micro-organisms and/or their toxins may track from the coronal aspect of the root to the root apex.
3. Chemical properties. Materials should be impervious to moisture, showing no solubility or corrosion.
4. Mechanical properties. These are comparatively unimportant, since the materials are not subjected to mechanical loading to any great degree.
5. Esthetic considerations. Obviously root canal filling materials are not visible, so there are no color and translucency requirements. But esthetic considerations are important, because staining of the tooth by the root filling should not occur. This is of particular relevance to silver-containing sealers, which may cause staining.
6. Practical considerations. Materials should be easy to introduce into the root canal with ample working time, and with ease of removal if re-treatment or post space preparation becomes necessary. A degree of radiopacity is essential for diagnostic purposes. In service no shrinkage should occur.

[‡‡] Adapted from ANSI/ADA Specification No. 57 for endodontic filling materials, 1983.

The above requirements are for the total system used for root canal obturation. In addition, some requirements for a sealer material should be noted. It should be easy to mix, ideally should adhere to the canal walls and the core material and should not set too rapidly, especially when used with heated obturation techniques.

29.2.3 Core filling materials

1. Gutta percha based products. Gutta percha is a naturally occurring polymer, being *trans*-polyisoprene, which is an isomer of rubber (*cis*-polyisoprene). Gutta percha is partially crystalline, with two different forms, termed α- and β-gutta percha. The α-form is naturally occurring. If this is heated above 65°C and cooled very slowly (< 0.5°/hour), the α-material recrystallizes. More rapid cooling leads to the development of the β-form (Figure 29.1)

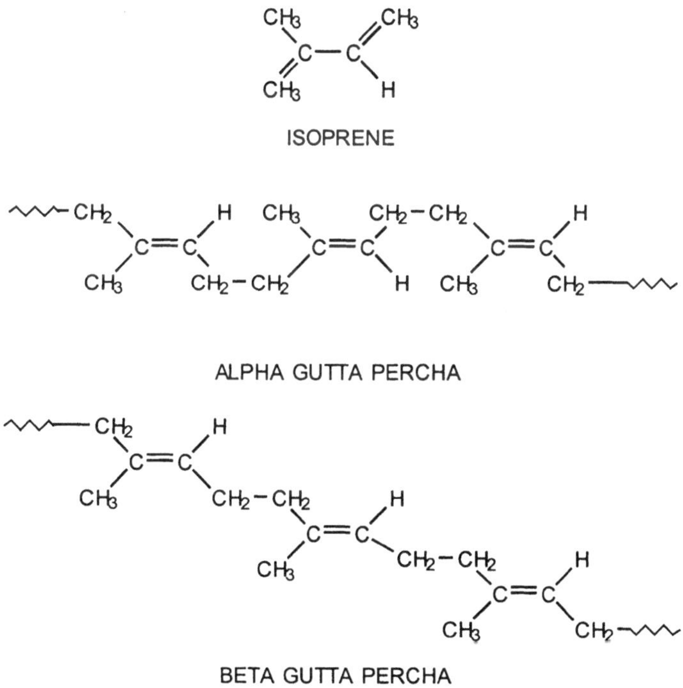

Figure 29.1. Isoprene and alpha and beta forms of gutta percha.

Core filling materials are blends of a number of constituents, the functions of which are detailed in Table 29.2

Table 29.2. Typical composition of gutta percha core filling materials

Constituent	%	Function
Gutta percha	20	Adaptability to the canal
Barium sulfate	11	To give radiopacity
Zinc oxide	66	Filler
Other components	3	Waxes and/or resins as plasticizers; coloring agent

Gutta percha cones have a number of advantageous properties, such as their ability to be adapted to the canal by a variety of techniques, including vertical and lateral condensation and heat softening. Limitations include the lack of adhesive qualitites and the ease by which they may be distorted during insertion.

2. Silver cones. In the past points of pure silver were used because of their ability to be shaped to the root canal. However, silver corrodes readily in the root canal and the cytotoxicity of pure silver may be considered problematical.

3. Other materials. Experiments have been carried out with cones of a titanium alloy (Ti-6Al-4V), which are more corrosion resistant than silver.

29.2.4 Sealers

1. Non-polymerizing materials. These are mostly cements based on the reaction between zinc oxide and eugenol, and containing other constituents, including:

- A radiopaque constituent such as barium sulfate, bismuth subcarbonate, bismuth trioxide or precipitated silver;
- Agents to modify the consistency and handling characteristics, such as resins, oils and waxes.

One of the best known traditional materials is *Grossman's sealer*, the formulation of which is given in Table 29.3.

Table 29.3. Formulation of Grossman's sealer

	Constituent	%
Powder	Zinc oxide	42
	Staybelite resin	27
	Bismuth subcarbonate	15
	Anhydrous sodium borate	1
Liquid	Eugenol	100

An alternative material (without eugenol) is based on the reaction of zinc oxide with carboxylic acids such as octanoic acid [$CH_3(CH_2)_6COOH$] and dodecanoic acid [$CH_3(CH_2)_{10}COOH$].

An adhesive glass-ionomer sealer is commercially available, but is not in widespread use owing to potential difficulty in removing it in the event that re-treatment is necessary.

In the past, materials containing chloroform have been advocated, but this chemical is now recognized to be carcinogenic.

Therapeutic sealers containing calcium hydroxide, aimed at improving periapical healing, are now available.

Two products were developed in the past containing formaldehyde. These are contraindicated because they are mutagenic and highly or extremely cytotoxic.

2. Polymerizing materials. An epoxy resin based sealer is available, a formulation of which is given in Table 29.4.

Table 29.4. Formulation of an epoxy resin sealer

	Constituent	%
Powder	Silver	10
	Bismuth oxide	60
	Hexamethylene tetramine	25
	Titanium oxide	5
Liquid	*Bis*-Phenol diglycidyl ether	100

29.2.5 Root canal filling systems

The above discussion relates to the use of a combination of core and sealer. Occasionally techniques advocating the use of a paste alone, injected into the root canal, or introduced by a Lentulo spiral, have been propounded. However, these techniques are little used due to the presence of voids and difficulty in controlling the paste. Some of these methods have employed formaldehyde-containing materials that are, as noted above, contraindicated.

29.3 ROOT END FILLING MATERIALS

When endodontic treatment fails, root end resection followed by root end filling may be indicated if a root canal re-treatment cannot be carried out. There is no consensus on the best material for this application, and numerous materials have been tested in the past, including calcium hydroxide cements, resin composites, gutta percha, silicones, gold leaf, orthopedic bone cement, cyanoacrylates, poly(tetrafluoroethylene) and titanium screws. Three materials are currently important.

1. Dental amalgam (Chapter 24) has been used for many years, but leakage may occur around the root end filling. There are presently concerns about the use of mercury-containing materials in these situations. Also long term corrosion products may be cytotoxic.

2. EBA cements (Chapter 25) are now being advocated, but they are not adhesive. Comparative *in vitro* leakage data are often conflicting.

3. A new material, probably the first to be designed specifically for this application, has been proposed. Mineral trioxide aggregate (MTA) is a powder which, when mixed with water, forms a colloidal gel then solidifes to a hard mass in under 3 hours. The material develops a high pH (around 12.5). The exact composition has not been published, but it is known that it contains calcium and phosphate ions. It has been claimed to give good resistance to leakage by dyes and bacteria, according to *in vitro* testing. This material may also be used for pulp capping and repair of perforations.

29.4 REPAIR OF ROOT CANAL PERFORATIONS

Root repair materials carry out a similar function to materials used for root-end filling – that is – they should seal a defect between the root filling and the periodontal tissues. Accordingly, the materials discussed in Section 29.3 may be appropriate.

FURTHER READING

Ørstavik D (1988). Endodontic materials. *Advances in Dental Research* **2**: 12-24.

VIII

IMPRESSION MATERIALS

Chapter 30

Impression Materials: General Considerations

Summary: A review of the requirements for dental impression materials, and a classification of the available materials and impression trays.

30.1 INTRODUCTION

The construction of the many types of restoration and appliance (for example, dentures, crowns, inlays, bridges and orthodontic appliances) requires the preparation of a replica of the patient's oral tissues. One out of a wide range of impression materials is used to obtain a reverse or negative form of the tissues. This is converted into a positive model, using one of the available cast and die materials (Chapter 51).

Impression materials, in the fluid or plastic state, are carried to the mouth in a suitably sized tray; hardening of the material takes place either on cooling or through chemical reaction. More viscous impression materials are called *mucocompressive* because they record the tissues in their compressed state.

30.2 REQUIREMENTS

A primary requirement for any impression material is dimensional accuracy and stability. This is clearly important, since a restoration or appliance fabricated in the laboratory cannot be more accurate than the impression from which a working cast is prepared. For greater accuracy, the following factors are important:

- Rheological properties; the material must be in a fluid or plastic state on insertion into the mouth; it must be sufficiently fluid to record fine

detail; it must have sufficient working time during which there is no significant increase in viscosity;
- There should be negligible dimensional changes associated with the setting reaction or process;
- Ideally the material should be elastic on removal from the mouth, so that undercuts can be recorded without distortion of the impression;
- It should adhere to the tray;
- There should be no dimensional changes as a result of the change in temperature from the patient's mouth to room temperature;
- There should be negligible dimensional changes on storage of the impression in the dental laboratory;
- It should be compatible with model and die materials.

Additional important requirements are that the materials should be non-toxic and non-irritant, with an acceptable odor and taste. Its setting time must be appropriate – the impression should not need to be in the mouth too long, to avoid fatigue to both operator and patients. It must have good resistance to tearing. The packaged product should have a long shelf life.

It has been demonstrated that pathogens can be transmitted to impressions and subsequently to gypsum casts prepared from them. It is thus important that a completed impression should be capable of being disinfected, prior to casting or transporting to a dental laboratory. Note that the impression tray may also be a source of contamination. Disinfectants are supplied as solutions containing iodophors, gluteraldehyde compounds or sodium hypochlorite, in which the impression and tray are immersed. An alternative is to use a spray disinfectant. It is clearly important that a disinfectant should not adversely affect the dimensional accuracy of the impression, nor its ability to give good surface detail on a cast or die.

30.3 CLASSIFICATION

The materials in common use can be classified as non-elastic or elastic, according to the ability of the set material to be withdrawn over undercuts. Ideally, of course, a set impression material should be elastic. That is, during setting it undergoes the conversion:

$$\text{plastic} \longrightarrow \text{elastic}$$

Table 30.1 classifies the currently available impression materials.

Table 30.1. Classification of dental impression materials

NON ELASTIC	ELASTIC Hydrocolloids	ELASTIC Elastomers (non-aqueous)
1. Plaster of Paris	1. Reversible (agar)	1. Polysulfide
2. Impression compound	2. Irreversible (alginate)	2. Polyether
3. Impression paste		3. Silicone – two types:
		a. Condensation
		b. Addition – (vinyl polysiloxane)

30.4 IMPRESSION TRAYS

These may be classified as:

- Stock trays, which are obtained in standard sizes;
- Custom or special trays fabricated from a cast of the mouth of the patient.

Stock trays may be:

- Reusable - made of metal, supplied either with or without perforations;
- Disposable - usually perforated, and made of a polymer such as nylon or polystyrene.

Custom or special trays are all disposable, and may be made of self-cured acrylic or shellac.

FURTHER READING

Chapters 31-33 deal with the various types of impression material in clinical use. Literature references follow these chapters.

Chapter 31

Non-elastic Impression Materials

Summary: Three types of non-elastic impression material are discussed in terms of composition, manipulation, properties and application.

31.1 PLASTER OF PARIS

31.1.1 Chemistry

The chief constituent of impression plaster is calcined calcium sulfate hemihydrate. On mixing with water this reacts to form a rigid mass of calcium sulfate dihydrate. The chemistry of this is given in detail in Chapter 51.

During the setting an expansion may be demonstrated; this is substantially reduced by the addition of potassium sulfate. However, as this accelerates the setting, borax is added to slow down the process. Another additive is alizarin red; this imparts a pink color to the impression enabling it to be distinguished from the model that is cast on it. A flavoring agent may also be added.

The additives may be blended with the plaster powder, or may be supplied as an aqueous solution to be mixed with plaster. In the latter case a suitable solution contains 4% potassium sulfate, 0.4 to 1% borax (the precise value being chosen to give a desirable setting time; this may vary for different batches of plaster) and 0.04% alizarin red. This solution is called 'A.E.' or 'anti-expansion' solution.

Some impression plasters may also contain additives such as gum tragacanth, to improve the cohesive properties of the mixed plaster. Starch is sometimes incorporated so that the set plaster will disintegrate due to the swelling of the starch when boiling water is poured over it - this facilitates removal of the impression from the cast model.

31.1.2 Manipulation

The plaster should be mixed with water or an A.E. solution in the ratio of 100 g to 50 to 60 ml. Care must be taken to ensure that the mix is free of air bubbles, since they may appear on the surface of the impression leading to inaccuracy in the cast.

31.1.3 Properties

In terms of accuracy:

- Plaster is excellent at recording fine detail since the mixed material is very fluid when inserted into the mouth;
- The dimensional changes on setting are small, due to anti-expansion additives;
- If there are undercuts present, the plaster impression will fracture on removal from the mouth;
- On storage of a plaster impression, the dimensional changes are small, though a small degree of drying shrinkage may occur.

Before preparing a cast in plaster or dental stone, the plaster impression must be treated with a separating agent. An alginate mold seal, a varnish or waterglass or soap solution is suitable.

In terms of other properties, impression plasters are non-toxic. However, they may be unpleasant for the patient, because they produce a dry sensation in the mouth. The setting time can be precisely controlled by use of the appropriate quantities of additives. Plaster is stable on storage over a long time, provided it is kept in a sealed container.

31.2 IMPRESSION COMPOUND (COMPOSITION)

31.2.1 Constituents and applications

These materials are generally composed of a mixture of natural resins (e.g. colophony and shellac and/or waxes), fillers (soapstone or talc) and lubricants (stearic acid or stearin). They are *thermoplastic* – that is, they soften when heated and harden when cooled, without the occurrence of a chemical reaction. The available materials may be classified into two types.

Type I – lower fusing materials – are used for recording prosthodontic impressions, such as preliminary impressions of edentulous patients, and are supplied in sheets about 4 to 5 mm thick. These materials have also been supplied in stick form for copper band impressions for inlays and crowns and marginal additions to special trays, etc. Today, inlay and crown impressions are most usually taken with an elastomeric material (Chapter 33).

Type II – higher fusing materials – are used as tray materials, which are sufficiently rigid to support other impression materials.

31.2.2 Manipulation

For prosthodontic impressions the compound is heated in a water bath at 55 to 60 °C. Since the material has a low thermal conductivity it must be immersed in the water bath for sufficient time to ensure complete softening. However, if it is left for an excessive time some of the constituents may be leached out into the water bath, so altering the properties of the material. If the composition is kneaded in the water bath, water will become incorporated in the material, and act as a plasticizer. If the composition is too cool, it will not flow properly in the mouth; if it is too hot, the material becomes sticky and can burn the patient's oral mucosa. In all cases the water bath should be lined with a napkin, otherwise the material will adhere to the bath.

31.2.3 Properties

In terms of accuracy, impression compound, though plastic on insertion into the mouth, is not sufficiently fluid to record all the fine detail of the mouth. It has a high coefficient of thermal expansion; thus, on cooling during setting, there is considerable shrinkage. This can be minimized in prosthodontic impressions by heating the surface of the set material in a flame and re-taking the impression. Since only a small quantity of composition is contracting, the actual magnitude of the contraction is small. Shrinkage also occurs on cooling from mouth temperature to room temperature (about 1.5% by volume). Impression composition will distort on removal over undercut areas. Dimensional changes can occur on storing the impression in the laboratory. Stresses can be set up within the material, particularly if it is manipulated or deformed when it is not fully softened. Subsequently distortion can occur due to relief of these stresses, particularly if the impression is left in a warm atmosphere before casting up the model.

Other properties include non-toxicity and non-irritancy. It hardens in a reasonably acceptable time in the mouth. Its shelf life is adequate, but changes in shellac may cause deterioration over a long period.

31.3 ZINC OXIDE-EUGENOL AND SIMILAR PASTES

31.3.1 Chemistry

The chemistry of the reaction between zinc oxide and eugenol is given in Section 15.5. The zinc oxide is supplied in paste form. This is achieved by the addition of an oil (e.g. olive oil, light mineral oil or linseed oil). The oil also acts as a plasticizer for the material. Hydrogenated resin can also be incorporated; it quickens the setting and makes the impression paste more cohesive. The eugenol contains talc or kaolin as a filler, to form a paste. Either or both pastes may contain accelerators, such as zinc acetate.

At least one proprietary paste contains a substitute for eugenol. This is a carboxylic acid, which can react with zinc hydroxide (possibly formed by the hydrolysis of zinc oxide) to form a salt as follows:

$$Zn(OH)_2 + 2RCOOH \longrightarrow (RCOO)_2Zn + 2H_2O$$

31.3.2 Manipulation

The two pastes, in tubes, are provided in contrasting colors. The correct proportions (usually equal lengths of the two) are mixed together on a slab or mixing pad with a flexible spatula until a homogeneous color is obtained.

31.3.3 Properties

In terms of dimensional accuracy and stability, these impression materials are sufficiently fluid to record the fine detail in the mouth. There is probably little or no dimensional change associated with the setting process. The set material is not elastic, so will not record undercuts. The set material appears to be stable on storage in the laboratory. Impression pastes are compatible with dental stone model materials. The paste can be removed from the stone by softening it in water at 60 °C.

Other properties include non-toxicity, but note that those containing eugenol can be irritant, giving a tingling sensation to the patient and leaving a persistent taste, which some people may regard as unpleasant. The paste can adhere to tissues, so the lips of the patient are usually coated with petroleum jelly before recording the impression. The setting time is acceptable if the manufacturer's instructions are followed and the correct ratio of pastes used. The presence of water and an increase in temperature both reduce the setting time. The shelf life of these materials is satisfactory.

31.3.4 Applications

This material is generally used in thin sections (2 to 3 mm) as a wash impression, in the production of complete dentures for patients whose ridges are no more than minimally undercut. A zinc oxide-eugenol impression can be taken using a close-fitting special tray, or in an existing denture, particularly one that is to be relined.

31.4 PERIPHERAL SEAL MATERIALS

A number of materials are available for outlining the denture-bearing area. These include impression composition (Section 31.2). Also used are monomer-polymer formulations, the monomer being n-butyl methacrylate containing a tertiary amine activator, and poly(ethyl methacrylate), with a peroxide initiator. On mixing together, polymerization occurs. The merits of this material are that it is simple and rapid to use. A conventional auto-polymerizing acrylic is unsuitable for this application because of the toxic effect of methyl methacrylate monomer and the heat evolved during the exothermic polymerization.

FURTHER READING

Craig R G (1988). Review of dental impression materials. *Advances in Dental Research* **2**: 51-64.

Olsson S, Bergman B, Bergman M (1982). Zinc-oxide-eugenol impression materials: dimensional stability and surface detail sharpness following treatment with disinfection solutions. *Swedish Dental Journal* **6**: 177-180.

Chapter 32

Hydrocolloid Impression Materials

Summary: The general nature of hydrocolloids is discussed, followed by details of both reversible (agar) and irreversible (alginate) hydrocolloids.

32.1 GENERAL NATURE OF HYDROCOLLOIDS

A *colloid* must be distinguished from a *solution* and a *suspension*. A *solution* is a homogeneous mixture. For example, in an aqueous solution the solute exists as small molecules or ions in the solvent. In contrast to this, a *suspension* is heterogeneous, consisting of particles of at least sufficient size to be seen microscopically, dispersed in a medium. Thus a suspension is a two-phase system.

Colloids fall between these two extremes. They are heterogeneous, (2-phase systems), like suspensions, but the particle size of the dispersed phase is smaller, usually in the range 1 to 200 nm. However, it is not always possible to distinguish between a colloid and a solution on the one hand and a colloid and a suspension on the other. When the dispersion medium of a colloid is water, it is termed a *hydrocolloid*.

Colloids may exist in the *sol* and *gel* state. In the *sol* state, the material is a viscous liquid. A sol can be converted into a *gel* - a material of gelatin-like consistency, due to agglomeration of the molecules of the dispersed phase, to form *fibrils*, or chains of molecules, in a network pattern. These fibrils enclose the dispersion medium, for example water.

A sol may be converted into a gel in one of two ways:

1. By a reduction in temperature. Such processes are reversible, since on heating, a sol is formed again; an example of this is agar (Section 32.2); in such a gel the fibrils are held together by Van der Waals forces.
2. By chemical reaction. Other materials can form a gel by a chemical reaction, which is irreversible (for example, alginates, Section 32.3).

The strength or toughness of a gel depends on the concentration of fibrils – the greater the concentration, the stronger the material. It also depends on the concentration of fillers. Chemically inert powders can be added to a gel to render it less flexible.

A gel can lose or take up water or other fluids. Loss of water can occur by evaporation. *Syneresis* can also occur; this happens when the gel molecules are drawn closer together, for example by continuation of the setting reaction. As a result a fluid exudate appears on the surface of the gel. Uptake of water is called *imbibition*.

In the use of hydrocolloids for dental impressions, the material is inserted in the mouth in the sol state, when it is sufficiently fluid to record detail. No gelation should have occurred at this stage. It is removed from the tissues after the gel is formed, when it exhibits elastic properties.

Clearly evaporation from, and imbibition by, the gel should be avoided, as the former is associated with shrinkage, and the latter results in expansion.

32.2 AGAR

32.2.1 Composition

This is recorded in Table 32.1. Figure 32.1 gives the chemical structure of agar.

Table 32.1. Typical composition of agar impression material

Constituent	Wt. %	Function
Agar	14	Colloid
Borax	0.2	Strengthens the gel but retards the setting of dental stone model and die materials
Potassium sulfate	2	Accelerates the setting of dental stone
Water	83.8	Dispersion medium

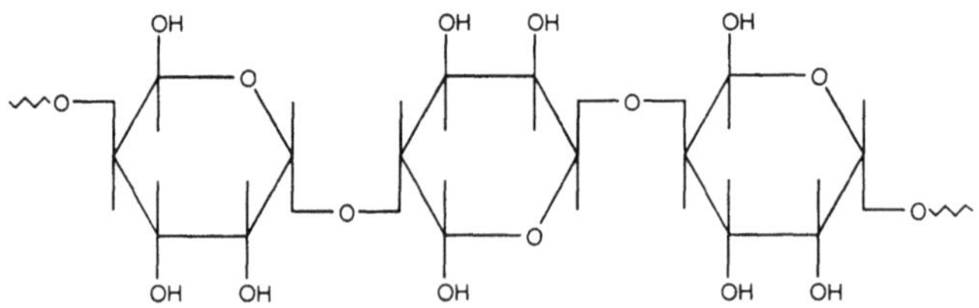

Figure 32.1. Simplified formula of agar, which is a sulfuric ester of a linear polymer of galactose.

32.2.2 Manipulation

The material is supplied in sealed containers to prevent evaporation of water. It is brought to a fluid state by heating the tube in boiling water in a processing unit for 10 - 45 minutes. After boiling, the material can be stored at 65 °C for up to 8 hours. It is important that the entire tube of material is softened. The material is extruded on to metal trays with mechanical interlocking. The filled tray is placed in a tempering bath at 45 °C for 2 minutes, before insertion into the patient's mouth. Water-cooled trays are often used to quicken the gelation of the agar. A higher temperature is required for the conversion of gel to sol than for the reverse reaction (hysteresis effect).

32.2.3 Properties

1. Dimensional accuracy. In terms of rheological properties, the material can be sufficiently fluid to record fine detail if it has been correctly manipulated. The first material to set is that which is in contact with the tray (contrast with alginates, Section 32.3.3) since this is cooler than the tissues. Thus the material in contact with the tissues stays liquid for the longest time, and can flow to compensate for any inaccuracy due to dimensional changes, or to inadvertent movement of the tray.

The set material can be withdrawn over undercuts. The adhesion of agar to metal is poor, so perforated trays are used.

Models should be cast up immediately from agar impressions, to avoid the possibility of evaporation or imbibition. If this is not possible, it has been claimed that stability is achieved by storage in 2% potassium sulfate solution or in a humidor.

The compatibility with cast materials depends on the chemical composition of the impression material. Without an accelerator for the setting of stone such as potassium sulfate, a soft surface may be obtained.

2. Other properties.

- These materials are non-toxic and non-irritant;
- Their setting time is rather slow, unless efficient cooling is achieved;
- Tear resistance is poor;
- Their shelf life is adequate;
- Agar materials can be reused; they are therefore cost-effective, but require facilities for the casting of models and dies to be close to hand;
- Loss of water, with an increase in viscosity of the sol, may occur. Water can be added if required;

- Agar can be disinfected by immersion for 10 minutes in dilute aqueous solutions of sodium hypochlorite or glutaraldehyde.

32.2.4 Applications

These materials may be used for crown and bridge work. They can be employed in the laboratory, for model duplication, since they can be re-used many times, because of the reversible nature of the reaction.

32.3 ALGINATES

32.3.1 Composition and setting

The composition of these materials is given in Table 32.2. Figure 32.2 gives the chemical structure of sodium alginate.

Table 32.2. Typical composition of an alginate impression material

Constituent	Wt. %	Function
Soluble salt of alginic acid (sodium, potassium or triethanol amine salt)	12	Reacts with calcium ions to give calcium alginate gel
Slowly soluble calcium salt (for example, calcium sulfate)	12	Releases calcium ions to reacts with salt of alginic acid
Trisodium phosphate	2	Reacts with calcium ions go give calcium phosphate and delay gel formation
Filler (for example, diatomaceous earth)	70	Increases cohesion of mix and strengthens gel
Silicofluorides or fluorides	Trace	Improves surface of stone model
Flavoring agents	Trace	Improves patient acceptability
Chemical indicator (present in some materials)	Trace	Changes color with pH change during setting to indicate correct timings for the impression procedure

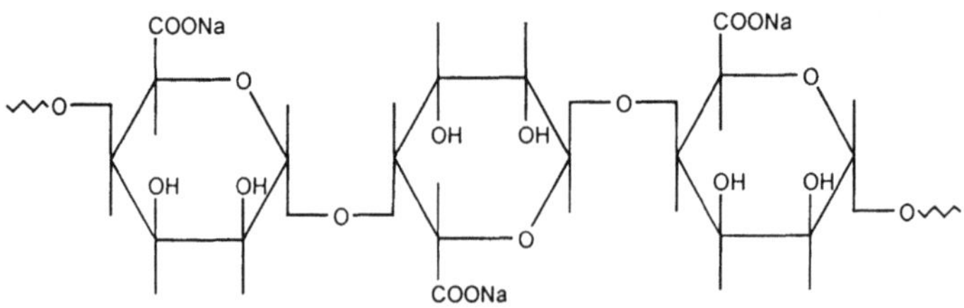

Figure 32.2. Formula of sodium alginate.

On mixing the powder with water a sol is formed, and the alginate, the calcium salt and the phosphate begin to dissolve. The following reaction, written in simplified form, occurs to form an elastic gel of calcium alginate:

$$Na_nAlg + n/2\ CaSO_4 \longrightarrow n/2\ Na_2SO_4 + Ca_{n/2}Alg \quad .....(1)$$

Only the outer layer of each particle of sodium alginate dissolves and reacts. However, the above reaction is liable to occur during the mixing and tray-loading procedures. This is obviously undesirable, since the material should deform plastically, not elastically, on insertion into the mouth. Gel formation is delayed by the presence of trisodium phosphate, which reacts with the calcium sulfate to give a precipitate of calcium phosphate, as follows:

$$2Na_3PO_4 + 3CaSO_4 \longrightarrow Ca_3(PO_4)_2 + 3Na_2SO_4 \quad .....(2)$$

This latter reaction does not contribute any elastic properties to the material.

Reaction (2) above occurs in preference to (1); no substantial quantity of calcium alginate gel is formed until the trisodium phosphate is used up. The manufacturer can therefore control the setting time of a product by adjusting the quantity of this constituent.

The fibrils of the set gel are linked together by the calcium ions; each divalent Ca^{2+} ion is linked to two carboxyl ($-COO^-$) groups, each from a different polysaccharide molecule.

32.3.2 Manipulation

The container of powder should be shaken before use to get an even distribution of constituents. The powder and water should be measured, as directed by the manufacturer. Room-temperature water is usually used; slower or faster setting times can be achieved, if required, by using cooler or warmer water respectively. Retention to the tray is achieved by one or both of two means: perforated trays and/or use of an adhesive such as molten sticky wax or a tray adhesive containing methylcellulose.

There should be vigorous mixing by spreading the material against the side of the bowl for the stipulated time, usually one minute. An alginate impression should be displaced sharply from the tissues; this sudden displacement ensures the best elastic behavior. The impression is removed about two minutes after it first appears to be elastic. On removal from the mouth, the impression should be washed with cold water to remove saliva, then disinfected (see below). The impression is covered with a damp napkin to prevent syneresis, and is cast up as soon as possible, preferably not more than 15 minutes after taking the impression.

32.3.3 Properties

1. Dimensional accuracy. In terms of accuracy, alginates are sufficiently fluid to record fine detail in the mouth. The viscosity-time curve shows a well-defined working time, during which there is no viscosity change (Figure 32.3).

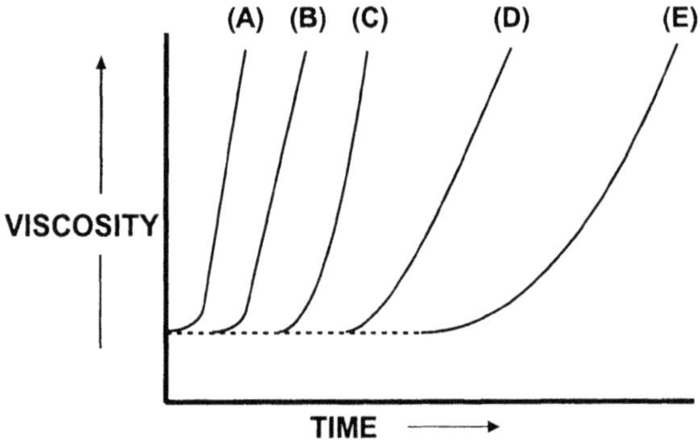

Figure 32.3. Viscosity-time curves for an alginate impression material at various temperatures: (A) 37°C, (B) 20°C, (C) 15.5°C, (D) 11.5°C and (E) 7°C. After Fish S F, Braden M (1964). Characterization of the setting process in alginate impression materials. *Journal of Dental Research* **43**: 107-117.

During setting of the material it is important that the impression should not be moved. The reaction is faster at higher temperatures (Figure 32.3) and so the material in contact with the tissues sets first (contrast with agar materials, Section 32.2.3). Any pressure on the gel due to movement of the tray will set up stresses within the material, which will distort the alginate after its removal from the mouth.

The material is sufficiently elastic to be withdrawn over undercuts; occasionally tearing of the impression material may occur with severe undercuts. Adhesion to the tray has already been considered above; the cellulose adhesives, though often effective, can be difficult to clean from the tray.

Alginates are not dimensionally stable on storage, because of syneresis. Compatibility with plaster and stone can be good; some alginates give a powdery surface on casts from some dental stones.

2. Other properties. The materials are non-toxic and non-irritant; their taste and odor is usually acceptable. The setting time depends on the composition (for example the trisodium phosphate content), and on the temperature of mixing. The alginate powder is not stable on storage in the presence of moisture or in conditions warmer than room temperature. Alginates are difficult to disinfect without harming the impression. Spray disinfectants diminish the sharpness of surface detail, whilst immersion in solutions may adversely affects dimensional accuracy.

32.3.4 Applications

These materials are not generally used for impressions for inlay, crown and bridge work, but are used with success for prosthetic and orthodontic purposes. Alginates are dimensionally less stable than the elastomers (Chapter 33).

FURTHER READING

Buchan S, Peggie R W (1966). Role of ingredients in alginate impression compounds. *Journal of Dental Research* **45**: 1120-1129.

Harris W T Jr (1969). Water temperature and accuracy of alginate impressions. *Journal of Prosthetic Dentistry* **21**: 613-617.

Miller M W (1975). Syneresis in alginate impression materials. *British Dental Journal* **139**:425-430.

Chapter 33

Elastomeric Impression Materials

Summary: The chemistry and properties of a range of synthetic rubber impression materials are presented, together with their comparative properties.

33.1 CHEMISTRY OF THE POLYSULFIDES

33.1.1 Composition

These materials are supplied as two pastes. The 'base' paste contains a polysulfide, the formula of which is given in Figure 33.1. This molecule contains three -SH groups; two of these groups are terminal, one is pendant.

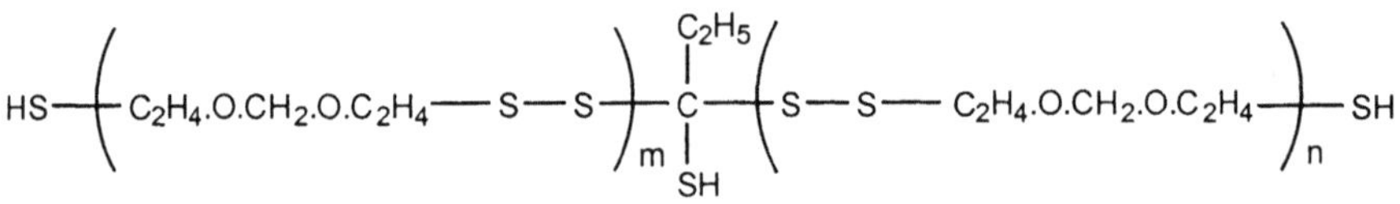

Figure 33.1. Polysulfide molecule with one pendant and two terminal –SH groups.

The base paste also contains a filler, between 11 to 54% for different materials, for example, TiO_2. This paste is usually colored white, because of the color of the filler.

The reactor paste (sometimes called 'accelerator' or 'catalyst' paste) contains lead dioxide (PbO_2) which causes polymerization and cross-linking, by oxidation of -SH groups (see below). Copper salts are present in one product. Sulfur is also present. An oil, (an ester or chlorinated paraffin) is included to form a paste of the correct consistency. This paste is brown colored due to the lead dioxide.

33.1.2 Setting

The -SH groups can be oxidized by PbO_2, giving S-S linkages, as shown in Figure 33.2.

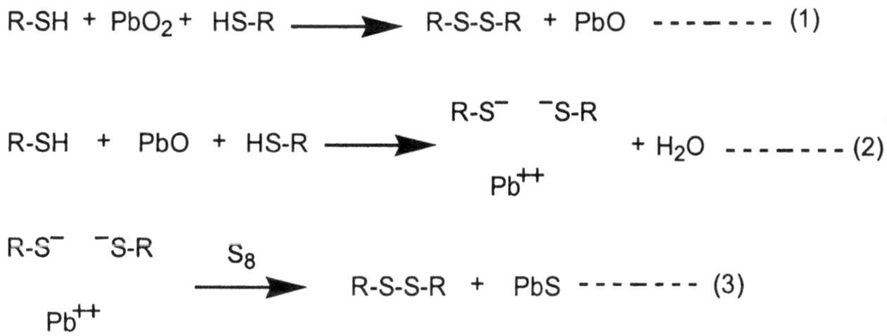

Figure 33.2. Setting reactions of a polysulfide.

In the second reaction in Figure 33.2, ionic cross-linking can occur. This is undesirable, because, under stress, such a structure can undergo exchange reactions leading to high permanent deformation. Thus sulfur is added, which can react as shown in reaction (3) in Figure 33.2.

In the above reactions, the polysulfide paste undergoes two reactions:

- Further polymerization takes place, due to oxidation of the terminal –SH groups.
- Cross-linking occurs due to oxidation of pendant –SH groups; it has already been shown that some cross-linking is necessary for an elastomer (Section 11.5.4).

The percentage of cross-links will depend on the values of m and n in the formula of the polysulfide (Figure 33.1) that is, on the initial chain length of the polysulfide.

33.1.3 Modifications

Alternative reactors to PbO_2 have been tried - for example, cumene hydroperoxide or t-butyl hydroperoxide. However, these constituents are volatile, and its loss by evaporation leads to shrinkage of the set mass. Another development replaced the PbO_2 by a zinc carbonate/organic accelerator system.

33.2 CHEMISTRY OF THE SILICONES

33.2.1 Condensation reaction

The base paste contains a silicone polymer with terminal hydroxyl groups (Figure 33.3A) and a filler. This is mixed with a reactor paste (or liquid) containing a cross-linking agent such as an alkoxy ortho-silicate or a polymer of it (Figure 33.3B). In the reactor paste there is also an activator, usually an organo-tin compound, such as dibutyl-tin dilaurate.

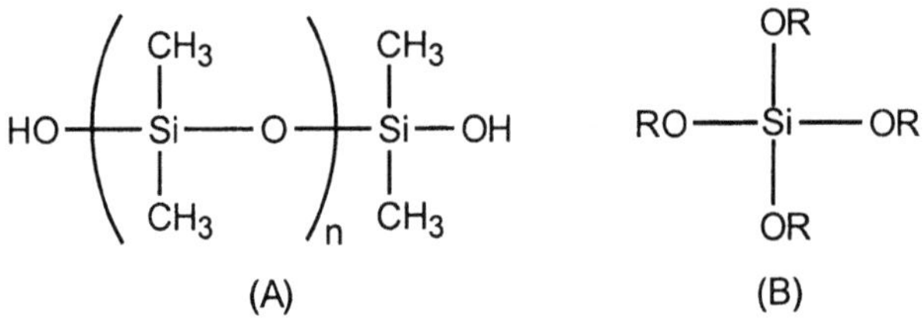

Figure 33.3 (A) Silicone polymer with terminal hydroxyl groups; (B) alkoxy ortho-silicate.

Cross-linking occurs on mixing the two materials together, as shown in Figure 33.4.

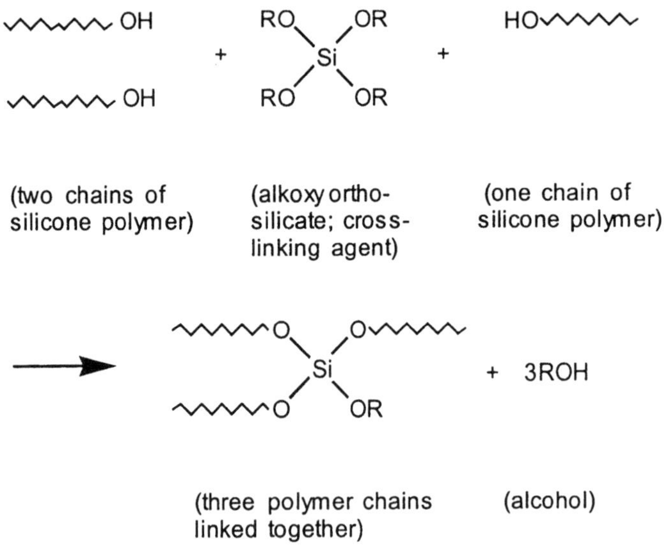

Figure 33.4. Condensation reactions in silicone formation.

The cross-linking reaction in Figure 33.4 occur with elimination of alcohol, volatilization of which can contribute to lack of dimensional stability (Section 33.6).

33.2.2 Addition reaction

Silicones that set by an addition reaction, avoiding the above problems, are now widely used, and are often termed vinyl polysiloxanes. The name polyvinyl siloxane is strictly not correct. These materials contain an organo-hydrogen siloxane, which can undergo an addition reaction with a siloxane compound containing a terminal vinyl group in the presence of a precious metal catalyst such as H_2PtCl_6 (Figure 33.5).

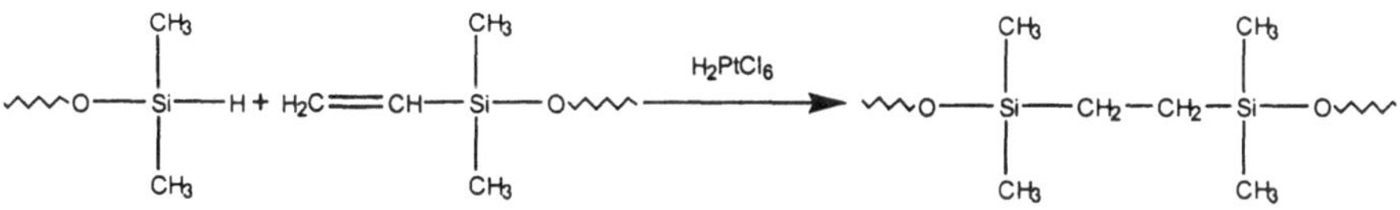

Figure 33.5. Addition reaction between a siloxane with a terminal hydrogen and a siloxane with a terminal vinyl group.

This type of reaction can lead to the formation of a cross-linked silicone rubber (Figure 33.6).

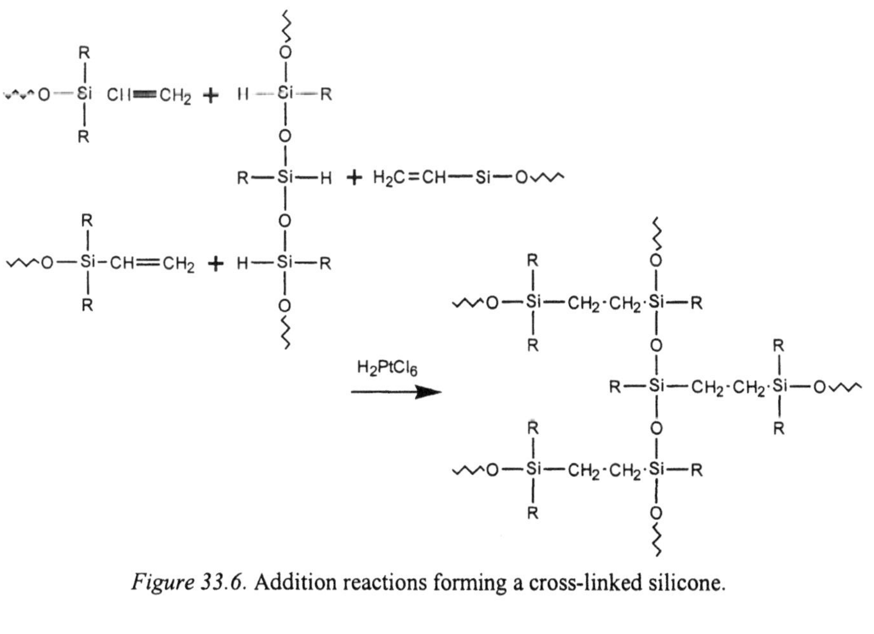

Figure 33.6. Addition reactions forming a cross-linked silicone.

33.2.3 Hydrophilic materials

Many current silicone impression materials are claimed to be hydrophilic. This may be achieved by the incorporation of a non-ionic surfactant. Such impression materials are more capable of wetting tooth surfaces during impression recording. Also, when set they are more easily wetted by water-containing die materials.

33.3 CHEMISTRY OF THE POLYETHERS

The base paste contains an unsaturated polyether with imine end groups (Figure 11.10), a plasticizer and a filler. The reactor paste contains an aromatic sulfonate, a plasticizer and a filler. Setting is by cross linking reaction of the imine groups by cationic addition polymerization (Section 11.4).

33.4 VISIBLE LIGHT CURE IMPRESSION MATERIAL

A visible light cure impression material has been marketed. As supplied, this material contained a polyurethane dimethacrylate resin with SiO_2 filler, and constituents to enable the resin to polymerize in the presence of light of around 480 nm wavelength. A plasticizer, coloring agent, stabilizer were also included. Conventional dental light curing units (see Section 27.3) with transparent trays were used. The operator had control over working and setting time.

33.5 MANIPULATION OF ELASTOMERS

Uniform mixing is required. Some products are now produced with an automatic mixing system, in which the two pastes are mixed as they are extruded together through a spiral in the nozzle of a syringe (Figure 33.7).

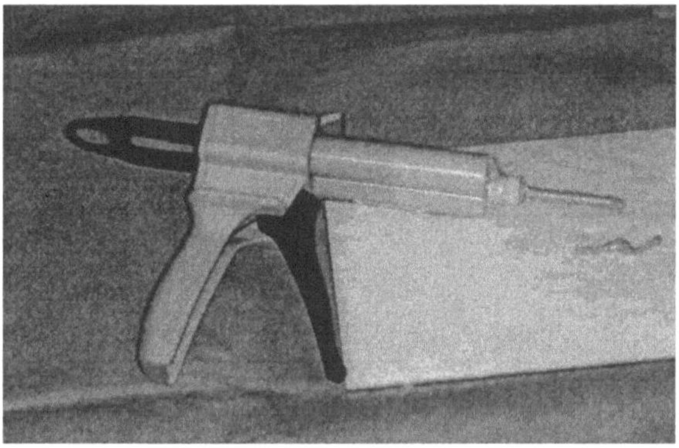

Figure 33.7. Automatic mixing system for elastomers.

Vinyl polysiloxanes are very sensitive to contamination, especially by contact with traces of sulfur compounds from disposable latex gloves, specifically dithiocarbamates which are used as accelerators in latex processing.

Retention of the material on the tray is achieved by use of an adhesive such as a rubber solution. Ideally there should be a uniform thickness (2 to 3 mm) of impression material.

Numerous techniques of impression taking have been reported. Two-step impressions (use of a fluid paste in a putty impression) can lead to dimensional distortion and problems of adhesion between the two materials. A single-step technique is usually favored, either with two mixes of material of different viscosity, or with a single mix of elastomer.

Set elastomers should be displaced sharply from the tissues to ensure elastic behavior.

33.6 PROPERTIES OF ELASTOMERS

1. Accuracy and dimensional stability. The fluidity of these materials depends largely on their composition. Some polysulfides are supplied in a range of viscosities, for example, light bodied for injection by a syringe, and medium and heavy bodied for use on a tray. Some materials are supplied with a diluent to enable the operator to alter the viscosity of the mixed material as required. Silicones are also supplied with a range of consistencies including putty type and lower viscosity materials. (Table

33.1). In general elastomers can record fine detail. Unmixed elastomers are usually pseudoplastic in nature.

Table 33.1 Apparent viscosities of unmixed impression pastes at a shear rate of 65 s^{-1} at 25°C

Grade of material	Typical range of apparent viscosity values (Pa.s)
Putty	400-700
Heavy bodied	200-300
Regular	40-150
Light bodied and wash materials	10-70

There is a small contraction on setting of these materials, because of polymerization shrinkage. Contraction also occurs on cooling the impression from mouth to room temperature. The coefficient of thermal expansion of these materials is in the order:

polyether > silicone > polysulfide

The magnitude of the thermal shrinkage is reduced by the adhesion of the material to the tray.

These materials are sufficiently elastic to be withdrawn over undercuts, and are usually tougher and less likely to tear than the alginates. Polyether materials are more stiff than the other elastomers, therefore are the most difficult to withdraw over undercuts.

On storage, contraction can result from further polymerization of the material. Evaporation of volatile by-products from a condensation reaction (e.g. alcohol) is another source of shrinkage. The dimensional stability of polyethers may be poor in the presence of moisture. In terms of dimensional stability, addition silicones are the optimum, followed by polyether, then polysulfides.

These materials are in general compatible with model and die materials, though they can cause a small degree of softening of a dental stone surface. In early addition silicones evolution of hydrogen from materials containing an organo-hydrogen siloxane caused pitting of stone surfaces. Present day silicones either do not use this system, or contain a compound to react with hydrogen as soon as it is generated. These impression materials can be electroplated to give metal coated dies.

2. Other properties. In general these materials are non-toxic and non-irritant as set. However, unmixed pastes can be irritant and produce tissue

reactions. The odor and taste of some pastes containing lead dioxide is not pleasant.

The setting time depends on the composition of the material (for example, the quantity of reactors, etc). Also the presence of water and high temperatures accelerate the setting of polysulfides.

In terms of tear energy:

- Higher viscosity materials are often better than lower viscosity products;
- Polysulfides are better than silicones, but distortion can occur instead of tearing;
- Polyethers are similar to regular grade silicones.

Stability on storage of the unmixed materials is not always ideal; some of the reactors are unstable over a two-year period, but keep better if stored in a refrigerator.

Elastomers can be disinfected by immersion in aqueous hypochlorite or glutaraldehyde solutions; short term immersion does not have any significant effect on dimensional stability.

A general comparison of the merits and limitations of dental elastomers is presented in Table 33.2.

Table 33.2. Merits and limitations of elastomeric impression materials

Material	Merits	Limitations
Polysulfide	Long working time – useful if impression is to include multiple preparations Good tear strength	Poor taste Messy to mix Permanent staining if inadvertently placed on clothing Increased chair time because of slow set Dimensional stability not as good as vinyl polysiloxanes
Polyether	High accuracy and good dimensional stability Poorer tear strength than polysulfides	Fast set – difficult for impressions of multiple units Low tear strength Difficult to remove from undercuts
Condensation silicone	Clean; minimal taste Lower cost than vinyl polysiloxanes	Hydrophobic, therefore a dry working field is required Dimensional stability poorer than vinyl polysiloxanes, therefore need to pour dies and casts early
Addition silicone (vinyl polysiloxane)	Excellent dimensional accuracy and stability	Low tear resistance of thin sections of material Some products are hydrophobic

33.7 APPLICATIONS

The chief use of elastomers is in impressions for inlays, crowns and bridges, or for partial dentures when the undercuts are so severe that alginate would tear on removal from the tissues. Because of their expense, these materials are not frequently used in impressions requiring large quantities of material.

FURTHER READING

Craig R G, Sun Z (1994). Trends in elastomeric impression materials. *Operative Dentistry* **19**: 138-145.

Salem N S, Combe E C, Watts D C (1988). Mechanical properties of elastomeric impression materials. *Journal of Oral Rehabilitation* **15**: 125-132.

IX

INDIRECT RESTORATIVE MATERIALS

Chapter 34

Dental Ceramics

Summary: The scientific principles of ceramics have already been outlined in Chapter 15. In this chapter, the clinical applications of ceramic materials are discussed, and many exciting recent developments are critiqued.

34.1 GENERAL PROPERTIES OF CERAMICS

A very general critique of ceramic materials can be made according to the principles of evaluation outlined in Chapter 2.

1. Biological properties. Often ceramics are inert in the body, with excellent biocompatibility. However, some dental ceramics are harmful because of their mechanical properties; abrasive wear of opposing tooth substance can occur.
2. Interfacial properties. It is difficult to obtain chemical adhesion to most ceramics because of their lack of chemical reactivity.
3. Chemical properties. In general ceramics do not undergo any chemical breakdown in the oral environment.
4. Mechanical properties. Though often strong in compression, ceramics have relatively low tensile strength and are subject to brittle fracture, related to crack propagation through the material.
5. Esthetic properties. Many ceramic materials are translucent and can be pigmented to give excellent esthetics. Furthermore, ceramics do not readily discolor, and do not stain if there is a reasonably smooth surface.
6. Practicability. When a powder-slurry ceramic is fired, there is a large volumetric shrinkage (of the order of 30%). Thus it is impossible to produce accurate ceramic inlays by this technique.

In summary, conventional ceramics offer many potential advantages for oral use. Many recent developments have attempted to overcome the problems outlined above. That is, there has been much research into development of improved mechanical properties and/or alternative fabrication techniques. In this chapter we are concerned with 'all-ceramic' systems. In Chapter 36 porcelain-fused-to-metal (PFM) techniques are discussed.

34.2 CLASSIFICATION ACCORDING TO FABRICATION PROCEDURE

Current materials can be classified according to their laboratory fabrication procedures:

- Powder-slurry formation, followed by firing (sintered ceramics);
- Use of a casting technique;
- Machinable ceramics;
- Pressable ceramics;
- Infiltrated ceramics.

Each of these is considered in turn.

34.3 POWDER-SLURRY CERAMICS

34.3.1 Introduction

Traditionally household porcelain is made from about 50% by weight, kaolin, 25% feldspar and 25% quartz. The functions of these ceramic raw materials are discussed in Chapter 15. Dental products differ from this in that little or no kaolin is present. They may thus be more accurately described as glasses than porcelains. The dental laboratory is supplied with a powdered material. This is a *frit*, which has been prepared by the manufacturer by blending the raw materials, melting them together in a refractory crucible, during which procedure the fluxes partially combine with the silica. These high temperature reactions are termed *pyrochemical reactions*. Quenching the red-hot glass is carried out to break it up, followed by grinding to the required particle size.

The porcelain powder is mixed with water to form a slurry, which is adapted as a plastic mass to the requisite shape prior to firing in an oven. According to standard specifications, the available materials may be classified according to their temperatures of fusion in the dental laboratory:

- High-fusing 1200 - 1400°C;
- Medium-fusing 1050 - 1200°C;
- Low-fusing 800 - 1050°C.

However, it is now rare to find a porcelain with a firing temperature in excess of 1200 °C.

Classification can also be made according to application:

- *Core porcelain* - the basis of a porcelain jacket crown, which must have good mechanical properties;
- *Dentin or body porcelain* - more translucent than the above, this largely governs the shape and color of the restoration;
- *Enamel porcelain* is used in areas requiring maximum translucency, for example, at the incisal edge.

Another difference between materials is in the method of firing. An alternative to firing at atmospheric pressure is to use vacuum firing.

34.3.2 Composition

A typical traditional porcelain, medium-fusing, for vacuum firing will contain the following oxide composition (figures are weight %): SiO_2 65%; Al_2O_2, 19%; fluxes (B_2O_3, K_2O, Na_2O, MgO, Li_2O, P_2O_5) 16%. These materials are *feldspathic* porcelains. They are also *non-aluminous.* Although Al_2O_3 is present, there is no free alumina, since it is part of the glass network.

Other components include pigments that are fused in the glassy material. These are typically the oxides of chromium, cobalt, nickel, titanium and iron (II) oxide. Oxides such as that of titanium can be used to increase the opacity of the material. Glazes and stains may also be used to achieve required esthetic effects.

34.3.3 Aluminous porcelain

In the 1960s, *aluminous porcelain* was developed. This is a material similar to the above, but strengthened by the incorporation of 40 to 50% by weight of crystalline alumina. Recrystallized alumina has a higher compressive, tensile and flexural strength than conventional porcelain. If added in sufficient quantities to porcelain it can strengthen the material by hindering crack propagation. For this to happen it is necessary for both phases to have identical coefficients of thermal expansion so that no stresses will be induced during heating or cooling. Addition of about 40% alumina to porcelain approximately doubles the flexural strength of the porcelain. However, the translucency of the porcelain is decreased by the addition of alumina, although this is to some extent overcome by careful selection of the grain size of the reinforcing phase.

34.3.4 Leucite-reinforced porcelain

Some contemporary feldspathic materials are reinforced by the presence of up to 45 volume % leucite, which has the formula $KAlSi_2O_6$. In terms of coefficient of thermal expansion, there is a considerable mismatch between that of leucite (22 parts per million per °C) and the glassy phase (8 parts per million per °C). On cooling, there are resultant compressive stresses in the glass around the leucite particles. Such stresses act as crack deflectors, resulting in a material with greater modulus of rupture. It should be noted that materials containing leucite might be abrasive to opposing tooth structure.

34.3.5 Zirconia based porcelain

Another idea for the potential reinforcement is to include fibers of zirconia (ZrO_2) into the material. Under stress, the zirconia can undergo a phase change accompanied by an increase in volume. This places compressive stresses on the crack surface, thus stopping crack growth. This is known as *transformation toughening.*

34.3.6 Manipulation

1. Compacting (or condensation). In the construction of a porcelain jacket crown, the plastic mass of powder and water (or modeling fluid, containing surfactants, supplied by the porcelain manufacturer) is applied to a platinum foil thimble that has been adapted to a stone die. Compacting is carried out to adapt the material to the requisite shape and to remove as much water from the material as possible. On firing there is a volumetric shrinkage of 30 to 40%; the more water removed, the less is this contraction.

A number of methods of compacting have been suggested for use. Dry powder can be sprinkled on to the surface of the wet material. This helps to remove water by capillary action. Excess water can be blotted off the material after condensing it, or whipping it with a brush. Vibration may be used to help the powder particles settle.

The success of compacting depends not only on the skill of the operator, but also on the range of sizes of the powder particles. It has been shown theoretically that if all the particles are of approximately the same size, 45% of a given volume will consist of voids. If a number of smaller particles are blended with larger ones, the void space is considerably reduced. Three or more particle sizes achieve an even greater degree of compaction (Figure 34.1).

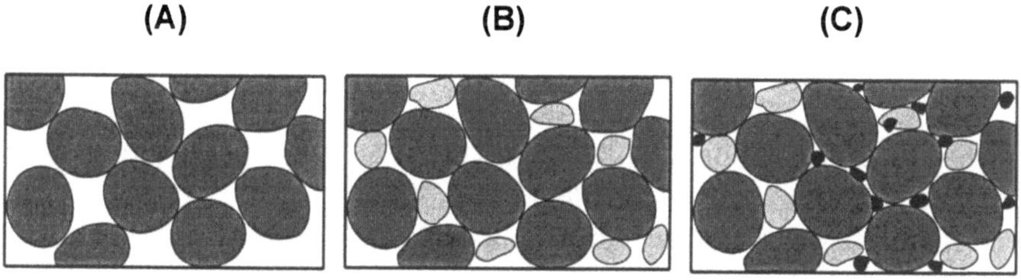

Figure 34.1. Packing of particles: (A) Particles of approximately same size with 45% volume of voids; (B) Two different particle sizes, lower volume of voids; (C) Three different particle sizes with much greater degree of compaction.

2. Firing. This is carried out in an electrically heated muffle furnace. The heating element may be made of either nickel-chromium alloys, suitable for the lower fusing porcelains, or platinum or platinum alloys, where higher temperatures are required.

The compacted porcelain should be placed on a fire-clay tray, and not be permitted to come into contact with the floor or walls of the furnace. The heating element will become brittle if porcelain fuses on to it. The initial rates of heating should be slow otherwise the water would be converted to steam so rapidly that the unfired restoration would crumble. Uniform heating is desirable. Since the thermal conductivity of porcelain is low, slow heating is desirable to give sufficient time for the interior of the porcelain to heat up. Initially the furnace door should be left open to allow steam and the combustion products of any binders to escape.

The following stages can be recognized in firing porcelain:

- *Low bisque* or *low biscuit* stage, when the material develops some rigidity and the fluxes have started to flow;
- *Medium bisque* or *medium biscuit* stage, when some shrinkage has occurred and there is greater cohesion between the particles;
- *High bisque* or *high bisque* stage - at this stage no further shrinkage will occur.

3. Cooling. This is ideally carried out slowly and uniformly, otherwise different portions will shrink to different extents, leading to stresses that can cause cracking and a loss in strength.

4. Re-firing. Adding more porcelain to the restoration and re-firing compensates for the firing shrinkage.

5. Glazes and stains. When the final desired shape is achieved, a smooth surface is desirable to prevent food clinging to the restoration. Polishing

may not achieve a satisfactory surface due to the presence of porosity. The desired surface finish can be achieved for some materials by heating under controlled conditions (rapid heat up to the fusion temperature, this temperature maintained for about five minutes) which causes the surface to flow and become smooth. This is termed *autoglazing*. Prolonged heating can result in *pyroplastic flow* - flow of the material at high temperatures, which causes rounding of sharp angles and edges of the restoration. Gross overheating may result in complete loss of form.

Alternatively, a *glaze*, an almost transparent ceramic, is applied to the surface, which is re-fired. A glaze is composed of low fusing fluxes and silica. Before glazing, a *stain* may be painted on to the porcelain surface, to imitate stains or developmental faults and features of the natural teeth. The stain is suspended in a liquid that evaporates during firing.

34.3.7 Properties

1. Shrinkage on firing. During firing any residual water is lost from the material, accompanied by loss of any binders which may be present. Volume shrinkage is of the order of 30 to 40%, principally due to elimination of voids during sintering. This is a particular problem in the fabrication of ceramic inlays.
2. Porosity. Inevitably in a fired porcelain there are present numerous air bubbles. This can weaken the material, and reduce its translucency. Research workers have suggested the following methods of reducing porosity, the first of which is frequently used in the dental laboratory:
- Firing in a vacuum to remove air;
- Firing in the presence of a gas which will be able to diffuse out of the porcelain;
- Cooling under pressure to reduce the magnitude of the pores.

3. Chemical properties. One of the chief attractions of porcelain as a dental material is that it is chemically indestructible in most environments.
4. Mechanical properties. Porcelain is essentially a brittle material; developments in ceramics over the last few years have been directed to the attainment of improved mechanical properties as in the aluminous materials.
5. Thermal properties. The thermal conductivity of porcelain is low. The coefficient of thermal expansion is close to that of enamel and dentin (Table 6.2).

6. Esthetics. The esthetics of porcelain itself are excellent. Nevertheless, if the luting cement dissolves, the crevice formed at the margin of the restoration may be discolored by debris.

34.3.8 Ion strengthening

One way of improving the properties of a ceramic object is to introduce compressive stresses into its surface layer, by replacing smaller ions by relatively larger ones. As a result, crack growth from surface flaws is more difficult.

This idea has been tested on dental porcelains immersed in molten potassium nitrate at 400 °C for 4 hours, which results in a significant strength improvement, as potassium ions replaced smaller sodium ions. An ion exchange paste product is available in which the ceramic is coated with the paste and heated in a conventional porcelain furnace.

34.4 CASTABLE CERAMICS

Glass-ceramic restorations can be prepared by lost-wax centrifugal casting techniques (similar to dental alloys, Chapter 54), followed by heat treatment to cause partial crystallization, which increases the strength of the material.

34.4.1 Mica-based glass ceramics

After casting, a mica-based glass ceramic is heated for 6 hours at 1070°C, to permit nucleation and growth of mica crystals (a tetrasilic fluormica, $KMg_{2.5}Si_4O_{10}F_2$). In addition to improving mechanical properties, this process also imparts some degree of opacity to the transparent glass. For better esthetics, stains are baked on the surface of the material, though these may not always be durable in clinical service.

34.4.2 Hydroxyapatite-based glass-ceramics

A castable glass-ceramic is available in which the crystalline component is oxyapatite, which forms hydroxyapatite in the presence of water.

34.5 MACHINABLE CERAMICS

CAD-CAM ('Computer Aided Design - Computer Aided Manufacture') systems are now being used in dentistry, specifically for the preparation of inlays, onlays, crowns and laminate veneers. Benefits of this approach include the ability to perform the treatment in one visit, avoidance of the costs of laboratory processing, and no need for a provisional restoration.

Following tooth preparation, an image of the tooth is acquired by a miniature three-dimensional video camera. This is stored in a computer. On a video display of the image, the margins of the preparation are outlined by the operator. The microprocessor deletes data beyond the margins of the restoration. Information is transferred from the microprocessor to a three-axis milling device that prepares a restoration from a standard ceramic block. The fitting surfaces of the restoration are then given a surface treatment with hydrofluoric acid to render them micromechanically retentive.

At this time, there is a limited choice of machinable ceramic materials. One product is a glassy matrix containing sanidine ($KAlSi_3O_8$). Alternatively, a mica-based product is available, similar to the castable ceramic described above.

34.6 PRESSABLE CERAMICS

34.6.1 Leucite-based materials

A refractory mold is prepared by a lost wax technique (similar in principle to the casting of alloys, Chapter 54). Ingots of a leucite-containing ceramic are heated to around 1150°C under a pressure of 300-400 kPa; the temperature is maintained for 20 minutes. The processed material contains about 40% by volume leucite crystals of size 1-5 μm.

34.6.2 Spinel-based materials

An alternative material for injection molding contains a magnesium spinel ($MgAl_2O_4$) as the crystalline phase.

34.7 INFILTRATED CERAMICS

These materials are composed or a porous core which is then infiltrated with a molten glass to give a dense solid. The core is prepared by *slip casting*. The mixture of fine grain particles (0.5 - 3.5 μm) of alumina mixed with water is called a *slip*. The slip is baked on a gypsum die at around 1100°C for 10 hours. This produces a fragile, opaque and porous core. To this is applied the desired shade of a lanthanum glass powder, which is fired at 1150°C for 4 hours. During this second firing the glass flows into the pores of the core by capillary action, giving a high strength material. The restoration is finished by applying a ceramic veneer.

An alternative material uses a core of a magnesium spinel which is then infiltrated with a glass, to give a more translucent restoration than the alumina-based material.

34.8 DENTAL APPLICATIONS OF MATERIALS

Given the potential for life-like esthetics from porcelain, there are a wide variety of techniques which utilize the rapidly increasing range of ceramic materials. These are principally full coverage restorations, veneers and inlays. Many types of porcelain are capable of being bonded to tooth enamel and/or dentin by the technique in which the ceramic fitting surface is etched with hydrofluoric acid or a hydrochloric acid/nitric acid mixture for approximately 2 minutes. This differentially dissolves the ceramic surface, producing a micromechanically retentive surface that will adhere to a light cure or dual-cure resin cement. Bond strength has been considered to be improved by up to 20% by the application of silane solution (Figure 27.5) to the etched ceramic. This improvement in bond strength appears to be optimal if the silane is applied between 30 minutes and 24 hours prior to the placement of the restoration. Other techniques rely on luting with conventional materials such as glass-ionomer or zinc phosphate cement. In full crown restorations in which the crown is bonded to the underlying dentin, it may be considered that the dentin acts as the 'core' in a manner similar to alumina in the aluminous porcelain crown, leucite in leucite reinforced ceramics, and metal in metal-ceramic restorations.

34.8.1 Dentin-bonded all-ceramic crowns

The *dentin-bonded crown* has been defined as a full coverage restoration in which an all-ceramic crown is bonded to the underlying dentin (and any available enamel) using a resin-composite based luting material, with the bond being mediated by use of a dentin bonding system and a micromechanically retentive ceramic surface. The fracture resistance of such restorations has been considered good and these crowns are therefore of value in situations where minimal preparation is appropriate, such as in teeth that have suffered tooth substance loss through erosion. The esthetic properties of dentin-bonded all-ceramic restorations have been also considered good because there is no opaque substructure such as metal, or an opaque cement. The technique relies on the application of a dentin bonding system of low film thickness to the dentin and any remaining enamel: this allows the bonding of the crown to the etched ceramic surface by way of a dual cure resin-composite luting system. The shade of the luting cement will affect the shade of the completed restoration if the preparation and the thickness of the crown is minimal. Any ceramic material that is capable of being etched to produce a micromechanically retentive surface may be appropriate for this technique. Feldspathic porcelain has been widely used for dentin-bonded crowns in the past, but reinforced ceramics are being used increasingly. One disadvantage is the need to carry out occlusal adjustments after rather than before placement, which means that the adjusted areas must be polished in the mouth, rather than at the chairside or in the laboratory.

34.8.2 Porcelain inlays

Porcelain inlays may provide restorations of excellent esthetics and good durability when placed using a similar technique to that described for dentin-bonded crowns, above. Restoration longevity is substantially diminished if a conventional non-adhesive luting materials is used. Occlusal cavity margins should not be bevelled as there is a risk of fracture of thin porcelain sections: for this reason the preparation should allow a thickness of at least 2 mm porcelain.

34.8.3 Porcelain veneers

Porcelain veneers are thin veneers (generally of 0.5 mm-1 mm section) of porcelain which are bonded to the facial surfaces of teeth, although veneers may also be placed on the palatal surfaces of teeth in cases of tooth substance loss. The placement technique may use a light-cured resin composite luting material rather than dual cure as described above, given that light penetration through the restoration does not present a problem except in cases where the veneers is of thicker than normal section or of dark shade. Indications include discolored, intrinsically stained or unsightly teeth and restoration of peg-shaped lateral incisors.

34.9 REPAIR OF FRACTURED CERAMIC RESTORATIONS

Regrettably, if ceramic is used as a restorative material, fracture of a small number of restorations will occur, often as a result of trauma. The ability to repair porcelain intra-orally would therefore be an advantage, given that the potential for trauma to the tooth by re-preparation is reduced, notwithstanding the reduced cost of a repair to the patient. Techniques for repairing porcelain have therefore been described, although none have been evaluated in the long term. Porcelain repair techniques require the roughening of the fractured ceramic using an intra-oral sandblaster, generally using 30-50 μm alumina grit. The intra-oral use of hydrofluoric acid has also been suggested, but has not gained widespread acceptance due to the highly corrosive nature of this acid. However, the surface obtained following etching with hydrofluoric acid is likely to be more micromechanically retentive than that following sandblasting (Figure 34.3). Following roughening of the porcelain, silane should be applied and application of a resin that bonds to ceramic is required. A number of dentin bonding systems list bonding to ceramic among their applications and the resin 4-META has shown demonstrable bond strengths to ceramic. Such a material is applied to the porcelain surface and the defect may then be restored using a composite restorative material. If a metal substructure of the restoration is exposed, the metal is roughened as above by sandblasting and a resin that demonstrates adhesion to metal utilized. Again 4-META containing materials may be of value.

Another concept in porcelain repair has been adopted by a system which uses a surface-coating 30 μm alumina grit which applies a silicate coating to the metal or ceramic surface on which it is used. This then allows bonding of the composite by means of a silane applied to the silicate impregnated metal or ceramic surface.

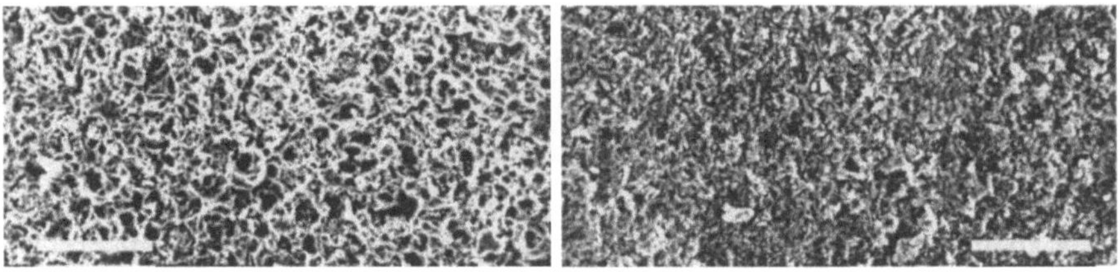

Figure 34.3. Surface of feldspathic porcelain; Left: after etching with hydrofluoric acid; Right: after roughening by abrasive grit The horizontal bars represent 100 μm.

34.10 OTHER DENTAL APPLICATIONS OF CERAMICS

In later chapters of the book, other ceramic applications are discussed:

- Orthodontic brackets (Chapter 41);
- Porcelain-fused-to-metals (Chapter 36);
- Denture teeth (Chapter 48);
- Implant materials, including bioactive ceramics (Chapter 50).

FURTHER READING

Appendix IV lists some current dental ceramics, classified according to Section 34.2.

Denry I L (1996). Recent advances in ceramics for dentistry. *Critical Reviews in Oral Biology and Medicine* **7**: 134-143.

Qualtrough A J E, Piddock V (1997). Ceramics Update. *Journal of Dentistry* **25**: 91-95.

Rosenblum M A, Schulman A (1997). A review of all-ceramic restorations. *Journal of the American Dental Association* **128**: 297-307.

Burke F J T, Grey N J A (1994). Repair of fractured porcelain units; alternative approaches. *British Dental Journal* **176**: 251-256.

Burke F J T, Watts D C (1994). Fracture resistance of teeth restored with dentin-bonded crowns. *Quintessence International* **25**: 335-340.

Burke F J T, Qualtrough A J E and Hale R W (1998) Dentin-bonded all-ceramic crowns: Current status. *Journal of the American Dental Association* **129**: 455-460.

Chapter 35

Alloys for Inlays, Crowns and Bridges

Summary: In this chapter, alloys for casting inlays, crowns and bridges are considered, including noble and base metal alloys. The correct choice of alloy for a given clinical procedure can make the difference between clinical success and failure.

35.1 INTRODUCTION

The principles of metallurgy have been described in Chapters 12 and 13. Of particular importance is the effect of alloying elements on gold (Section 13.5.2) and the nature and properties of chromium-containing alloys (Section 13.8). The principles of metal casting, and faults that can occur in this procedure are described in Chapter 54.

35.2 REQUIREMENTS

There are a number of stringent requirements for casting alloys for the fabrication of inlays, crowns and bridges.

1. Biocompatibility. Alloys should be non-allergenic to patient and technician, and should not contain toxic components that can be dangerous in the dental laboratory during grinding and polishing procedures.
2. Good corrosion and tarnish resistance are essential.
3. Mechanical properties. These include:
- High yield stress if the cast restoration is to be subjected to large forces *in situ*;
- Sufficient ductility to resist fracture during burnishing procedures;
- Hardness: this is an indication of the difficulty of grinding and finishing of the alloy.

4. Ease of casting. Alloys of high density and good fluidity when molten are easier to cast.
5. Economic considerations. Ideally, alloys should be inexpensive, both in terms of material and labor costs.

35.2 GOLD ALLOYS WITH AT LEAST 75% NOBLE METALS

35.2.1 Introduction

The proportion of gold in alloy may be designated in one of two ways:
1. The *carat rating* expresses the number of 24th parts of gold in the alloy: for example, 24 carat gold is pure gold, 18 carat gold contains 18/24ths or 75% gold.
2. The *fineness rating* is the parts per thousand of gold; for example, 24 carat gold is 1000 fine, and 18 carat gold is 750 fine.

35.2.2 Classification and composition

Table 35.1 shows the approximate compositions of the various types of dental gold alloys.

Table 35.1. Composition of dental gold alloys**

Type	Noble metals (%)	Au (%)	Ag (%)	Cu (%)	Pt (%)	Pd (%)	Zn (%)
I (or A), soft	≥ 83	80-90	3-12	2-5	Little or none	little or none	little or none
II (or B), medium	≥ 78	75-78	12-15	7-10	0-1	1-4	0-1
III (or C), hard	≥ 78	62-78	8-26	8-11	0-3	2-4	1
IV (or D), extra hard	≥ 75	60-70	4-20	11-16	0-4	0-5	1-2

35.2.3 Dental uses

Type I alloys are used in situations where they are not subjected to great stress, as in Class III and Class V cavities. Type II alloys are widely used

* *Data adapted from Crowell W S (1961). Gold alloys in dentistry. *Metals Handbook*, 8th edn. Vol I. pp 1188-1189. Metals Park, Ohio. American Society for Metals.

for most types of inlay. Type III alloys are used for crowns and bridges, and in situations where there may be great stresses involved. Type IV alloys are used for cast partial dentures and clasps; these are discussed further in Chapter 47.

35.2.4 Heat treatment

As outlined in Chapter 13, the properties of an alloy depend on:

- Composition, as in Table 35.1;
- Mechanical history, for example, the extent to which it has been work hardened;
- Thermal history, for example, the temperature to which it has been heated, and its rate of cooling.

Heat treatments can be performed on some gold alloys to improve their mechanical properties. This is carried out for class IV alloys, and is discussed in detail in Chapter 47. Type I and II alloys, in the as-cast condition, have usually adequate mechanical properties for their various applications. The properties of type III alloys can be improved by heat treatment.

35.2.5 Mechanical properties

Table 35.2 gives the mechanical properties of types I, II and III alloys. For comparison, data are given for heat hardened alloys of type III. Similar data for type IV alloys are in Table 47.1.

Table 35.2. Mechanical properties of gold alloys[§§]

Type	Proportional limit (MPa)	Ultimate tensile strength (MPa)	Elongation (%)	Hardness (BHN)
I (as cast)	85	200	25	40-75
II (as cast)	160	345	24	70-100
III (softened)	195	365	20	90-140
III (hardened)	290	445	10	120-170

35.2.6 Some practical precautions

To obtain a successful cast restoration, attention must be given to manipulative variables associated with the impression and die materials (as in the indirect technique), inlay wax (in both the direct and indirect

[§§] See Crowell W S (1961). *Op cit.*

technique) and investment materials. The following points in relation to the manipulation of gold alloys are important:

1. Melting can be carried out by a gas/air torch. It is important that the alloy is sufficiently heated to render it completely molten, otherwise an incomplete casting may result. Overheating should be avoided to reduce the likelihood of contamination of castings as a result of oxidation. The reducing zone of the flame is used. Flux should be applied to prevent oxidation.
2. Re-use of surplus alloy. Inevitably there is surplus alloy removed from a casting. This alloy can be re-used, provided that surplus alloys of different types are not mixed and that the alloy is not melted more than two or three times, otherwise zinc (a scavenger for oxygen) may be lost by volatilization. A mixture of new and used alloy is commonly used.

35.2.7 Critique

In most respects, gold alloys are ideal for oral use. However, in recent years, economic considerations have led to the development of less expensive materials as detailed in the Sections below.

35.3 OTHER ALLOYS

35.3.1 Medium and low gold alloys

Medium gold alloys contain around 50% gold, with palladium, silver, copper and zinc. Other alloys contain lesser amounts of gold. There is an approximate linear relationship between gold content and density. The alloys with less gold content are more prone to show tarnish, although few comparative data are available.

35.3.2 Silver-palladium alloys

These alloys contain silver, palladium (at least 25%), and gold, copper, indium and zinc. They are more difficult to cast than gold alloys, owing to their density, and to the dissolution of oxygen by molten alloys, resulting in porosity in casting.

35.3.3 Nickel-chromium alloys

These alloys contain about 75% nickel and 20% chromium. They are used in resin bonded techniques, and can also be used in metal–ceramic restorations; a critique of them is given in Section 36.2.6.

FURTHER READING

Cruickshanks-Boyd D W (1981). Alternatives to gold 1. Non-porcelain alloys. *Dental Update* **8**:17-23.

Leinfelder K F (1997). An evaluation of casting alloys used for restorative procedures. *Journal of the American Dental Association* **128**: 37-45.

Chapter 36

Porcelain-fused-to-metal

Summary: Alloys and ceramics designed for porcelain-fused-to-metal techniques are discussed, as is the mechanism of ceramo-metallic bonding.

36.1 INTRODUCTION

In general, alloys have good mechanical properties, and porcelain can have excellent esthetics. Techniques are available in which porcelain is fired on to a surface of a cast restoration, in attempts to obtain a strong and esthetic restoration. This chapter should be read in the context of the material Chapters 34 and 35, where ceramic and metallic restorations have been discussed.

36.2 TYPES OF ALLOY

36.2.1 Requirements

Good corrosion resistance is essential. The alloys should have a high melting range, so that no melting or permanent deformation will occur during fusion of the porcelain. Close matching of thermal properties of alloy and porcelain is important. High modulus of elasticity (minimum elastic deformation) and high yield stress (no plastic deformation) are important, to avoid excess stress on the porcelain, which is brittle.

Also the alloy should not impart color to the ceramic. Discoloration of the ceramic can occur due to the presence of copper in certain alloys. Also, greening of porcelain is a problem sometimes encountered with alloys containing silver.

36.2.2 High gold alloys

1. Composition. These alloys contain 80 to 90% gold, with platinum and/or palladium to provide hardening, but no copper. Small amounts of silver, iron, tin and indium may be present. Iron can produce a precipitate of $FePt_3$, which has a strengthening effect. Tin and indium migrate to the surface on heating and produce oxides that aid chemical bonding of porcelain to alloy.
2. Merits. These alloys have excellent corrosion resistance. They also bond well to porcelain.
3. Limitations. Creep of alloy may occur during firing of porcelain, since alloys have a comparatively low melting range. Also they have a comparatively low modulus of elasticity, thus minimum alloy thickness of 0.5 mm is required.

36.2.3 Gold-palladium alloys

1. Composition. These alloys contain 50% (approximately) gold, 30% palladium, 10% tin and indium, the remainder being silver.
2. Properties. These alloys have better resistance to creep, and are more economical than high gold alloys.

36.2.4 Palladium-silver alloys

1. Composition. These alloys contain 60% palladium, 30% silver and 10% indium and tin.
2. Properties. Their mechanical properties similar to high gold alloys. They may be difficult to cast owing to their ability to occlude gases, their low density and high shrinkage. Further, problems with 'greening' can occur when used with certain porcelain products.

36.2.5 High palladium alloys

1. Composition. At least 80% palladium is present, with 10 to 12% tin. The alloys also contain gallium, but do not contain gold or silver.
2. Properties. These alloys are considerably less expensive than high gold alloys: the absence of gold from the composition gives a stable price. They are silver-free, so no greening problems with porcelain. Their density is lower than that of gold alloys. They are somewhat technique sensitive in obtaining a good bond with porcelain.

36.2.6 Nickel-chromium alloys

1. Composition. 70% to 80% nickel (which may be partially replaced by cobalt), and 10% to 25% chromium are present. These alloys may also contain molybdenum, tungsten, manganese and beryllium and other minor components.
2. Merits. Corrosion resistance is good, owing to the passivating effect of chromium. They show low creep during porcelain firing. They have a high modulus of elasticity, so can be used in thin sections (e.g. 0.3 mm). They have high yield strength values.
3. Limitations. Nickel is well known to be allergenic. Beryllium is toxic, so hazards arise in the laboratory when casting the alloys, and also when grinding the cast alloys. Many nickel chromium alloys do not now contain beryllium. They may be difficult to cast because of their low density and high shrinkage on cooling. They are difficult to finish because of their hardness. Adhesive failure of porcelain bond has sometimes been observed.

36.3 CHOICE OF CERAMIC MATERIAL

When a porcelain (or more correctly, a glass) is used to veneer a restoration, it is important that the porcelain should fuse at a temperature lower than the melting point of the alloy.

Because it is not possible to obtain an exact match of coefficients of thermal expansion between porcelain and alloy, the latter should contract slightly more than the former, giving a degree of compressive bonding. This is controlled by composition, that is, increase in network modifiers resulting in formation of high expansion leucite crystals. *Leucite* is a crystalline phase in the SiO_2-Al_2O_3-K_2O system of formula $KAlSi_2O_6$.

36.4 NATURE OF THE CERAMO-METALLIC BOND

36.4.1 Gold-porcelain bond

The observed bond between gold alloys and porcelain is believed to result from a combination of three factors:
1. Mechanical bonding. If the fused porcelain is able to wet the metal surface efficiently, it will flow into small irregularities on the surface, resulting in mechanical interlocking.

2. Chemical bonding. Evidence suggests that if tin or indium is present in the alloy, it will form a surface film of oxide that can react with porcelain to give a chemical bond. In contrast to this, poorer bonding results from treating the alloy surface by acids that remove elements capable of being oxidized.
3. Compressive bonding. If the porcelain contracts less than the alloy on cooling, in the resultant restoration the ceramic material will have a residual compressive stress. Consequently a higher applied stress is necessary to cause tensile failure of the bond.

In practice, with careful attention to detail strong bonds can be formed between gold alloys and porcelain. In testing such bonds, cohesive failure of the ceramic is usual, indicating the presence of good adhesion between the two materials.

36.4.2 Base metal alloy-porcelain bond

Strong bonds can also be formed between nickel-chromium alloys and porcelain. In contrast to the above, however, failure of such bonds occurs at the interface between metal and ceramic (that is, adhesive failure). Sudden failure of such restorations may occur because of the high degree of residual stress at the bond, or due to excessive oxidation of the alloy at the interface with the porcelain.

36.5 PRACTICAL POINTS

To obtain good bonding between gold and porcelain, it is essential that the metal surface is degassed and free of grease and other contaminants. Strong acids should not be used to clean the casting. The surface is sandblasted to aid mechanical bonding.

36.6 PORCELAIN BONDED TO PLATINUM FOIL

As an alternative to the techniques described above, porcelain can be bonded to platinum foil. The die is covered with a layer of platinum foil. Then a second layer of foil is placed over all the die surfaces except the shoulder. This second layer is bonded to the porcelain, the following procedures being carried out to both outer and inner surfaces of the foil:

- Light abrasion to increase surface area;

- Degreasing using sodium hydroxide solution;
- Neutralization of the caustic solution and thorough washing;
- Tin plating, using a stannous sulfate solution;
- Heating in a vacuum up to 1000°C so that the tin will alloy the platinum;
- Oxidation of the tin by permitting air to enter the furnace.

A porcelain crown is constructed over the double foil matrix, using a special core material developed for this procedure. The dark color of the platinum is effectively masked by this opaque core porcelain.

The oxidized tin coating has a number of functions. On the outer surface, it improves wettability by the porcelain. It enhances strength of the restoration by hindering crack propagation. On the inner surface, it enables adhesion to occur between the restoration and a cement containing poly(acrylic acid) such as the polyalkenoate cements.

The technique of bonding porcelain to platinum can lead to the production of single unit crowns of good mechanical properties.

An alternative technique uses a gold-coated fluted foil matrix that is burnished on to a die. Heating causes melting of the gold coating which solders the folds to give a stable coping for the build-up with porcelain.

FURTHER READING

Jones D W (1988). Coatings of ceramics on metals. *Annals of the New York Academy of Sciences* **523**: 19-37.

Bagby M, Marshall S J, Marshall G W Jr (1990). Metal ceramic compatibility: a review of the literature. *Journal of Prosthetic Dentistry* **63**: 21-25.

Chapter 37

Indirect Resin Composites

Summary: A discussion of resin composite materials designed for indirect techniques, to be utilized for load-bearing restorations in posterior teeth.

37.1 INTRODUCTION

The expanding patient demand for tooth-colored restorations in the late 1980s led to an increased use of resin composite as a restorative material in load-bearing situations in posterior teeth. Initially the material was placed using instruments, devices (including matrices) and techniques designed for amalgam placement, but eventually it was realized that specially designed matrices, wedges and instruments were essential, as too were placement techniques. The performance of the composite material in small-to-medium sized cavities has been considered satisfactory; however, there have been doubts regarding the effectiveness of composite materials as a restorative for large cavities. Additionally, composites as restorative materials for posterior teeth may be considered to have a number of problems and limitations. Among these are:

- Control of polymerization shrinkage (see Chapter 27). This necessitates incremental build-up and/or other measures;
- Difficulties in achieving adequate polymerization in deep proximal cavities;
- Difficulties in achieving a firm contact point, especially in cavities with a wide proximal box;
- Difficulties in achieving a bond where the cavity margin is located on dentin;
- Absorption of water by some materials.

A tooth-colored restorative material or system that could overcome these difficulties, completely or in part, would therefore be of value. Two such systems are the ceramic inlay (Chapter 34) and the composite inlay. In the latter, an inlay of composite is cemented into the cavity as a solid mass, the inlay having been formed directly in the mouth, or, more commonly, by an indirect procedure. By this means, the polymerization shrinkage occurs during the fabrication of the inlay. The inlay is placed using a dual-cure resin luting material. It therefore follows that the only polymerization shrinkage that may occur in the mouth is in the layer of luting material, typically 50 μm to 100 μm in width. It may be considered that this is likely to cause less stress than the shrinkage of a thick layer of composite cured in bulk. However, the possibility remains that stresses may arise within the layer of luting cement as it shrinks, given that:

- The polymerization shrinkage of the luting material layer is likely to be greater than that of more heavily-filled composite restorative materials;
- The luting cement layer is enclosed (above by the restoration and below by the bonded dentin) other than for a thin layer at the margins of the restoration, which is the only position that shrinkage may occur.

37.2 METHODS OF CURING

In directly placed resin composite restorations only about 70% of the double bonds react in the polymerization process. Given that indirect resin composite restorations are formed in the laboratory, it is therefore possible to subject the restoration to additional curing. This additional, or secondary, curing may take the form of additional light curing, heat curing or curing under pressure, or a combination of these. Accordingly, manufacturers developed and manufactured equipment that could carry out these functions (Figure 37.1). These additional methods of curing generally increase the resin conversion of the composite to over 90%.

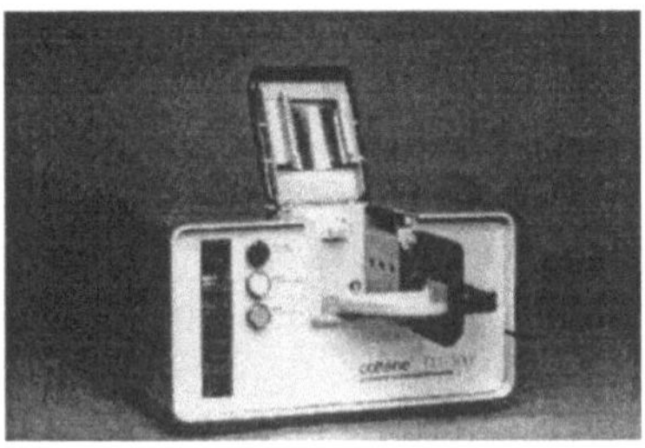

Figure 37.1. Curing equipment for indirect resin composites.

37.2.1 Light and heat cure

Research had demonstrated that the greatest improvements in a number of physical properties (tensile strength, compressive strength, wear resistance, hardness and color stability) occurred after heating at 120°C for 7 minutes. Accordingly, manufacturers have developed a light/heat curing oven, additional light curing units and light units which provide the additional curing under vacuum (Figure 37.1).

37.2.2 Heat and pressure

Other manufacturers developed materials that achieve optimum properties when subjected to additional curing at a temperature of 120°C, and pressure of 6 bar for 10 minutes - this has been described as *supercuring*.

37.3 CLINICAL CONSIDERATIONS

The cavity preparation must be withdrawable, with undercuts being blocked out using a glass-ionomer cement or resin composite. For direct inlays the inlay is built up in increments in the tooth and withdrawn from the cavity for addition of more composite as required and additional curing. For indirect techniques, this procedure is carried out in the laboratory. Final stains may be added before additional curing is carried out by one of the methods above. Although, in theory, bonding should be achieved between the composite inlay and the resin composite luting material, the high degree of resin conversion of the cured inlay means that little uncured resin is available for bonding. Accordingly, it is necessary to treat the fitting (internal) surface to provide mechanical retention. This cannot be achieved using hydrofluoric acid in a similar method to that used for ceramic fitting surfaces, because the acid does not differentially dissolve the surface – the whole surface is dissolved. Accordingly, the surface is roughened by sandblasting.

The inlay is placed using a dual-cure resin composite luting material, having treated the enamel and dentin of the cavity using a dentin bonding system. Dentin bonding systems of minimal film thickness are appropriate so that full seating of the restoration is not prevented. The restoration is finished and polished in the same way as a direct placement composite restoration. Results of clinical trials are positive.

37.4 CRITIQUE

Advantages of an indirect composite when compared with a direct composite include:

- Control of polymerization shrinkage;
- Less difficulty in achieving optimum restoration contour, especially with regard to the contact area,
- Possible improvement in marginal adaptation, especially at the gingival margin.

Disadvantages include:

- The need for two patient visits;
- Increased cost;
- The need for preparation of a withdrawable cavity, with the resultant potential for loss of tooth substance in achieving this.

The additional curing to which indirect composites are subjected has been shown to improve some physical properties such as diametral tensile strength, wear resistance, hardness and color stability. However, there is little indication that these improvements can be translated to improved wear resistance and general performance in the clinical situation.

In comparison to ceramic inlays, indirect composites offer easier handling with less potential for breakage of the completed inlay, a simpler laboratory procedure and possible lower cost, and easier chairside adjustment, finishing and polishing.

37.5 RECENT DEVELOPMENTS

Ceramic-polymer (ceromer) and polyglass materials are a diverse group of laboratory materials, cured by light, light/heat or heat and pressure, for construction of crowns and inlays. One material uses a novel xenon strobe light unit for curing which emits light of wavelength range of 320 to 500 nm. Another is based on a resin system similar to Bis-GMA but is polymerized under pressure in nitrogen. This oxygen-free atmosphere allows a higher level of polymerization, given that oxygen interferes with the curing process of resin-based materials. Some have been termed *polyglass* materials because they contain a glass filler (in one material this is porous) and a synthetic glass matrix. They are highly filled or fiber-reinforced polymers which may be used with or without a metal substructure. One material is marketed with a fiber-reinforcing sub-structure that is cured in vacuum by pressure, heat and light in specially designed apparatus. The molecular structure is more highly cross-linked than Bis-GMA, and, in comparison to conventional resin composites containing bifunctional molecules, these materials may contain molecules with up to six functional groups. Esthetic properties are good, wear resistance appears to be acceptable and there is little potential for wear of the opposing dentition. These properties may be attributed to the incorporation of multifunctional monomers and a narrow range of filler particles (generally 0.7 - 1.0 μm). However, there is a paucity of data on clinical effectiveness.

Another development is the provision of a machinable polymer-ceramic material, which can be used with CAD-CAM equipment, as described in Section 34.5. This material is based on a 'continuum filled' resin composite (Table 27.1).

FURTHER READING

Wendt S L (1987). The effect of heat used as a secondary cure upon the physical properties of three composite resins. I. Diametral tensile strength, compressive strength and marginal dimensional stability. *Quintessence International* **18**: 265-271.

Wendt S L (1987). The effect of heat used as a secondary cure upon the physical properties of three composite resins. II. Wear, hardness and color stability. *Quintessence International* **18**: 351-356.

McCabe J F, Kagi S (1991). Mechanical properties of a composite inlay material following post curing. *British Dental Journal* **171**: 246-248.

Burke F J T, Watts D C, Wilson N H F, Wilson M A (1991). Current status and rationale for composite inlays and onlays. *British Dental Journal* **170**: 269-273.

Burke F J T, Qualtrough A J E (1993). Aesthetic inlays: Composite or ceramic? *British Dental Journal* **176**: 53-60.

van Dijken J W V (1994). A 6-year evaluation of a direct composite resin inlay/onlay system and glass ionomer cement-composite resin sandwich restorations. *Acta Odontologica Scandinavica* **52**: 368-376.

Leinfelder K L (1997). New developments in resin restorative systems. *Journal of the American Dental Associaton*. **128**: 573-581.

Chapter 38

Provisional Crown and Bridge Materials

Summary: A wide range of materials can used to form provisional restorations, including preformed polymeric and metallic crowns and polymerizing temporary crown and bridge materials.

38.1 INTRODUCTION

Provisional crown and bridge materials are required during the interval between tooth preparation and placement of the final restoration. The provisional restoration is necessary for the following reasons:

- Protection of the prepared tooth or teeth from thermal stimuli and irritant effects of chemicals;
- Maintenance of esthetics;
- Maintenance of masticatory function;
- Maintenance of the relationship between the prepared teeth and other teeth.

The available materials may be either pre-formed, such as polycarbonates, or fabricated from chemically activated or visible light curing polymerizing materials.

38.2 REQUIREMENTS

1. Biological considerations. Materials must be non-irritant to soft tissue and the pulp.
2. Mechanical properties. The materials must be sufficiently strong to withstand the forces of mastication for a short period of time.
3. Thermal properties. Low thermal diffusivity is desirable.

4. Manipulative characteristics. The material must be easy to manipulate in a crown former.
5. Dimensional changes on setting should be low, and the reaction should not be highly exothermic.

38.3 POLYCARBONATE CROWNS

Pre-formed crowns are supplied which are made of polycarbonate resin. This is a polymer with high impact resistance. These temporary crowns can be cemented in place with a self-cured acrylic polymer. Only one shade of material is normally available.

38.4 METALLIC CROWNS

Pre-formed metallic crowns are available, which may be used as provisional, or in some cases, permanent crowns. They can provide a low-cost alternative to the provision of a cast restoration.

These crowns may be made of stainless steel or aluminum.

38.5 POLYMERIC PROVISIONAL CROWN AND BRIDGE MATERIALS

There are a number of types of material currently available:
1. Poly(methyl methacrylate) – (PMMA) – a mixture of monomer and polymer which contains benzoyl peroxide and a tertiary amine to give room temperature polymerization.
2. Some systems are based on higher methacrylates, containing, for example, ethyl or butyl methacrylate. Some products are chemically activated; others utilize visible light activation.
3. Resin composite systems can be used. One such product is a resin composite based on a visible light cured urethane dimethacrylate with 35 weight % filler.
4. At one time an epimine resin system was used, but this is no longer being marketed.

Some general comments can be made about the properties and performance of these materials, as guidelines for selection. The problems with PMMA systems are:

- Methyl methacrylate monomer is potentially irritant;
- There is a large degree of shrinkage on polymerization;
- There is a high degree of exotherm.

The above three problems are much less if a higher methacrylate monomer, such as ethyl, propyl or butyl methacrylates, is used. The same is true if a resin composite system is used. Visible light curing systems offer advantages in terms of ease of handling.

FURTHER READING

Gough M (1994). A review of temporary crowns and bridges. *Dental Update* **21**:203-207.

Tjan A H L, Castelnuovo J, Shiotsu G (1997). Marginal fidelity of crowns fabricated from six provisional materials. *Journal of Prosthetic Dentistry* **77**:482-485.

X

MISCELLANEOUS CLINICAL MATERIALS

Chapter 39

Post and Core Build-up Materials

Summary: Posts are considered in terms of their shape, length, surface configuration and diameter. The types of restorative materials which are suitable for core build-ups are assessed, noting the merits and limitations of each type of material.

39.1 POSTS

As increasing numbers of teeth are being restored using endodontic therapy, it follows that the restoration of the crowns of some of these teeth will require restoration using a post. Posts may be preformed or may be constructed using an indirect technique. However, the difficulties associated with achieving an accurate impression of the root canal have led to an increased use of preformed systems. Among these are, non-threaded cast posts and cores, non-threaded wrought posts with cast-on cores, threaded wrought posts with solid cores and threaded wrought posts with direct build-up cores. New examples of these types are introduced regularly. In the past, preformed posts were often constructed in stainless steel, but the improved biocompatibility and corrosion resistance of titanium alloys has led to their increased use. Carbon fiber posts have also become available.

Four factors are of importance in the retention of posts. These are, shape, length, surface configuration and diameter.

1. With regard to shape, in general, there are two categories, tapered, and, cylindrical. Both shapes may be obtained as cast posts by the use of burn-out patterns, while the tapered variety may also be constructed using the conventional lost wax technique. Both shapes are also available as prefabricated or manufactured posts which are appropriate to core build-ups. Although there is not general agreement, the retentive properties of cylindrical posts are considered superior to tapered posts.

2. With regard to length, it is generally accepted that the post length should be at least as long as the crown it is to support. However, due to factors such as curves in root canals and the increased length of tooth crowns in patients of advanced years, it may not always be possible to adhere to this ideal.
3. With regard to surface configuration, it is generally accepted that a smooth surface post is less retentive that a post with a sandblasted surface. Some preformed posts are supplied with threads and these may be subdivided into pre-threaded and self-threading types.

Pre-threaded posts. These have a thread cutter or tap that usually has three sharp blades with flutes or spaces between the blades into which debris can collect. By the use of a separate thread cutter, the preparation of the thread may be made 50 μm wider in diameter than the mating post, leaving 25 μm space on each side, into which the cement lute may flow. This space may also act as a vent during placement of the post.

Self-threading posts do not have the sharp blades of a thread cutter. Such systems compress the thread into the dentin, leaving a space of identical diameter as the thread crests, that is, there is no space for the luting cement. Cement, however, is an important element in making the threaded shank integrate into one unit with the root. There is not universal agreement as to the potential for such systems to generate stresses in the root tissue but there are considerations that pre-threading systems may result in a post with maximum retention and least stress distribution.
4. With regard to diameter, this must be sufficient to provide sufficient strength, while leaving sufficient tooth substance to avoid weakening or perforation of the remaining tooth, that is, clinical judgement is required.

It is also relevant to state that the success of the overall restoration is dependent upon the provision of an adequate root filling prior to placement of the post.

In addition to the above factors, retention of indirect posts is dependent on whether an anti-rotational device or ferrule effect is incorporated, and the luting material used. Suitable metals for cast posts constructed by an indirect technique include gold alloys.

39.2 CORE BUILD-UP MATERIALS

The success of a core build-up is dependent on a number of factors, principally,

- The properties of the core material;

- The means whereby the core is retained in the tooth;
- The clinical techniques used.

39.2.1 Ideal properties

A core build-up material ideally should possess the following properties:

1. Biocompatibility. The material should not be irritant to tooth tissue, and ideally should be capable of exerting a cariostatic effect on surrounding tooth substance.
2. Interfacial properties. The material should have the ability to bond to tooth structure and pins and/or posts. It should be capable of bonding to the luting cement.
3. Mechanical properties. Adequate strength in compression, tension and flexure is important.
4. Thermal properties. Low thermal diffusivity and coefficient of thermal expansion similar to that of dentin are both desirable.
5. Other important points include:

- Radiopacity similar to or greater than enamel;
- Ease of mixing and placement without the use of special equipment;
- Short setting time, in order to allow preparation at same visit as core placement;
- There should be no adverse reaction to temporary crown materials or cements;
- Sufficiently low in cost;
- Contrasting color to tooth;
- Capable of being added to.

39.2.2 Materials

Three core build-up materials appear to be used predominantly, namely, amalgam, composite and glass-ionomer. More recently, compomers have also been suggested as being suitable. Each material has its advantages and disadvantages. In clinical use, the core build-up material will be used in conjunction with pins or posts, or, alternatively, retention will be gained by extending the material into the pulp chamber in root filled teeth.

1. Amalgam (Chapter 24). The physical properties of amalgam make it suitable as a core build-up material. It is simple to use, it is radiopaque and has a contrasting color to tooth. However, it has high thermal conductivity and a higher coefficient of thermal expansion than tooth. It does not adhere

to tooth substance, although methods of bonding amalgam to tooth substance are now commonplace. A major disadvantage of amalgam as a core build-up material is the need for separate appointments for core build-up and crown preparation because of the slow set of conventional amalgam materials.

2. Composite/Compomer (Chapter 27). Composite materials also possess satisfactory physical properties for use as a core build-up material, although the only types which should be considered suitable are those which are radiopaque. They may be of contrasting color to tooth. These materials may be reliably bonded to tooth substance, and they may be command set to allow immediate crown preparation, although an incremental technique should be employed during placement to ensure complete polymerization at the base of the core. However, composite materials have a substantially higher coefficient of thermal expansion than tooth substance, which may increase the potential for microleakage if the core is exposed near the margin of the restoration.

More recently, compomers have also been suggested as core build-up materials. Their physical properties, although less good in some respects than composite, appear adequate. They are also capable of being bonded to tooth substance and may be command set.

3. Glass-ionomer cement (Chapter 26). Glass-ionomer materials are increasing in popularity because of advantageous properties such as adhesion to tooth substance and fluoride release. Their coefficient of thermal expansion is similar to that of tooth substance and they may be radiopaque and of contrasting color to tooth. However, although the compressive strengths of these materials may be considered suitable for a core build-up material, the flexural strength of conventional glass ionomer materials is low, making these materials unsuitable as core build-up materials unless they are well supported by tooth substance or pins and/or posts. Glass-ionomer variants such as cermets (Section 26.2) have been suggested as being suitable but have only minimal improvement in flexural strength as compared with conventional glass ionomers. Cermets are radiopaque.

More recently introduced glass-ionomer variants may overcome the deficiencies of the conventional glass-ionomers and cermets. Resin modified glass ionomers (RMGIs) have an increased flexural strength and adequate compressive strength. They bond reliably to tooth substance, may be of contrasting color to tooth and are capable of being command set, although they should be placed in increments so that they may be light cured and their physical properties thereby maximized. Some RMGIs are as radiopaque as enamel. These properties appear to make RMGIs suitable for use as core build-up materials.

Most recently, higher viscosity glass-ionomer materials have been introduced (Section 26.5). Their physical properties are also significantly improved as compared to conventional glass-ionomer materials, their setting time is short and colors that contrast to tooth are available. They may be placed in bulk rather than in increments. Little information is available as to their radiopacity. Notwithstanding this, these materials would also appear to hold promise as core build-up materials.

39.2.3 Choice of material

Most importantly, the ideal core build-up material should possess adequate physical properties to withstand applied forces, they should be capable of a one-visit core build-up and preparation, and should be capable of being bonded to tooth substance. The materials, RMGI, higher viscosity glass-ionomer, composite and compomer would appear to fulfil these criteria. It is then for the clinician to decide which material handles most easily in his/her clinical practice and to consider other aspects such as cost and time required for placement. If it is not necessary for the material to set sufficiently rapidly to allow crown preparation at the same visit as core build-up, amalgam may also be considered, provided that environmental considerations are acceptable, both to clinician and patient.

Table 39.1 presents a summary of comparative properties.

FURTHER READING

Edmunds D H, Dummer P M H (1993). Root canal retained restorations revisited. *Dental Update 20*: 14-20.

Bradigan T W (1988). Guidelines for the selection and insertion of posts: A review of the literature. *General Dentistry* **36**: 232-235.

Manning K E, Yu D C, Kwan E W (1995). Factors to consider for predictable post and core build-ups of endodontically treated teeth:

Part I: Basic theoretical concepts. *Journal of the Canadian Dental Association* **61**:685-686, 690, 693-695.

Part II: Clinical application of basic concepts. *Journal of the Canadian Dental Association* **61**: 696-701, 703, 705-707.

Table 39.1. Comparison of core build-up materials

Amalgam → AML; Resin composite → RC; Glass-ionomer → GI; Cermet → CER; Resin-modified glass-ionomer → RM GI; Viscous glass-ionomer → VGI; Compomer → CPR

Property	AML	RC	GI	CER	RM GI	VGI	CPR
Fluoride release	X	X	√	√	√	√	?
Bonding to tooth and pins	X	√**	√	√	√	√	√**
Bond to luting cement	X	√*	√*	√*	√*	√	√*
Adequate compressive strength	√√	√√	√	√	√	√	√√
Adequate flexural strength	√√	√√	X	?	√	√	√
Low thermal diffusivity	X	√	√	√	√	√	√
Coefficient of thermal expansion similar to tooth	X	X	√	√	√	√	X
Radiopacity greater than or equal to enamel	√	√*	X	√	√*	√	X
Ease of mixing and placement	√	X	√	√	√	√	√
No need for special equipment	√	√	√	√	√	√	√
Short setting time	X	√	√	√	√	√	√
No adverse reaction to temporary materials	√	X	√	√	√	√	√
Low cost	√	√	√	√	√	√	√
Contrasting color to tooth	√	√*	X	√	√*	√*	√*

√* - possible

√** - with intermediate system

Chapter 40

Tooth Bleaching Systems

Summary: The materials and techniques for bleaching both vital and non-vital teeth are considered.

40.1 INTRODUCTION

Interest in procedures that may improve the appearance of teeth, in particular their whiteness, appears to be increasing, and there is substantial media attention concerning such techniques. The majority of techniques which may improve esthetics are invasive to some degree, such as porcelain veneers, but bleaching may represent a variety of techniques which may be non-invasive. Indeed, bleaching of vital teeth has been a recognized technique in dentistry since the middle of the 19th century, when chloride of lime was used to bleach a non-vital teeth and 1864 when oxalic acid was used on a vital tooth. Bleaching techniques may be considered under two headings:

- Internal bleaching of discolored endodontically treated teeth;
- External bleaching of intrinsically discolored teeth.

40.2 INTERNAL BLEACHING

The most popular nonvital bleaching technique is the 'walking bleach' technique in which the coronal root filling is removed, rubber dam is applied, the root filling sealed with a base (of glass-ionomer, for example) and the internal dentin surfaces are etched with 35% phosphoric acid. A combination of 35% hydrogen peroxide and sodium perborate is mixed to a paste and this is sealed into the pulp chamber. The bleaching effect occurs while the patient is carrying on their normal daily activities and the dressing is changed at weekly intervals. The bleaching effect usually occurs after 2 to 3 changes of the bleaching solution. Alternatively, a thermocatalytic technique may be used. In this technique, the coronal root filling is removed, the root filling sealed with a base and 35% hydrogen peroxide is placed in the pulp chamber and the bleaching action activated by the placement of a heating instrument into the peroxide. Alternatively, sodium perborate may be used as it also releases oxygen, but more slowly. Some workers consider that when perborate is used, the risk of post-operative root resorption is reduced.

40.3 EXTERNAL BLEACHING

There are three methods of external bleaching:

- Thermocatalytic bleaching;
- Enamel microabrasion;
- Patient applied vital nightguard bleaching.

40.3.1 Thermocatalytic bleaching

In thermocatalytic bleaching, two approaches are possible – electric heating units and bleaching lights. Each method produces heat which causes the decomposition of hydrogen peroxide and the release of oxygen. In turn, the oxygen causes an oxidation reaction that causes release of discolored matter from the tooth. The tooth/teeth to be treated are isolated with rubber dam, cleaned with pumice and water, etched with 35% phosphoric acid and 35% (100 volumes) hydrogen peroxide applied in a gauze to the teeth. The heating tip is applied – it achieves a temperature of 35 - 55^0C – in bursts of up to 5 minutes over a 30 minute period. Alternatively, a bleaching light positioned in front of the patient directs a bright beam of light at the affected teeth for periods of up to 30 minutes, with the bleaching solution being replenished on the tooth surface as required. Up to six such visits may be required; successful results may be obtained but may be difficult to predict and regression may occur within a year. This form of bleaching has been considered to be most successful in treatment of yellow-brown tetracycline staining rather than with grey staining. The heat has a potential for pulp damage if applied too vigorously. Disadvantages of this technique include the need for *complete* isolation using rubber dam, the dangers of handling the extremely caustic 35% hydrogen peroxide solution and the unpredictability of the results.

40.3.2 Enamel microabrasion

This technique is used for the removal of superficial blemishes in the enamel, such as brown or white areas of fluorosis. It involves the application of a thick paste of 18% hydrochloric acid/pumice on to the blemish, usually by means of a wooden tongue blade. Up to 15 five-second applications may be required to eliminate the discoloration — such applications may remove up to 25% of the labial enamel. Following washing of the tooth with air/water, a non-acidulated fluoride gel should be applied. A product is now available which contains a low concentration of hydrochloric acid in an abrasive water-soluble gel for rotary instrument application.

40.3.3 Nightguard vital bleaching

Nightguard vital bleaching was introduced in 1989. This is a less hazardous and less complicated treatment than that described above. In this technique, 10%-15% carbamide peroxide is placed in a custom-made, close-fitting soft plastic prosthesis which has been constructed (usually by means of a vacuum forming technique) to cover the teeth which are to be treated. This is worn for several hours per day for several weeks. Carbamide peroxide is composed of approximately 3% hydrogen peroxide and 7% urea. The hydrogen peroxide degrades into water and oxygen and the urea degrades to ammonia and carbon dioxide. Some materials contain a high molecular weight resin polymer called Carbopol which thickens the bleach, making it more adherent to the teeth and prolonging its action. Carbamide peroxide has been used in the past as an oral antiseptic with no reported adverse effects but there is a small incidence of reported tooth sensitivity following treatment. No differences between enamel treated with carbamide peroxide and untreated enamel have been noted. Some increase in softness of resin composite specimens has been recorded following contact with carbamide peroxide for 4 hours per day for periods of up to 4 weeks. The release of urea from carbamide peroxide materials has also been considered to provide an anti-cariogenic effect.

40.3.4 Over-the-counter home bleaching systems

Soon after the introduction of dentist-applied/prescribed carbamide peroxide systems, a number of over-the-counter systems were introduced. These systems often had an acidic pre-rinse, a reduced concentration peroxide mouthwash and a titanium dioxide toothpaste. Their safety and efficacy is unproven.

FURTHER READING

Croll T P (1989). Enamel microabrasion: the technique. *Quintessence International* **20**: 395-400.

Fisher N L, Radford J R (1990). Internal bleaching of discoloured teeth. *Dental Update* **17**: 110-114.

Haywood V B, Heymann H O (1991). Nightguard vital bleaching: how safe is it? *Quintessence International* **22**: 515-523.

Haywood V B (1992). History, safety and effectiveness of current bleaching techniques and applications of the nightguard vital bleaching technique. *Quintessence International* **23**: 471-488.

Haywood V B (1996). Achieving, maintaining, and recovering successful tooth bleaching. *Journal of Esthetic Dentistry* **8**: 31-38.

Haywood V B (1997). Nightguard vital bleaching: current concepts and research. *Journal of the American Dental Association* **128** Supplement: 19S-25S.

Haywood V B (1997). Historical development of whiteners: Clinical safety and efficacy. *Dental Update* **24**: 98-104.

Chapter 41

Materials in Orthodontics

Summary: A wide range of materials for use in orthodontics is considered, including wires, brackets, bands, screws and polymers.

41.1 INTRODUCTION

Orthodontic appliances are employed to cause tooth movement for the treatment of malocclusion. An appliance is composed of active and reactive components. An active component applies a force to a tooth which is to be moved. This force should not be large enough to adversely affect the periodontal tissues, nor should it be too small. A reactive component anchors the appliances to teeth which are not to be moved.

Appliances may be classified as either removable or fixed. Removable appliances usually consist of a polymeric framework. This supports the active part which may consist of springs or rubber bands to apply a continuous force, or adjustable screws for the application of intermittent forces. Fixed appliances are secured in place by one or both of two techniques:

- By direct bonding of brackcts to acid-etched enamel;
- By using bands which are cemented around the clinical crown of a tooth.

41.2 TOOTH MOVEMENT

Tooth movement can be achieved by the application of a force to the tooth by an orthodontic appliance. In studying forces, it is necessary to specify the magnitude of the force, and the direction and point of application.

Tooth movement may be classified into the following five types:

1. Tipping movement, where force is applied to a single point on the crown of the tooth.
2. Rotational movements achieved by applying a force couple. Two equal (and opposite) forces F, separated by a distance d produce a moment $M = Fd$. For example, 2 forces of 0.3 N, 4 mm apart, produce a moment of 1.2 N mm.
3. Translation, or bodily, movement can occur if a force is applied to a large area of the crown of the tooth.
4. Extrusion of a tooth from its socket can be achieved.
5. Intrusion can also be carried out.

The magnitude of the applied force is important. Very heavy force can damage periodontal tissues. The correct force depends on which type of movement is required, and also on the geometry of the tooth roots. For bodily movements, forces of up to 3 N have been quoted, other procedures require typically 0.25 to 0.5 N.

41.3 INTRODUCTION TO FORCE MECHANICS

Basically a wire in an appliance can be considered as a beam. From an orthodontic viewpoint, three parameters need to be considered:

- The rigidity, often referred to as the load-deflection rate;
- The maximum load, or allowable working load, related to the elastic limit;
- The maximum deflection; related to the maximum amount of elastic strain.

41.3.1 Rigidity

For the flexure of a cantilever beam, the flexural rigidity = $E\pi r^4/4$, where E = modulus of elasticity and r = radius of the wire. Thus flexure depends both on material properties (E) and geometry (r).

The load-deflection rate also depends on the length L of the wire; it is universally proportional to L^3. For a rectangular wire, load-deflection rate is proportional to bh^3, where h is the dimension of the wire in the direction of bending and b is the width of the specimen.

Doubling the modulus will double the rigidity, but doubling the radius has a considerably greater effect. Consider two wires, of the same material, of modulus E, one with radius x, one with radius $2x$. The flexural rigidity of the first wire = $E\pi x^4/4$. For the second wire, flexural rigidity = $16E\pi x^4/4$. Thus wire 2 has a rigidity 16 times greater than wire 1.

When a material is in torsion the load-deflection rate is proportional to $1/L$, where L is the length in torsion.

41.3.2 Allowable working load.

Allowable working load is proportional to the elastic limit. For a circular wire, it is proportional to r^3 and $1/L$. For a rectangular wire, it is proportional to bh^2.

41.3.3 Maximum deflection

Maximum deflection depends on the elastic limit divided by modulus of elasticity. For a circular wire, this parameter is proportional to $1/r$, and to L^2. For a rectangular wire, it is proportional to $1/h$.

41.3.4 Geometry of wire

The above discussion is designed to introduce the subject, showing how mechanical properties and geometrical design are both important. Many other factors can be studied from the references at the end of the chapter, such as the use of braided wires, loops, etc.

41.4 WIRES

41.4.1 Desirable mechanical properties

Separate consideration must be given to the requirements for active and reactive components. Reactive components, which anchor the appliance to teeth that are not to be moved, should not deform. Thus high values of both yield stress and modulus of rigidity are important.

Active components must ideally have great flexibility. A more flexible component will be able to apply lower and a more constant force over a greater distance. Note that flexibility is a function both of mechanical properties and the geometry of the material, as discussed above. High resilience is also required; the material should be able to store and release elastic energy.

41.4.2 Materials

Since inert corrosion resistant alloys are required for oral use, only a limited range of materials can be used, as detailed below.

1. Stainless steel. The method of production of wires has been discussed in Section 12.2.2. Figure 12.13 shows the type of fibrous structure that results from such cold working. As well as a change in structure, the properties of the alloy are altered; cold working increases the tensile strength and hardness, but reduces the ductility.

Dental stainless steel wires are made from the austenitic (18-8) material (Section 13.7). During the working of the wire to the required form in the dental laboratory, further work hardening occurs. If a considerable amount of such working is necessary the ductility may be reduced to the point where fracture occurs. To avoid this risk it is necessary to choose a material that will withstand the required degree of working. Three grades of stainless steel wire are usually required: 'soft', 'half-hard' and 'hard'. If much cold working is to be carried out, a softer material should be selected, as it will work harden during manipulation. Conversely, a harder material can be selected if there is to be little cold-working.

With stainless steel wires it is not possible to apply heat treatment to restore the ductility of the wire during the working procedure. This is because a minimum temperature of around 500 °C is necessary to produce any degree of stress relief annealing. However, if some wires are heated for a prolonged period in the temperature range 500-900 °C, a reaction occurs between chromium and carbon, with the formation of chromium carbide and its precipitation at the grain boundaries. This should be avoided in practice because the alloy becomes more brittle due to slip interference of the precipitated carbide, and because the corrosion resistance is reduced because there is less chromium left in the grains to produce the required passivating effect.

The above phenomenon is called *weld decay*. It can be avoided by either having an alloy of very low carbon content, so that carbides will not be precipitated. In practice it is difficult and expensive to completely remove carbon from steel. Alternatively *stabilized stainless steel* may be used, which contains small quantities of either titanium or columbium. These constituents form carbides more readily than chromium, leaving the latter metal in solid solution.

Full restoration of ductility necessitates heating the wire to a temperature above 950 °C, when recrystallization occurs. This gives a fine

equiaxed grain structure, but destroys the fibrous structure of the wire, on which its 'springiness' depends.
2. Cobalt-chromium. The composition and properties of such materials are discussed in relation to their use for cast partial dentures (Section 13.2). The wrought materials can be heat-treated by an age hardening process, though the wires are usually pre-treated by the manufacturer.
3. Nickel-chromium. Wires are supplied in an alloy containing 80% nickel and 20% chromium. These wires are also used in the manufacture of heating elements because of their comparatively high electrical resistivity.
4. Nickel-titanium. These alloys contain nickel and titanium in the ratio 55/45 by weight, giving the intermetallic compound NiTi. They undergo a transition from a martensitic to an austenitic structure when heated above a transition temperature range. Below this temperature range, the alloys can readily be deformed plastically. On heating the alloy above this temperature range, the alloy recovers its original shape. This is called a 'shape-memory' effect, and can be used in orthodontics where mouth temperature activates this effect. A small quantity of cobalt may be present to lower the temperature transition range. Some nickel-titanium alloys also contain copper (about 1.6-1.8 atomic percent).
5. Beta-titanium. Titanium can exist in an α-form (hexagonal close packed structure) below 885°C and a ß-form (body centered cubic structure) at higher temperatures (Section 13.9.1). With the incorporation of alloying elements, α-titanium is stable at room temperature. A typical composition of such an alloy (weight %) is 79% Ti, 11% Mo, 6% Zr, 4%Sn. Titanium has excellent corrosion resistance.
6. Gold alloys. The functions of alloying elements on the properties of gold are discussed in Section 13.5.2. Gold alloy wires may be of the following types:
- Simple ternary alloys of gold, copper and silver;
- Platinized alloys, with 10 to 20% platinum and palladium;
- Highly platinized alloys, with up to 50% platinum and palladium.

As with stainless steel wires, these materials have a fibrous structure. Sufficient heating to cause recrystallization must be avoided if the resilience of the wire is to be retained. The more highly platinized alloys have higher recrystallization temperatures, so are indicated for use when soldering is to be carried out.

41.4.3 Properties

From Table 41.1, it can be seen that, in general, the chromium-containing alloys (stainless steel, nickel-chromium and cobalt-chromium) have higher moduli of elasticity than gold and titanium alloys. The flexibility of the modern titanium alloys is a useful property, as they can apply an active force to a tooth over a greater distance than a stainless steel wire of similar geometry.

Table 41.1. Mechanical properties of wrought alloys

Material	Condition	Modulus of elasticity (GPa)	Pro-portional limit (MPa)	Ultimate tensile strength (MPa)	Elong-ation (%)	Hardness (BHN)
Cobalt-chromium	Work hardened	240	1000	1800	2	250
Gold alloy	Work hardened	95	550	825	3	220
Nickel-chromium	Work hardened	210	900	1350	1	225
Stainless steel	Soft	200	280	620	50	170
	Medium	200	1050	1250	6	250
	Hard	300	1450	1700	1	350
Titanium	Work hardened	100	500	750	30	200
Ti alloy (6Al/4V)	Work hardened	120	1100	1200	12	300

41.5 BRACKETS, BANDS AND SCREWS

Prefabricated components such as brackets, bands and screws are usually made from stainless steel. Brackets for direct bonding techniques (see below) are designed to bond mechanically to the resin; this is achieved either by a metal mesh on, or by perforation in, the bracket. Polymeric brackets (e.g. polycarbonate) have not proved to be particularly successful, owing to their inadequate strength properties.

Ceramic brackets are preferred from an esthetic viewpoint, but some limitations should be noted. Bracket fracture can occur. Hard ceramics can abrade opposing natural dentition. Tooth damage during bracket removal can also occur.

Almost exclusively bands are cemented to the crowns of molar teeth, using, for example, a glass-ionomer cement.

41.6 ORTHODONTIC BASE POLYMERS

Autopolymerizing acrylic resins, similar to those used for denture repair, are available for this purpose. The main constituents of these materials are as follows:

1. Powder. Predominately poly(methyl methacrylate), some products with lesser amounts of polystyrene, poly(ethyl methacrylate) or poly(butyl methacrylate). At least one product is mainly poly(ethyl methacrylate).
2. Liquid. This is methyl methacrylate, with 0 to 6% ethylene glycol dimethacrylate.

In addition, peroxide and amine components will be present in powder and liquid respectively. The materials are formulated to facilitate their handling by the technician. These resins are in general softer and less rigid than denture materials.

Visible light cure acrylic resins are also advocated for orthodontic use.

41.7 ELASTIC MODULES

Elastic modules can be made either from natural rubber, or from synthetic polyester-urethane elastomers. These modules exhibit stress relaxation, owing to their viscoelastic nature (Section 5.7.1, Figure 5.12). Thus, the force exerted by a module will decrease as a function of time.

41.8 DIRECT BONDING MATERIALS

The bonding resins are often filled dimethacrylates, similar in principle to composite restorative materials (Chapter 27). These resins bond mechanically to the brackets and to acid etched enamel. The procedures for acid etching should be followed carefully (Section 19.3, Table 19.2). Alternative orthodontic cementing media are also available including glass-ionomers, resin-modified glass-ionomers and compomers.

Some advantages of direct bonding techniques include better esthetics, the ability for precise placement of brackets and the ability to bond on to unerupted and partially erupted teeth.

Following orthodontic treatment, the mechanical debonding of brackets may damage the enamel surface of teeth. There may be loss of natural luster and a roughened surface.

FURTHER READING

Burstone C J (1994). Application of bioengineering to clinical orthodontics. *Orthodontics—Current Principles and Techniques.*(editors: Graber T M, Vandersall R L) 2nd edn., Mosby, St Louis. pp 235-267.

Kusy R P (1997). A review of contemporary archwires: their properties and characteristics. *Angle Orthodontist* **67**: 197-207.

Kusy R P (1998). The future of orthodontic materials: the long-term view. *American Journal of Orthodontics & Dentofacial Orthopedics.* **113**: 91-95.

Baty D L, Storie D J, von Fraunhofer J A (1994). Synthetic elastomeric chains: a literature review. *American Journal of Orthodontics & Dentofacial Orthopedics* **105**: 536-542.

Karamouzos A, Athanasiou A E, Papadopoulos M A (1997). Clinical characteristics and properties of ceramic brackets: A comprehensive review. *American Journal of Orthodontics & Dentofacial Orthopedics* **112**: 34-40.

Zachrisson B U (1994). Bonding in orthodontics. *Orthodontics — Current Practice and Techniques.* (editors: Graber T M, Vanarsdall R L) 2nd edn., Mosby, St Louis. pp 542-626.

Chapter 42

Mouth Guards

Summary: Polymeric materials are available which reduce or eliminate orofacial injuries in sports players. These mouthguard materials are described, classified and critiqued.

42.1 INDICATIONS

Dental injuries are the commonest type of orofacial injury sustained during participation in sports. Many are preventable through wearing a professionally fitted (custom made) mouthguard.

Principal causes of dental trauma are sporting accidents and accidents at home. The maxillary central and lateral incisors are the teeth most affected by trauma, accounting for four-fifths of all cases, with the central incisors being involved over four times as frequently as the lateral incisors. The risk of injury in contact sports is greater than in non-contact sports, and the dental profession therefore has an important role to play in advising patients of the risk and on how to reduce the potential for injuries to teeth and supporting structures. Mandatory dental protection for all players involved in contact sports would have major effects in preventing unnecessary dental injuries and associated life-long discomfort, as well as reducing the high treatment costs involved. Furthermore, there may be a significant reduction in the risk of concussion injury following an impact to the mandible if a mouthguard is worn.

42.2 HISTORICAL DEVELOPMENT

Protective mouthguards were first developed in the early 1900s and consisted of a piece of rubber suitably trimmed and hollowed out. This was worn on the upper teeth in the sport of boxing but had no adaptation to the teeth, so retention could only be achieved by clenching the teeth together. Mouthguard technology developed rapidly in the 1950s and 1960s when extensive field studies and material testing were undertaken. Early work identified that mouthguards should be worn on the maxillary teeth, as it was evident that the maxillary anterior teeth were the most prone to injury except in a Class III malocclusion when the mouthguard should be worn on the mandibular teeth. In 1962 a mandatory mouthguard rule was adopted in the USA by the National Alliance Football Rules Committee, with a recommendation that the mouthguard should be constructed from a model made from an impression of the athlete's teeth.

42.3 MATERIAL REQUIREMENTS

Ideally, a mouthguard should be made of resilient material and should cover all the remaining teeth of one arch, customarily the maxilla. To provide effective protection, a mouth protector should:

- Be impact absorbing;
- Be fitted to the individual's mouth and accurately adapted to the mouth structures;
- Have smooth well contoured edges;
- Should be retained comfortably and securely;
- Should be capable of being cleaned easily and should not remit any unpleasant odors or tastes.

From the player's viewpoint, the most important qualities of a mouth protector are retention, comfort and fit, ease of speech, resistance to tearing, ease of breathing and protection of the teeth, gingiva and lips.

42.4 CLASSIFICATION

Mouthguards fall into three categories, stock, mouth-formed and custom-made. Typical stock mouthguards (unfitted) can be bought at sports stores. These may only be considered to provide a low level of protection and little retention.

The mouth-formed mouthguard is relatively inexpensive and can be replaced more frequently over time. They are available from sports shops and are softened in hot water and molded to fit the teeth of the individual.

Custom-made mouthguards are normally constructed from vacuum formed poly(vinyl acetate-ethylene) co-polymer – see Figure 42.1 – in a variety of colors and thicknesses, from 3 mm to 5 mm on the labial and incisal aspects of the anterior teeth to 1 mm across the palate. Colored versions were originally developed for water sports as they are easier to locate if they accidentally fall to the bottom of the pool.

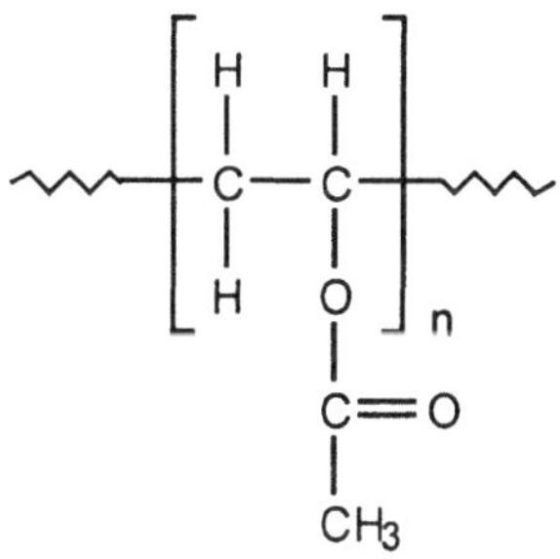

Figure 42.1. Poly(vinyl acetate).

42.5 ADVANTAGES AND DISADVANTAGES OFDIFFERENT MOUTHGUARD TYPES

Stock mouthguards, while comparatively inexpensive, are often loose, cumbersome, and may interfere with speech and breathing. Furthermore, they may require the jaws to be closed to keep them in position. Mouth-formed protectors may be either the shell-liner device or thermoplastic types. The shell-liner mouthguard consists of an outer poly(vinyl chloride) shell, which is filled with a soft liner made from plasticized acrylic gel or from silicone rubber. Disadvantages of this type include decreased retention because of repeated biting into the liner material, hardening of the soft liner as a result of exposure to oral fluids, increased vertical dimension, decreased comfort and bulkiness. Thermoplastic types have several advantages. They may be refitted if not properly made at the first attempt, they have comparatively low bulk, and all necessary fitting procedures are accomplished in one session. Disadvantages include the possibility of distortion of the buccal flange with time, and hardening of the mouthguard material from continued exposure to oral fluids.

Custom-made mouthguards have a number of advantages over other types. These include best retention, fit, comfort and acceptance, with the ability to adapt such mouthguards to orthodontic appliances or erupting teeth. The mouthguards do not deteriorate rapidly with use. The protective functions afforded by such mouthguards include prevention of laceration of the tongue, lips and cheeks against the sharp edges of the maxillary teeth, substantial reduction of the risk of injury to the anterior maxillary teeth.

The latest type of mouthguard, the bimaxillary mouthguard, was designed in the early 1980s. It covers both dental arches with the mandible fixed at a predetermined maximum breathing position, which allows the athlete to maintain adequate oral ventilation during strenuous exertion. The bimaxillary design allows the mandible to be stabilized in a position which increases the degree of protection against fractures and temporomandibular joint capsule injuries, and makes the wearer less susceptible to concussion.

42.6 FABRICATION

Mouthguards are usually made from a poly(vinyl acetate) co-polymer, adapted by compressed air or vacuum. After outlining the periphery on the cast with a marking pencil and spraying the model with a silicone spray, the poly(vinyl acetate) is heated and placed over the cast by a pressure forming method, using pressure of around 550 kPa, or a vacuum forming procedure. The mouthguard is then cooled in water and trimmed and the cut margins smoothed using a micro-torch. The mouthguard should be adjusted so that there is even contact between its occlusal surface and the lower dentition on closure of the mandible. This may be carried out using burs, or alternatively, the occlusal surface of the mouthguard may be gently heated and the patient asked to close into the softened surface. This will help to more evenly distribute impact forces to the maxilla following traumatic closure of the mandible, thereby reducing the risk of injury.

The bimaxillary mouthguard is constructed in a manner similar to that of the custom made maxillary mouthguard. The maximum breathing position is simulated using a cycle of different duration of inspirations and exhalations. An occlusal record is then taken and used to articulate the patient's models on a fully adjustable articulator. The two custom mouthguards are then fused together by flasking, or more conveniently with heat. The cost of such a mouthguard is higher, but it provides excellent fit and retention, no noticeable impairment of oral breathing, excellent orofacial protection and high player acceptance when compared to other types.

42.7 CARE OF MOUTHGUARDS

The mouthguard should be kept moist to maintain flexibility and resilience and should therefore be kept in a rigid sealable container containing a dilute antiseptic mouthrinse. After use, the mouthguard should be washed with clean water then replaced in the container. Soap and a toothbrush may be necessary for adequate cleaning. It is generally accepted that children should be provided with mouthguards when they commence playing in organized contact sports. Deciduous teeth may be blocked out on the cast to extend the life of the custom mouthguard.

FURTHER READING

Scott J, Burke F J T, Watts D C (1994). A review of dental injuries and the use of mouthguards in contact team sports. *British Dental Journal* **176:** 310-314.

Chapman P J (1989). Mouthguards and the role of the sporting team dentists. *Australian Dental Journal* **34:** 36-42.

Sane J, Ylipaavalniemi P (1988). Dental trauma in contact team sports. *Endodontics and Dental Traumatology* **4:** 164-169.

American Dental Association Bureau of Health Education and Audiovisual Services and Council on Dental Materials, Instruments and Equipment (1984). Mouth protectors and sports team dentists. *Journal of the American Dental Association* **109:** 84-87.

XI

THE SELECTION OF RESTORATIVE MATERIALS

Chapter 43

Choice of Materials for the Restoration of Teeth

Summary: For many tooth restorations the operator is faced with a wide choice of materials and techniques. In this chapter the various materials are assessed, and principles of material selection are provided.

43.1 INTRODUCTION

The correct choice of a material to restore a cavity or defect is central to the provision of a successful long-term restoration. A quarter of a century ago, the clinician had a meager variety of materials from which to chose, among those being amalgam, silicate, early resin composites, cast gold, acrylic/gold and early porcelains. Today the clinicians' restorative armamentarium is enormous – amalgam, resin composites of many types, compomers, glass-ionomers of various types, ceramics of many types constructed in a variety of methods, metal-ceramic, reinforced composite and a range of cast alloys. There are often therefore a variety of materials appropriate to a given clinical problem. The requirements for materials for oral use have been outlined in Section 2.2. These include the biological, interfacial, chemical, mechanical and esthetic properties of the material as well as its practicability and ease of use.

However, the choice of material for a given clinical situation is complex because many factors need to be considered. Data obtained from *in vitro* testing of materials are of value, but they do not predict a material's performance *in vivo*. Cost effectiveness is related not only to material cost and time of placement, but also to long term durability.

In addition there are other factors to take into consideration. The choice of material is also related to patients' needs and preferences. Operator preference must also be taken into account.

There is no perfect substitute for tooth substance, and no material has all the ideal requirements for any particular clinical application. One of the problems is that so many materials are of recent origin, thus long-term clinical data are not available. The aim of this chapter is to critique materials in such a way that the reader can develop a systematic approach to making informed personal choices.

Factors to be considered can be summarized in the following questions:

- What laboratory evidence is available, following the pattern set out in Chapter 2?
- What will be the clinical performance of the material?
- Are esthetic considerations important?
- Are there any specific factors relating to the patient's clinical needs?
- Does the patient have specific preferences for (or against) a specific material?
- Does the operator have specific preferences? Are there any risks to dental staff associated with the use of a particular material?
- How cost effective is the treatment?
- Are there any environmental factors to be taken into consideration?

Each of these questions is explored, followed by the application of these principles to selected clinical situations.

43.2 FACTORS TO BE CONSIDERED

43.2.1 Evidence from laboratory data

1. Effect on tissues. The clinician should be aware of the potential effect of a given material on the periodontal and pulpal tissues. For example, if a material is to be placed subgingivally, the surface must be capable of being polished to minimize the potential for plaque accumulation, and if the material is being placed close to the pulp, it should be of a material that is unlikely to exert an inflammatory response. The clinician should also be aware that certain restorative materials are implicated in the pathogenesis of mucosal lesions such as lichen planus but that the risk of true allergy to materials is low.

2. Caries resistance. The ability to resist the recurrence of caries around a restoration is an ideal requirement of any restoration. Cariostatic activity was a property of the previously used silicate cement because of the high levels of fluoride ions which leached from the material and which were in solution around the restoration. Other restorative systems, such as the glass-

ionomer cement family, also release fluoride, but whether the amount of fluoride released is sufficient to inhibit caries at the restoration margin is currently a matter for discussion. However, it may be considered that some fluoride release is better than no fluoride release. Fluoride releasing materials may therefore be considered appropriate for high caries-active patients.

3. Margin quality. The achievement of a margin of good quality with no leakage is an ideal requirement for a satisfactory restoration. However, for example, the achievement of a good marginal seal may be difficult at the margin of a deep approximal cavity in all cases but more difficult with a resin-based restoration and an alternative should be considered in such a situation.

4. Chemical durability. Consideration must be given to a material's ability to withstand the hostile effects of the oral environment – for example, dissolution and corrosion effects must be considered.

5. Mechanical properties such as compressive, tensile and flexural strength. In general, the forces on a small restoration may be less than on a large restoration. The pre-operative assessment of the potential forces on a restoration is therefore central to success in restoring a lesion of caries by examining the number and severity of the occlusal contacts on the site to be restored. Situations in which the contacts are few in number and light may be restored in a material which demonstrates less than optimal resistance to wear. Notwithstanding this, however, all restorations in occlusal contact will be subjected to forces of a compressive, tensile and shear nature (Figure 43.1) and these physical properties must be adequate if the restoration is not to fail prematurely.

6. Wear resistance. This should, ideally, be similar to that of tooth substance, yet the material should not abrade or wear the opposing dentition. The operator should be aware of the wear resistance of the material, with highest wear resistance being required for a patient with parafunctional habits, and lower wear resistance being required for the elderly patient with reduced muscle strength, or in situations where the restoration is opposed by a denture. Forces on molar teeth are generally greater than forces on bicuspids and anterior teeth so the wear resistance of restorations in molar teeth should be optimal.

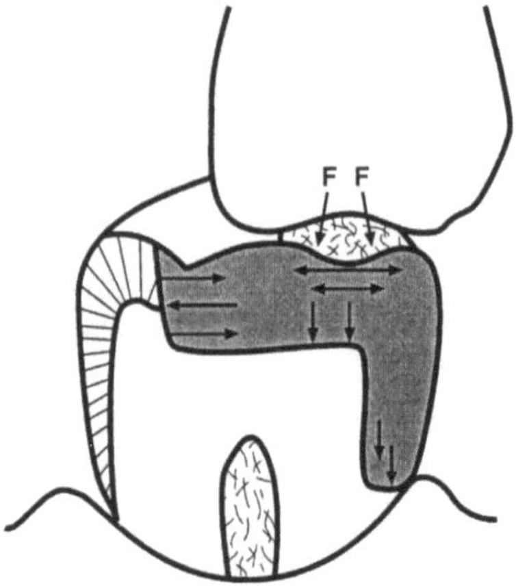

Figure 43.1. Compressive, tensile and shear forces on a dental restoration.

7. Other physical properties – coefficient of thermal expansion. A material with a different coefficient of thermal expansion to tooth substance will expand and contract at different rates to the tooth when hot and cold foods or liquids are applied. This may lead to marginal leakage. This is of particular relevance for materials used for core build-ups where there could be potentially differences in coefficient of thermal expansion between not only the core and the tooth but also between the core and the material from which the crown is constructed.
8. Dimensional changes. Polymerization shrinkage stresses the bond between the restoration and the tooth. The adhesion of the restorative either *per se* or by means of an intermediate bonding system, must be sufficient to withstand this stress.

43.2.2 Clinical performance

It has been considered that physical properties of a material cannot reliably predict the performance of a material in a given clinical situation. It is therefore a responsibility for clinicians to have evidence that the material being used is adequate and appropriate for the purpose for which it is used. This evidence, ideally, should be in the form of results from clinical trials or systematic reviews or meta-analyses of the literature. However, such data in dentistry are limited, possibly because of the cost of mounting such trials, and because advances in materials often lead to the development and production of a new version or a new material by the time the results of the clinical trails have become available. However, this is the era of 'evidence-based' dentistry and, with the increasing computerization of dental offices and the increased availability of information via that route, the time is approaching when clinicians (and patients) will routinely request information as to the likely success of a given restoration or restorative technique before the placement of a restoration.

43.2.3 Esthetic considerations

Patients are increasingly requesting tooth-colored restorations and are therefore likely to expect that esthetic restorations can be provided for both anterior and posterior teeth. In this respect, tooth-colored materials (resin composite) are now available which have been shown to perform satisfactorily in posterior teeth.

43.2.4 The patient's clinical needs

All patients present with differing problems and different materials will therefore be appropriate for different patients. The patient factors which require consideration therefore include:

1. Dental status. If the dentition is well supported, the forces on a load-bearing restoration will be less than if the dentition is not well supported.
2. Oral hygiene. If oral hygiene is inadequate and the patient is failing to respond to oral hygiene advice:
   - A restoration with some potential for cariostatic activity should be considered;
   - A restorative material that will not accumulate plaque should be used.
3. Size and nature of the caries. A large cavity is likely to have greater applied forces than a small cavity, a cavity with a wide contact will provide a greater challenge in restoring the contact area satisfactorily than a cavity with a narrow isthmus.
4. The function of the tooth to be restored. A restoration in a molar is likely to receive higher loading than a restoration in a bicuspid or anterior tooth, and the forces exerted on a restoration in a patient with parafunctional habits are likely to be greater than those in a patient without such habits.
5. Access to the cavity. If easy access to a cavity is possible, then the clinician may chose any of the restorative materials at his/her disposal, notwithstanding the other factors involved. However, if access is limited or difficult because of poor patient compliance, then the clinician will be

forced to choose only those materials which are technique insensitive and quick to place.

6. The ability to isolate the cavity. An inability to isolate the cavity will again limit the materials which may be used and it may be that the patient in this category will be forced to accept a transitional restoration or a restoration of reduced longevity.

7. Patient cooperation. The comments in the previous sections also apply to the uncooperative patient.

43.2.5 The patient's personal preferences

Patients are increasingly well informed on dental techniques and materials, and there appears to be increasing anxiety, expressed by some patients, concerning the use of materials containing mercury. It is for the operator to inform the patient about what techniques and materials are available for a particular restorative situation and for the patient to make an informed decision on the potential longevity of the restoration and its cost effectiveness.

43.2.6 The operator's preferences

Clinicians have preferences in materials. These preferences will be based upon his/her ability to manipulate the material, that is. its handling characteristics, including the time required to use the material or technique. The operator's preference will also be based upon their perception of the performance of the material in their own office. In the past, this was based on an anecdotal observation of patients at recall. However, with the increasing computerization of dental offices, it will become possible for the dentist to assess the longevity of the restorations that he or she places. Furthermore, the operator who is informed about the results in the research dental literature will be in a position to assess a preference of a material or technique in a given situation.

43.2.7 Cost effectiveness

The increasing cost of dental treatment has inevitably led to discussions on cost-effectiveness of a given material or technique, or health economics when a health system is examined in its entirety. Discussions with patients may therefore relate to the potential longevity of a material and the comfort of the restoration in a given situation with respect to the cost of the alternatives, for example the different costs and effectiveness of a direct placement composite *versus* an indirect restoration.

Another concept is that of the interim restoration, in which the operator and patient elect to place a restoration which lacks the necessary physical properties for ideal longevity, but which may provide a low-cost compromise. In such cases, it may be possible to employ a more conservative approach to cavity design, and thereby to retain as many options as possible for the future management of the tooth. This may include the re-surfacing of a glass-ionomer restoration with, for example, resin composite after a period in function. This approach would appear to hold the attraction of low initial cost, but can only be sanctioned if it is certain that the interim restoration will not cause irreparable problems. The concept of interim restorations still necessitates a life-long management strategy for teeth for patients, for whatever reason, are unable or unwilling to accept or fund the ideal restorative solution.

43.2.8 Environmental considerations

Regarding the use of amalgam, while there is sufficient evidence to demonstrate that its use is not unsafe for the patient, the environment suffers if quantities of amalgam or mercury are discharged into the dental surgery effluent or when mercury vapor is discharged from crematoria.

43.3 SUMMARY OF COMPARATIVE PROPERTIES

Based on the above considerations, the properties of the most frequently used restorative dental materials may be summarized in Tables 43.1 and 43.2.

Table 43.1. Comparison of direct restorative materials

	Amalgam	Resin composite	Glass-ionomer	Cermet	Resin-modified glass-ionomer	Viscous glass-ionomer	Compomer
Property	AML	RC	GI	CER	RM GI	VGI	CPR
Fluoride release	X	X	√	√	√	√	?
Adequate compressive strength	√√	√√	√	√	√	√	√√
Adequate flexural strength	√√	√√	X	?	√	√	√
Low thermal diffusivity	X	√	√	√	√	√	√
Coefficient of thermal expansion similar to tooth	X	X	√	√	√	√	X
Esthetics	X	√√	√	X	√	√	√√
Radiopacity greater than or equal to enamel	√	√*	X	√	√*	√	X
Ease of mixing and placement	√	X	√	√	√	√	√
No need for special equipment	√	√	√	√	√	√	√
Short setting time	X	√	√	√	√	√	√
Low cost	√	√	√	√	√	√	√

√* - possible

Table 43.2. Comparison of indirect restorative materials

	Compomer	Ceramic	Cast gold	Indirect resin composite
Property	CPR	CRM	Au	RC
Cariostatic	?	X	X	X
Bonding to tooth substance	√	√*	X	√
Adequate compressive strength	√	√	√	√
Adequate flexural strength	√	X	√	√
Low thermal diffusivity	√	√	X	√
Coefficient of thermal expansion similar to Tooth	X	√	X	X
Radiopacity greater than or equal to enamel	√*	X	√	√
Ease of mixing and placement	√	?	√	?
No need for special equipment	√	√	√	√
Low cost	X	X	X	X

√* - possible

43.4 THE SELECTION OF RESTORATIVE MATERIALS

43.4.1 What should I use for permanent restorations in anterior teeth?

Based on the properties summarized in Table 43.1, the material of choice for direct restoration of anterior teeth is resin composite, bonded in place using an enamel and dentin bonding system. Its esthetic properties, an important factor for an anterior restoration, are superior to compomer or glass-ionomer as also are its physical properties and resistance to wear and degradation in oral fluids. However, if the patient has high caries activity, a restoration in glass-ionomer may be indicated as an interim restoration, which could then be reduced and the surface 1.5-2.0 mm replaced with resin composite if and when the patient's caries activity has been controlled. Compomers may be preferred by a number of clinicians because of the ease of handling of these materials and because they release a small amount of fluoride. However, their wear resistance and esthetic properties are not as good as resin composite, and they may be less stain resistant.

If a crown is required due to the extent of loss of tooth tissue, the materials of choice are ceramic or metal/ceramic, depending on:

- The occlusal clearance;
- Occlusal forces which are likely to be applied;
- The esthetic result which is required.

Metal/ceramic provides a more fracture resistant restoration but has potentially poorer esthetics because of the need to mask the underlying metal framework. Reinforced ceramics are also available. Dentin-bonded all-ceramic crowns are increasingly providing long-term, fracture resistant, minimal preparation restorations of good esthetics.

43.4.2 What should I use for permanent load-bearing restorations in posterior teeth?

Based on the properties summarized in Table 43.1, the material of choice for direct restoration of all classes of cavity in posterior teeth remains amalgam in view of its good physical properties, ease of handling and low cost. However, increasingly, patients are requesting tooth-colored restorations in posterior teeth and environmental concerns have been expressed over the use of amalgam. For small to medium restorations, therefore, directly placed resin composite, bonded in place using an enamel and dentin bonding system, is an increasingly good alternative. The wear resistance of most contemporary resin composite materials may now be considered satisfactory for all but the more extreme occlusal situations and a good esthetic result may be provided. However, restorations of posterior teeth in resin composite may take up to three times as long to complete as similar restorations in amalgam. They are also more technique sensitive to place both in respect of the achievement of a good contact with the adjacent tooth and in the need for incremental placement. Thus the cost of resin composite restorations in posterior teeth is substantially greater than equivalent amalgam restorations.

More recently introduced materials such as compomer, heavily-filled glass-ionomer and resin-modified glass-ionomer lack the necessary wear resistance for the majority of load-bearing restorations in posterior teeth. However, these restorations are less technique sensitive than resin-composite and may therefore provide cost-effective long-term transitional restorations provided that the patient is prepared to accept the suboptimal physical properties.

For large restorations, cast gold may provide a long-lasting restoration, while for patients requiring a tooth-colored restorations, ceramic or composite inlays are indicated.

43.4.3 What should I use for permanent non-load-bearing restorations in posterior teeth?

These are predominantly Class V carious cavities or non-carious lesions. Adhesive techniques are indicated in view of the difficulties in preparing retentive cavities in these situations and in view of the need to conserve tooth substance.

The materials suggested are therefore:

1. Resin composite in situations where esthetics is the prime consideration, with some operators preferring to use 'flowable' composites for these situations. The latter materials have the advantage of being sufficiently flexible to deform as the tooth flexes under loading.
2. Compomer materials are also suitable where esthetics is less critical. These materials have gained widespread acceptance and are easier to use then glass-ionomer.
3. Traditional glass-ionomer materials where fluoride release is considered of value. These materials also are sufficiently flexible to flex with the tooth, a factor considered to be of importance in Class V situations.

4. Resin-modified glass-ionomer materials also have moderate popularity in many countries, again with the advantage of fluoride release.

Metallic restorative materials such as amalgam or compacted gold may be used for restoration of Class V cavities but these materials will require the preparation of a retentive cavity, with the potential need for removal of sound tooth structure.

43.4.4 What should I use for the restoration of deciduous teeth?

Restorations in deciduous teeth differ from those in posterior teeth in that it is not necessary for them to provide such a long-lasting restoration given the reduced life span of deciduous teeth. Considerations of relevance in the choice of material include the co-operation of the patient, the need for fluoride release and the smaller occlusal forces on these restorations as compared with those placed on permanent teeth. While amalgam has been used for many years as a restorative for deciduous teeth, it is necessary to cut a retentive cavity preparation and this may not always be possible due to less-than-optimum patient co-operation, let alone the need to remove sound tooth substance. Glass-ionomer materials, in particular the recently-introduced heavily-filled 'condensable' materials would appear to have benefits over amalgam in terms of their adhesion to enamel and dentin and their release of fluoride, while compomer materials provide ease of handling and rapid command set.

Preformed stainless steel crowns have been shown to provide good long-term restorations in deciduous teeth which have large cavities.

43.4.5 What material(s) should I use in conjunction with amalgam?

Amalgam is a poor thermal insulator. A base is therefore indicated beneath amalgam restorations if it is considered that insufficient dentin is present beneath the restoration to provide insulation from hot and cold stimuli. Bases currently used beneath amalgam restorations include calcium hydroxide-containing liners that provide good thermal insulation but do not bond to the underlying tooth. Resin-modified glass ionomer materials appear to possess the necessary physical properties for bases under amalgam restorations and have advantages of fluoride release and reliable adhesion to tooth substance. These would therefore appear to be the material of choice if a base is indicated.

An alternative concept is that amalgam restorations produce sensitivity because they leak at the margins and that this gives rise to the sensitivity. This problem may be addressed by the use of a dentin bonding system or adhesive cement to bond the amalgam in place, thereby preventing leakage at the restoration margin. This approach is increasingly being used, but there is little long-term data on its effectiveness (Section 24.7.2). A disadvantage is the increased time taken by the bonding procedure and the associated increased cost.

Cavity varnishes have been used in the past, but there is little evidence to indicate that they are effective in reducing leakage or sensitivity.

43.4.6 What should I use for pulp capping?

Calcium hydroxide, in the form of a suspension of calcium hydroxide in either distilled water or Ringer's Solution, has been suggested as the ideal material for use in pulp capping, because the pH of circa 10 prevents of growth of caries-forming bacteria and is close to the optimum pH of the enzyme alkaline phosphatase which has been considered to be nvolved in hard tissue formation. Many papers in the literature report the effectiveness of calcium hydroxide in formation of dentin bridges over exposure sites and radicular pulps following vital pulpectomy. More recently, calcium hydroxide-containing liners have been suggested as materials suitable for pulp capping. However, there is little data on the long-term effectiveness of pulp capping with calcium hydroxide or calcium hydroxide-containing materials.

In the search for an alternative pulp capping agent, there has been considerable interest in the use of dentin bonding agents. The concept is that the exposure site can be totally sealed by the bonding system, and, given that microleakage has been considered to play a major part in pulp death following pulpal exposure, the sealing of the exposure may allow for healing and possible dentin bridge formation. It may be considered that such cases have only a chance of success when the pulp, prior to treatment, is not inflamed or damaged. A number of successfully treated cases have been reported but no long-term studies are available.

Another suggested approach is to apply mineral trioxide aggregate (MTA) as a pulp capping material. MTA was developed as a root end filling material (Section 29.3).

43.4.7 What should I use for temporary (provisional) restorations for direct restorations?

The ideal provisional material should provide a good marginal seal, be insoluble or relatively insoluble in the oral fluids, be strong enough to withstand occlusal forces, yet be easy to remove when the definitive restoration is to be placed or when a root treatment visit is to be carried out.

The choice of a provisional restorative material is related to the length of time for which the restoration is planned to be *in situ*, and also to the functional requirements of the restoration. For temporary restorations that are required to remain in place for an extended period, for example, 4 weeks, the use of a more robust material such as glass-ionomer may be indicated. In a number of such cases, the surface 2 mm of the glass-ionomer may be removed and the restoration placed, using the glass-ionomer as a base. However, if the cavity is to be restored with an indirect restoration, glass-ionomer is not suitable, as the cavity margins could be damaged during its removal. In such cases a temporary inlay is indicated, constructed in a resin-based temporary crown and bridge material. Glass-ionomer materials, because of their reliable adhesion to tooth substance, are of value as a temporary restoration replacing fractured cusps of posterior teeth.

In situations in which the potential longevity of the provisional restoration is less than 4 weeks, a modified zinc oxide/eugenol (ZOE) material should provide adequate service, although the use of ZOE is considered to be contraindicated by some clinicians if a resin-based restoration is to be placed, given the potential for eugenol to plasticize resin-composite materials: however, there is not universal agreement on this matter. An alternative material, a proprietary calcium sulfate hemihydrate, has also been shown to provide good service as a provisional material.

The ability to seal a cavity is of special importance when the tooth is being endodontically treated. Recent research has indicated that a ZOE material provided a better marginal seal than a material based on calcium sulfate hemihydrate; it is likely that a glass-ionomer material could provide a satisfactory seal in such circumstances, but with the disadvantage of less easy removal.

The increasing use of ceramic and composite inlays in non-retentive cavities has produced difficulties in the provision of provisional restorations for such cavities during the construction of the inlay. Adhesive cements such as glass-ionomer are contra-indicated as they are difficult to remove from the cavity without the potential for damage to the cavity margins. Accordingly, the use of a medium/thick mix of zinc phosphate cement may be suggested. This has certain mechanical adhesion properties and has adequate physical properties, but may easily be removed in sections from the cavity.

FURTHER READING

Brown D (1997). The status of restorative dental materials. *Dental Update* **24**: 402-6.

Brown D (1998). The status of indirect restorative dental materials. *Dental Update* **25**: 23-28, 30-32, 34.

Dietschi D, Magne P, Holz J (1994). Recent trends in esthetic restorations for posterior teeth. *Quintessence International* 25: 659-677.

A symposium entitled: 'Current concepts and controversies in vital pulp capping' was held in Orlando, Florida on March 16, 1997. The proceedings of this symposium have been published in a special issue of the *American Journal of Dentistry* **11** (special issue), January 1998.

Pittford T R, Torabinejad M, Abedi H R, Bakland L K, Kariyawasam S P (1996). Using mineral trioxide aggregate as a pulp-capping material. *Journal of the American Dental Association* **127**: 1491-1494.

Chapter 44

Choice of Cements for Luting

Summary: Many materials, previously discussed in Chapters 25-27 are available for luting indirect restorations. This chapter discussed the advantages, disadvantages and applications of each type of material.

44.1 INTRODUCTION

Dental luting materials fill the space between an indirect restoration and the prepared tooth and therefore have an important function in the retention of the restoration and in the prevention of leakage at its margins. However, other than the group of truly adhesive materials, luting materials play only a passive role in the retention of restorations.

The ideal luting material should:

- Be biocompatible with the tissues that it contacts;
- Be cariostatic;
- Adhere to both tooth substance and restoration;
- Prevent leakage;
- Be insoluble in the dilute organic acids that may be found in plaque;
- Resist water absorption;
- Have sufficient compressive and tensile strengths to resist the forces of occlusion;
- Be available in a range of shades if it contributes to the overall restoration shade;
- Allow easy removal of excess and easy clean-up;
- Have sufficiently low film thickness so that the restoration seats fully.

The materials reviewed in this chapter have all been discussed in detail in earlier chapters, namely:

- Zinc phosphate (Chapter 25);

- Glass-ionomer (Chapter 26);
- Resin-modified glass-ionomer (Chapter 26);
- Resin-based cements (Chapter 27).

Here, indications for currently available materials are suggested, with a summary of the advantages and disadvantages of each type of material

44.2 ZINC PHOSPHATE

This is the oldest of the currently available luting materials. Despite less than ideal characteristics, especially in respect of its high solubility, it has been a very popular material with high documented success rates. Indications for use are metal crowns, metal ceramic crowns, aluminous porcelain and reinforced porcelain crowns and cast metal cores and posts.

Advantages of this material include:

- Documented reliability;
- Ease of use;
- Easy removal of excess.

Disadvantages include:

- High solubility;
- Potential for leakage;
- Potential for pulpal irritation.

44.3 ZINC POLYCARBOXYLATE

These materials possess adequate physical properties, show some adhesion to tooth substance, have good biocompatibility but have high solubility. Indications for use are metal crowns, metal-ceramic crowns, aluminous porcelain and reinforced porcelain crowns and cast metal cores and posts.

Advantage – the principal advantage is low potential for pulpal irritation.

Disadvantages include:

- High solubility;
- High potential for leakage;
- Difficult clean-up.

44.4 GLASS-IONOMER

These materials have high compressive strength, release fluoride, adhere to tooth substance, and have less solubility than phosphate or polycarboxylate cements. Indications are therefore for luting of metal crowns and inlays, metal-ceramic crowns, aluminous and reinforced porcelain crowns and cast gold cores and posts.

The adhesion of these materials to tooth substance may help retention of restorations and reduce the potential for microleakage. The principal disadvantages are:

- The potential for pulpal irritation if the material is mixed to a low powder/liquid ratio;
- Difficult clean-up.

44.5 RESIN-MODIFIED GLASS-IONOMER

This recently introduced group of luting materials has excellent physical properties, low solubility and retains the characteristic glass-ionomer properties of fluoride release and adhesion to tooth substance. Clean-up is easy. Indications are for luting of metal crowns and inlays, metal-ceramic crowns and cast gold cores and posts. The reported fracture of porcelain crowns luted with these materials has resulted in this indication being deleted from suggested uses until more research is carried out.

The adhesion of these materials to tooth substance may help retention of restorations. Potential for microleakage is low. The principal disadvantage is their limited indications for use.

44.6 RESIN COMPOSITE-BASED CEMENTS

Some formulations show adhesive properties without the use of an intermediate bonding system. Physical properties are excellent, solubility is low, potential for microleakage is low. When used in combination with a dentin bonding system, biocompatibility is high. These materials may contribute to the shade of ceramic restorations and are therefore, often available in a range of shades. Resin-based cements are therefore indicated for all indirect restorations.

Advantages include excellent physical properties, low solubility and potential for adhesion to tooth substance. The principal disadvantage is the need to finish restoration margins, the increased time that that may take, and difficulties with premature set when placing posts in prepared root canals.

Despite these disadvantages, the use of resin cements to place restorations is increasing alongside the rapidly expanding range of techniques which have been developed with the properties of resin cements in mind.

FURTHER READING

Rosenstiel S F, Land M F, Crispin B J (1998). Dental luting agents. A review of the current literature. *Journal of Prosthetic Dentistry* **80**: 280-301.

XII

MATERIALS FOR REMOVABLE PROSTHODONTICS

Chapter 45

Acrylic Denture Base Materials

Summary: The requirements for polymeric denture base materials are listed, and heat cured acrylic materials are discussed in terms of composition, manipulation and properties. A critique is given of available denture materials. Self-cured materials are also discussed, as are materials for denture repair, rebasing and relining.

45.1 REQUIREMENTS OF POLYMERIC DENTURE BASE MATERIALS

Ideally a denture base material should possess the following properties:

1. Biological properties. It should be non-toxic and non-irritant.
2. Chemical properties. It should be unaffected by oral fluids, that is, it should be insoluble, non-absorbent and inert.
3. Mechanical properties. It should have adequate mechanical properties, for example:
   - High modulus of elasticity, so that greater rigidity can be achieved, even in comparatively thin sections of material;
   - High proportional limit, so that the denture will not easily undergo permanent deformation when stressed;
   - High strength - this is frequently measured as the transverse strength;
   - Sufficient resilience;
   - High impact strength, so that the denture will not fracture if accidentally dropped, or fracture if the wearer is involved in an accident;
   - High fatigue strength;
   - Hard and with good abrasion resistance, so that the material will not wear appreciably, but will take and retain a high polish.
4. The other physical properties such materials should have are:
   - The thermal expansion of the denture base should match that of the tooth material;

- The thermal conductivity should be high;
- The density should be low, to assist in the retention of an upper denture;
- The softening temperature should be higher than the temperature of liquids and foods in the mouth.

5. Esthetics. As a matter of prime importance, the material should be esthetically satisfactory. The material should be transparent or translucent, and easily pigmented. The color should be permanent.

6. Other considerations for denture base materials are:

- Radiopacity - if a denture or a fragment of a broken denture is accidentally inhaled or ingested, it should be capable of detection on radiographs;
- A denture base material should be easy to process with the minimum of expense and equipment;
- It should be easy to repair if accidentally fractured;
- There should be no dimensional changes (expansion, contraction or warpage) either on processing the denture, or while it is in service;
- The material should be easy to clean.

No known denture material adequately fulfills all these requirements.

45.2 FORMERLY USED MATERIALS

In the past, a wide range of synthetic polymers has been used, including vulcanite (vulcanized rubber), Bakelite (phenol-formaldehyde), cellulose nitrate, nylon, epoxy resins and vinyl polymers such as poly(vinyl chloride), poly(vinyl acetate) and polystyrene.

Polycarbonates containing up to 10% glass fibers of 150 μm length and 10 μm diameter have been used for denture construction. These polymers have remarkably good impact properties – up to nine times better than poly(methyl methacrylate). These materials are more difficult to mold dentally than acrylics, since injection molding is required.

45.3 HEAT-CURED ACRYLIC MATERIALS

45.3.1 Introduction

These are the most widely used polymeric denture materials today. The chemistry of their free radical addition polymerization is discussed in Chapter 11.

45.3.2 Composition

Acrylic denture base materials are supplied as a powder to be mixed with a liquid, which is then molded under heat and pressure to form dentures.

The powder contains principally poly(methyl methacrylate) usually as beads produced by polymerizing methyl methacrylate in water, or irregular particles ground from a block of polymer. Benzoyl peroxide initiator is present (0.2 to 0.5%). A pigment (about 1%), ground into the polymer particles is also present.

The liquid is predominantly methyl methacrylate monomer, together with a stabilizer - for example about 0.006% hydroquinone - to prevent polymerization on storage. A cross-linking agent may sometimes be present, such as ethylene glycol dimethacrylate.

Figure 45.1 shows the strucutre of poly(methyl methacrylate) formed from beads of polymer and polymerized monomer.

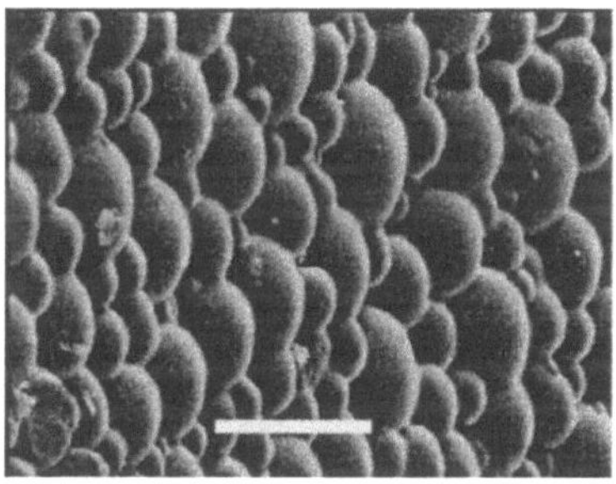

Figure 45.1. Poly(methyl methacrylate) prepared from monomer and beads of polymer. The horizontal bar represents 100 μm.

45.3.3 Manipulation

1. Polymer/monomer ratio. This is usually 3 to 3.5/1 by volume, or 2.5/1 by weight. Use of the correct ratio is important because if it is too high, not all the polymer will be wetted by monomer, and the cured acrylic will be granular. Neither should the ratio be too low. There is shrinkage on polymerization of about 21% by volume for pure monomer. In correctly proportioned acrylic dough this is about 7%. If there is too much monomer there will be greater shrinkage.

2. Mixing. The correct proportions are mixed and allowed to stand in a closed container until the dough stage is reached. After mixing monomer

and polymer, the consistency of the mixed material goes through the following stages:

- Initially a wet sand-like mixture is formed;
- The material becomes tacky as the polymer begins to dissolve in the monomer;
- A smooth dough-like material then results, which does not stick to the mixing jar; this is the correct dough stage for the packing material;
- If the mix is left too long it becomes too rubbery and stiff to be molded properly.

The dough time depends on the particle size of the polymer; the smaller the particles, the more rapid is the dissolution and dough formation. It also depends on the molecular weight of the polymer; the lower this is, the faster is the dough formation. Also a plasticizer is present in some materials – this reduces the dough time. Temperature affects the rate of dough formation; for example, dough formation can be delayed by refrigeration of the mix. Also a high polymer/monomer ratio gives a shorter dough time.

3. Mold lining. After the wax pattern is completely removed from the mold by flushing with boiling water and detergent, the walls of the gypsum mold must be lined to prevent monomer penetrating into the mold material and polymerizing there, producing a rough surface with adherent mold material. A lining should also prevent water from the mold entering into the acrylic resin.

Formerly tin foil was widely used to line the molds. This is a time consuming and difficult process. Tin foil substitutes are mainly used today. These are usually a solution of an alginate, such as potassium, sodium or ammonium alginate. They react with the calcium of the plaster or stone mold material to form a film of insoluble calcium alginate. These substitutes are used with great success, though they are not entirely satisfactory in preventing water from the mold entering the acrylic. This may lead to crazing.

4. Packing. It is important to ensure that the mold is full. There must be sufficient pressure on the mold; this is achieved by packing excess dough into the mold causing it to deform. On polymerization there is contraction which reduces the pressure in the mold. Under-packing can lead to shrinkage porosity.

5. Polymerization. The packed mold is heated in an oven or water-bath; both the temperature and time of heating must be controlled. If the material is under-cured the denture may have a high residual monomer content. As will be shown, it is important that this is avoided. Also the rate of temperature rise must not be too high. Monomer boils at 100.3°C. The resin

must not reach this temperature while there is a substantial quantity of unreacted monomer left. The polymerization reaction is exothermic. Thus if a large mass of uncured material is suddenly plunged into boiling water, the temperature of the resin may rise above 100.3°C, so vaporizing the monomer. This causes gaseous porosity.

The material should be heated at 72°C for at least 16 hours. Alternatively, heating at 72°C for 2 hours, by which time most of the monomer has reacted, although the residual monomer content is still above acceptable limits; the temperature is then raised to 100°C and heating continued for a further 2 hours. This latter technique obviously enables a denture to be produced in a shorter time, but there is more likelihood of distortion of the denture on deflasking (see below).

Microwave curing techniques have been advocated using specially designed non-metallic flasks.

6. Cooling. The flask should be cooled slowly on the bench, or in the oven or water bath. Sudden cooling should not be allowed. On cooling, there is a difference of contraction between the mold material and acrylic, which causes stresses within the polymer. Slow cooling permits relief of these stresses by plastic deformation. Materials cured at higher temperatures will have greater residual stresses, and will be more likely to warp.
7. Deflasking. This has to be done with care to avoid flexing and breaking the denture.
8. Finishing and polishing. A suspension of finely ground pumice in water is commonly used. Final polishing is done with, for example, whiting, used as a suspension on a wet soft mop. Sometimes dry polishing techniques are used but care must be taken not to overheat the denture.

45.3.4 Properties

The molecular weight of polymer powder, as supplied, is up to 500,000 to 1,000,000 (in the literature lower values, for example, 3,500 to 36,000 have been wrongly quoted). The molecular weight of the monomer is 100. For the cured polymer, figures up to 1,200,000 (again lower values have sometimes been quoted, for example, between 10,000 and 40,000).

Residual monomer has a pronounced effect on the average molecular weight. Even in a properly cured acrylic, 0.2 to 0.5% remains. Processing at too low a temperature or for too short a time gives higher residual monomer values. This should be avoided because free monomer may be released from the denture and irritate the oral tissues. Also residual monomer will act as a plasticizer and make the resin weaker and more flexible.

Porosity may have undesirable effects on the strength and optical properties of the acrylic. Shrinkage porosity appears as irregular voids throughout, and on the surface of the denture. Gaseous porosity shows as fine uniform bubbles, particularly in thicker sections of the denture remote from the external heating source.

Water absorption and desorption characteristics must be considered. Immediately after processing, a denture produced in a mold with tin foil substitutues contains some water. In service, further water absorption can occur up to an equilibrium value of about 2%. It has been claimed that each 1% increase in weight of the resin due to water absorption causes a linear expansion of 0.23%. Similarly, drying out of the material is associated with shrinkage. For this reason, dentures should at all times be kept wet when not in service.

Cracks may appear on the surface of the resin; this is termed *crazing*. This is believed to be due to tensile stresses causing separation of the polymer molecules. Such crazing can result from mechanical stresses on repeated drying and wetting of the denture, causing alternate contraction and expansion. The use of tin-foil substitutes for mold lining permits the cured denture to contain water. Subsequent loss of this water may lead to crazing. Stresses due to differences in the coefficients of thermal expansion between porcelain teeth or other inserts, such as clasps, and the acrylic denture base may cause crazing, in which cracks may appear around the inert. Solvent action may cause crazing, for example, when a denture is being repaired, some monomer comes in contact with the resin. Crazing has a weakening effect on a denture. Cross-linked resins are less likely to craze.

The dimensional accuracy of dentures is complex, and the following factors must be taken into account:

- The mold expansion on packing;
- Thermal expansion of the acrylic dough;
- Polymerization shrinkage - approximately 7% by volume for the polymerization of the dough, or over 2% linear contraction;
- Thermal shrinkage on cooling - the coefficient of thermal expansion of acrylic is 81 x 10^{-6}/°C, it can be shown that there is 0.44% shrinkage on cooling from 75 to 20°C. This may be a cause of palatal discrepancies in upper dentures;
- If excess heat is generated during polishing the denture, this may cause distortion due to release of stresses within the material.

The dimensional stability of acrylic dentures is related to water absorption/desorption, as discussed above. Also, relief of internal stresses may occur while the denture is in service. This effect is probably small and is unlikely to be of clinical significance.

Fracture of dentures can occur by different mechanisms. Dentures may break on impact, for example, if dropped on a hard surface. Fatigue fracture can also occur, from repeated bending of the denture in service. It is possible to determine the cause of fracture by observing the fracture surfaces with a magnifying glass. If there are parallel cracks within the material the breakage was probably due to fatigue.

The 'strength' of a denture depends on the design of the denture, as discussed in texts on dental mechanics and prosthodontics; for example, stress concentration around a notch may occur (e.g. the frenal notch) leading to midline fracture. Surface irregularities also lead to stress concentration. The strength of the resin itself is also important; this depends on the molecular weight of the cured polymer, the residual monomer content, porosity and inclusions of foreign matter.

Acrylic resin is radiolucent. Several experimental approaches have been tried to solve this problem, with as yet little success. The incorporation of metal wire or mesh into acrylic weakens the material by causing stress concentration. The addition of compounds containing halogens (bromine and iodine) and heavy metal (bismuth and barium) has not yet been fully successful.

45.3.5 Assessment

How do these materials compare with the list of ideal properties given in Section 45.1?

1. They are non-toxic, and, if properly manipulated, non-irritant.
2. They are insoluble and inert in oral fluids, though they show a degree of water absorption.
3. In terms of mechanical properties the impact and fatigue properties of acrylic are not ideal. Also, although the material can take a good polish, its abrasion resistance is not good.
4. The other physical properties of acrylic are:

- The coefficient of thermal expansion is 81 x 10^{-6}/ °C, similar to that of acrylic teeth, but very much greater than that of porcelain teeth (Chapter 48);
- The thermal conductivity is low, in common with other polymers;
- Its density is 1.18 g/cm^3 - this is comparatively low;
- The softening temperature is about 75°C, higher than the temperature of hot foods and liquids.

5. One of the chief merits of acrylic is that it can provide good esthetics; the polymer is translucent and easily pigmented. Color stability is good (in contrast to self-cured acrylics, Section 45.4).
6. Other factors are:
- Acrylics are radiolucent as discussed above;
- They are easy to process with simple equipment; no expensive injection molding equipment is required;
- Acrylic dentures are easy to repair if accidentally fractured;
- Dimensional changes can occur, as outlined above.

45.4 SELF-CURED ACRYLIC MATERIALS

45.4.1 Introduction

The chemistry of these materials is given in Chapter 11. Their composition is similar to heat-cured materials except that the liquid contains an activator, such as N,N-dimethyl-*p*-toluidine (Figure 11.7). They are sometimes called cold-curing, auto-polymerizing or chemically activated materials.

45.4.2 Comparison with heat-cured materials

The porosity of self-cured materials is greater, though this is not easy to see in pigmented resins. This may be due to air dissolved in the monomer that is not soluble in the polymer at room temperature.

In general, self-cured materials have lower average molecular weights, and higher residual monomer contents - of the order of 2 to 5%.

Self-cured materials are not as strong; the transverse strength is about 80% of that of the heat-cured materials. This may be related to their lower molecular weight.

In terms of rheological properties, self-cured materials are less satisfactory, since they show greater distortion in use. In measurements on creep of poly(methyl methacrylate), heat-cured polymers had less initial deformation, less creep and quicker recovery than self-cured materials (Figure 45.2).

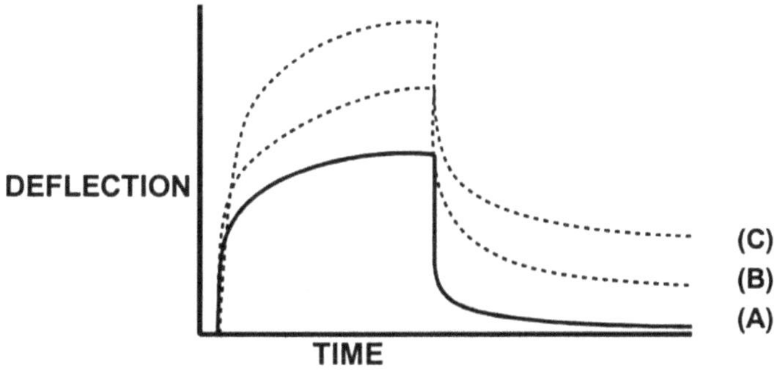

Figure 45.2. Creep of denture base materials. (A) heat-cured avrylic; (B) self-cured acrylic; (C) 'pour-and-cure' resin

The color stability of self-cured materials is poorer; if a tertiary amine activator is used, yellowing over a period of time can occur.

45.4.3 'Pour-and-cure' resins

A technique is available whereby a fluid mix of a self-curing acrylic is poured into an agar mold to form a denture. Such dentures may be dimensionally less accurate, more porous and weaker and show greater creep (Figure 45.2) than those prepared from conventional heat-cured materials.

45.4.4 Other applications

Self-cured acrylics are used:

- With inert fillers, for the construction of special trays for impression taking;
- For denture repair, relining and rebasing;
- In removable orthodontic appliances;
- For adding a post-dam to an adjusted upper denture.

45.5 DENTURE REPAIR, REBASING AND RELINING

45.5.1 Denture repair

For self-cured repairs, the parts of the broken denture are held together with sticky wax and wires, and a model cast up in plaster. When the denture parts are removed from the model, the fracture surfaces are finished with a smooth rounded contour with 3 to 5 mm separation. V-shaped edges should be avoided, as they will lead to stress concentration. Alginate separating medium or tin foil is applied to the model, and the denture parts replaced on it. The self-curing acrylic repair material is mixed to a fluid consistency and applied to the repair area. The porosity of the self-curing acrylic will be less if it is polymerized under a hydraulic pressure of up to 250 kPa and at a temperature of 40 to 45°C.

Heat-cured repairs are often advocated for all but minor repairs. A problem is that distortion of the denture base is liable to occur. This can be overcome by replacing the palate of the denture with new heat-cured material.

45.5.2 Rebasing and relining

Dentures sometimes require adjustment of their fitting surfaces to accommodate changes in the soft tissue. This may be carried out by constructing a new denture base (rebasing), or a new fitting surface for the denture (relining). The use of soft or resilient lining materials is discussed separately in Chapter 46.

45.6 MODIFIED ACRYLICS

There is a need for materials with greater impact and fatigue strength. These materials include vinyl co-polymers and rubber-acrylic graft co-polymers. Several such products are available, some of them requiring injection molding. The graft co-polymers have better impact resistance properties than conventional acrylic materials.

One group of such materials is essentially emulsion polymerized beads of poly(methyl methacrylate) to which are grafted a rubbery butadiene-styrene layer that are then coated with poly(methyl methacrylate). These beads are then mixed with monomer that is composed of methyl methacrylate, a cross-linking agent and an inhibitor. These materials show a greater resistance to crack formation, causing deceleration of the crack when it reaches the rubber phase. Rubber modified resins have better impact and fatigue properties.

One experimental approach to the development of stronger denture base materials is to incorporate high modulus fibers into the material.

45.7 LIGHT-CURED DENTURE BASE MATERIALS

Free radical addition polymerization can be initiated by visible light. This technique has become widely used for composite restorative materials and is now available for denture base applications. The system comprises of a denture base material with acrylic copolymers, microfine silica and high molecular weight acrylic monomers; no methyl methacrylate is present. A coating for the denture base material is supplied. This helps to eliminate surface inhibition of polymerization by oxygen. A bonding agent which is cured by visible light, to aid bonding between base and teeth, is included. This agent contains a mixture of acrylic monomers, including methyl methacrylate. Polymerization takes place in a curing unit, with four tungsten halogen lamps, giving light of wavelength 400-500 nm.

FURTHER READING

Takamata T, Setcos J C (1989). Resin denture bases: review of accuracy and methods of polymerization. *International Journal of Prosthodontics*. **2**: 555-562.

Eichhold W A, Woelfel JB (1990). Denture base acrylic resins: friend or foe? *Compendium* **11**: 720-735.

Chapter 46

Denture Lining Materials

Summary: A range of denture lining materials, intended for temporary and permanent application, is considered and assessed.

46.1 INTRODUCTION

46.1.1 Classification

Denture lining materials can be classified into a number of types:

- Hard reline materials;
- Soft reline materials for temporary use;
- Soft reline materials, intended for permanent use;
- Patient-administered lining materials.

Hard reline materials have already been considered in Chapter 45. Patient administered materials such as denture adhesives are discussed in Chpater 49. This chapter is concerned with soft or resilient material, that is, materials with low glass transition temperature (T_g). The basic concept of T_g has been discussed in Section 11.5.3.

46.1.2 Indications and applications

An acrylic denture may have a soft lining, either as a temporary measure, or intended for permanent use.

A temporary lining may be used for one of two purposes. Firstly, it may be a *tissue conditioner*; this may be defined as a soft material that is applied temporarily to the fitting surface of a denture in order to allow a more equal distribution of load, to permit the mucosal tissues to assume a more normal position.

Secondly, temporary lining materials may be used as *functional impression materials*; these are applied to the fitting surface of dentures in order to secure impressions under functional stresses.

A permanent resilient lining may be used in a number of clinical situations. Where the tissues of the denture bearing area show evidence of atrophy, a soft lining may be used to avoid pain through pressure from, or movement of, the denture under masticatory load. A resilient material can utilize undercut areas to achieve maximum retention of the denture. These resilient materials can also be used for obturators and other prostheses such as facial prostheses.

46.1.3 General principles

The above applications require polymers that are soft at mouth temperature - in other words, their glass transition temperature (T_g) must be below 37°C. The following type of materials are used:

1. Acrylic polymers with a solvent.
2. Acrylic polymers or co-polymers with an inert ester as plasticizer. Poly (ethyl methacrylate) is frequently used, as it has a lower glass transition temperature than poly(methyl methacrylate), so requires less plasticizer.
3. Silicones, including both heat cured and room temperature vulcanizing materials.
4. During the 1990s a polyphosphazine-based material was available for permanent soft linings. At the time of writing it has been withdrawn from the market, but may be reintroduced at a later date.

46.2 TISSUE CONDITIONERS AND FUNCTIONAL IMPRESSION MATERIALS

46.2.1 Requirements

These materials should have no irritant or toxic effect. The set materials for each of the two applications being considered have different requirements:

1. A tissue conditioner must be soft, and it must not undergo substantial permanent deformation – that is, it must be elastic. The softness and elasticity must be maintained for a sufficient length of time.
2. A functional impression material should also be soft, but must deform plastically to record the impression.

It should be noted that many of the materials used for these applications are viscoelastic – that is, they flow under steady pressure, but are resilient under dynamic forces such as chewing.

46.2.2 Composition and properties

Powder/liquid materials contain an acrylic polymer, for example, poly (ethyl methacrylate) or co-polymers, to be mixed with a liquid that is usually a mixture of ethyl alcohol and an aromatic ester (for example, butyl phthalyl butyl glycolate).

On mixing the two together, a slurry is formed. The liquid then penetrates between the molecules of the powder, a process accelerated by the ethyl alcohol present, and the whole material becomes stiffer, until a gel is formed. The setting, therefore, is a physical process, there being no chemical reaction involved. Note that these materials do not contain any monomeric substances.

Preformed sheets of acrylic gel are also available, which can be adapted to the surfaces of the denture.

The available commercial materials vary considerably in their precise composition and properties. Some of them are more suitable for tissue conditioning, others for functional impressions.

46.3 RESILIENT LININGS

46.3.1 Requirements

The following is a list of desirable properties of resilient linings:

1. They should be non-toxic, non-irritant, odorless and tasteless.
2. Interfacial properties. There should be a good bond formed between lining and denture base, which will not be adversely affected by the conditions of the oral environment.
3. They should be unaffected by the oral environment. Gel type materials should not imbibe water and undergo excessive swelling; the percentage water absorption should be the same as that of the denture base. There should be no absorption of constituents of foods and drinks. Plasticizers (where present) should not be leached out of the materials.
4. In terms of mechanical properties, the set material should be soft and permanently resilient, and resistant to abrasion.

5. Esthetics. There should be a natural appearance, and no discoloration or staining should occur.
6. Other desirable properties include the need for stability on storage of the unmixed material, simplicity in manipulation and dimensional stability during processing and in use. Ease of cleaning is important.

46.3.2 Classification and composition

Early materials, not widely used today because of their inferior properties, included natural rubbers and poly(vinyl chloride) or poly(vinyl acetate) plasticized with dibutyl phthalate or dioctyl phthalate.

Present-day materials include heat-cured acrylics. The powder of these materials contains acrylic polymers such as poly(ethyl methacrylate) or acrylic co-polymers, and benzoyl peroxide. The liquid is an acrylic monomer (e.g. ethyl, butyl, or 2-ethoxyethyl methacrylate) and plasticizers. Alternatively these materials may be supplied as a preformed sheet, which is soaked in a monomeric material which causes it to swell, and then processed against the acrylic dough.

Self-cured acrylics are also available, which are supplied in powder/liquid form of composition similar to the above, except that they are polymerized by a peroxide-tertiary amine system.

Silicone polymers provide an alternative to the acrylic type systems. These contain a polysiloxane material and silica as a filler. They are processed against acrylic dough. One commercial product has a methacrylate group to aid bonding with the acrylic denture base.

Self-cured room temperature vulcanizing (RTV) silicones are similar in composition and setting to the silicone impression materials (Chapter 33). Bonding to the acrylic denture base is helped by applying a special primer to the acrylic.

46.3.3 General properties

1. In general these materials are non-irritant and are not unpleasant in the mouth.
2. Interfacial properties. In general, acrylic materials bond durably to acrylic denture bases. However the silicone materials may show failure of bonding, which can create a potential surface for bacterial growth and plaque and calculus formation.
3. Water absorption of the heat-cured acrylic soft liners is closest to that of the acrylic denture base. In general the silicones have the best all-round

resistance to the effects of constituents of foods and drinks. This has been demonstrated in laboratory tests with olive oil and peppermint oil.

However the effects of the oral environment can be considerable. The plasticizers of the acrylic materials are lost by being leached out into the saliva, causing hardening of the lining, and dimensional change. Growth of the fungus *Candida albicans* has been found to occur with some silicone materials.

4. In terms of mechanical properties, the silicones are the most elastic, but have poorer abrasion resistance than the acrylics.
5. Esthetic properties of soft linings may be lost by deposits of calculus, or by use of the wrong denture cleansers (Chapter 49).
6. These materials are often adversely affected by denture cleansers.

46.3.4 Conclusions

Soft linings are intended to be permanently attached to the denture. However, their general properties are often so poor that they must be considered as semi-permanent.

In practice, a number of failings are commonly seen. Some materials develop a rough surface after wear, with food being embedded in the surface. Some linings split under stress and/or peel away from the denture base. There may be a change of color due to staining and deposits of calculus. The linings may become hard due to loss of plasticizer. The surface may become bubbled if an oxygenating type of denture cleanser is used. If a bleach is used to clean the denture, the lining becomes white and hard.

FURTHER READING

Mack P J (1989). Denture soft lining materials: clinical indications. *Australian Dental Journal* 34: 454-458.

Braden M, Wright P S, Parker S (1995). Soft lining materials - a review. *European Journal of Prosthodontics & Restorative Dentistry* **3**: 163-174.

Nikawa H, Iwanaga H, Hamada T, Yuhta S (1994). Effects of denture cleansers on direct soft denture lining materials. *Journal of Prosthetic Dentistry* **72**: 657-662.

Chapter 47

Partial Denture Casting Alloys

Summary: Gold, cobalt-chromium and titanium-based casting alloys and wrought wires are reviewed and assessed.

47.1 INTRODUCTION

A cast partial denture is a complex structure which includes saddles to carry the artificial teeth, retainers such as clasps, rests to provide resistance to displacement of the denture in a direction towards the tissues, and connectors to link together the other components of the structure. Figure 47.1 shows a cast metal framework with these components and Figure 47.2 shows a completed partial denture.

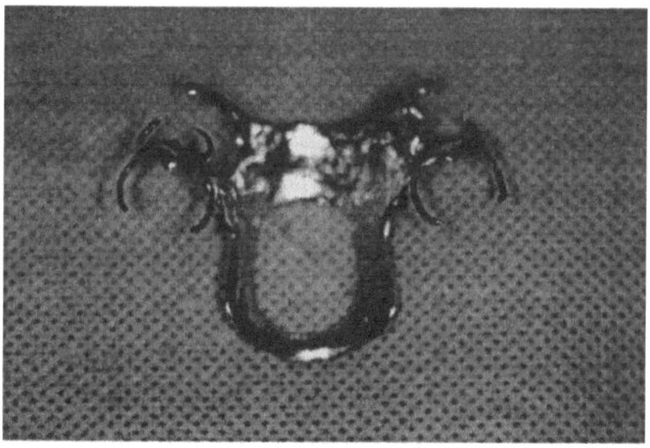

Figure 47.1. Example of a cast metal partial denture framework.

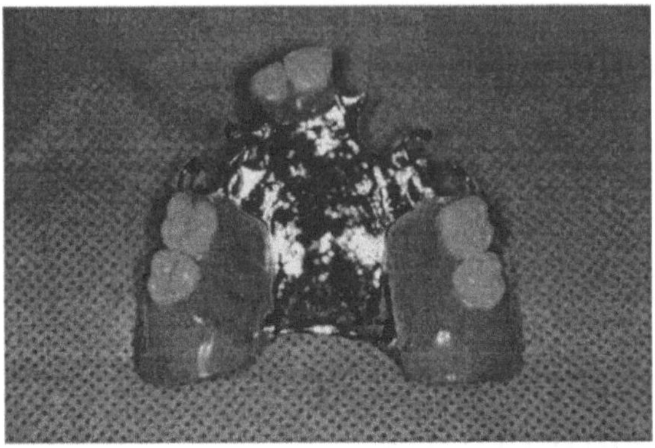

Figure 47.2. Partial denture.

Mechanical property considerations are important in the design of partial dentures. The material for the connectors of a partial denture should have the following mechanical properties:

- High modulus of elasticity, so that it is rigid in thin sections;
- High proportional limit, so that permanent deformation is unlikely.

For clasp construction a high proportional limit is also important. However a lower modulus of elasticity would be desirable, so that the clasp is flexible enough to be withdrawn over undercuts, without either the tooth or the clasps being overstressed.

Traditionally gold and cobalt-chromium alloys have been the materials of choice. More recently titanium and its alloys have become available.

47.2 GOLD ALLOYS

Type IV gold alloys are used for partial denture construction; their composition is in Table 35.1. The effect of each metal constituent has been discussed in Section 13.5.2. The properties of these alloys are in Table 47.1, where they are compared with alternative materials.

These alloys are designed to be heat treated, which increases hardness, yield strength and tensile strength. Typical heat treatment procedures include the following stages:

Stage 1. The alloy is usually quenched after casting.

Stage 2. Homogenization is carried out since coring occurs with alloys containing platinum. This is achieved by heating to 700°C for 10 minutes, followed by quenching.
Stage 3. If any cold working is done to the alloy, for example, adjustment of clasps, a stress-relief anneal is carried out.
Stage 4. Heat hardening is achieved by heating and maintaining the alloy at an elevated temperature for a sufficient time for diffusion of atoms to occur, to permit order and precipitation hardening. This can be achieved by one of the following methods:

- Cooling the alloy slowly from 700°C;
- Cooling the alloy from 450 to 250°C over 30 minutes, followed by quenching;
- Maintaining the alloy at between 350 and 450°C for around 15 minutes, followed by quenching.

The effect of this heat treatment on the mechanical properties of these alloys can be seen in Table 47.1

47.3 COBALT-CHROMIUM ALLOYS

These alloys are hard, rigid and corrosion resistant, and their composition is presented in Section 13.8.1. Because of their corrosion resistance at high temperatures, other applications have been for car sparking plugs and turbine blades. This type of alloy is often referred to as *stellite*.

The casting technique for these alloys is similar in principle to that of gold alloys, but the following differences in manipulation should be noted:

1. The melting point of these alloys is in the range 1250 to 1450°C, hence gypsum-bonded investments should not be used. A silica-bonded or phosphate-bonded material should be chosen (Chapter 53).
2. Because of the high melting range, gas/air torches cannot raise the alloy temperature sufficiently to melt it. There is a choice of using either an oxy-acetylene flame or induction heating. The former method is not usually used because it requires careful control to use the correct ratio of oxygen to acetylene. Too much of the former gas may result in oxidation of the alloy; too much acetylene will result in carbon pick-up by the alloy, which must be avoided (see below). Induction heating, by which the alloy is heated electrically, is usually preferred, as it avoids the problems mentioned above.

3. Because of the great hardness of the alloy, special polishing and finishing techniques are required. Sand blasting can be used to smooth the surface of the casting and remove adherent investment materials. Electrolytic polishing is then applied. The principle is the same as for electroplating, except that the appliance is made the anode of an electrolytic cell. When a current is applied, the surface layer is dissolved.

Comparative data are presented in Table 47.1. The proportional limit of cobalt-chromium alloys is less than that of the hardened gold alloys, and the ultimate tensile strength of the former is slightly lower than that of the latter material. The cobalt-chromium alloys have a modulus of elasticity about twice that of gold alloys, that is, they are stiffer. This is very desirable for connectors and it means that sections of cobalt-chromium alloys of about half the thickness of gold alloys can be used to achieve the same degree of rigidity. Gold alloy clasps, however, are more flexible, and can be withdrawn over a greater degree of undercut (that is, a deeper undercut can be engaged) than clasps of cobalt-chromium. The cobalt-chromium alloys are more brittle (lower percentage elongation) than gold alloys.

The higher melting range, and greater hardness, of cobalt-chromium alloys, have already been discussed in terms of the significance of these properties in the handling of the materials.

The casting shrinkage of cobalt-chromium alloys is greater than that of the gold-containing materials, but the available investment materials appear to give satisfactory compensation for this contraction.

The density of cobalt-chromium is about half that of gold. This together with the fact that cobalt-chromium dentures can be made of thinner cross-section, means that lighter dentures can be made.

47.4 TITANIUM AND ITS ALLOYS

47.4.1 Titanium ('commercially pure')

Titanium has a number of important merits as a potential material for the fabrication of cast partial dentures. Its biocompatibility is excellent. Its corrosion resistance is good since it forms a stable oxide passive layer of thickness about 1 nm. Its mechanical properties (except modulus of elasticity) are very similar to cobalt-chromium. It has a very low specific gravity. Titanium is inexpensive.

However, the material is difficult to manipulate for a number of reasons. It has a high melting temperature (near 1700°C). Its low density (4.5 g/cm^3) makes it difficult to cast. Titanium has a strong affinity for gases, especially oxygen, nitrogen and hydrogen. It also reacts with most investment materials at the temperature of casting. It is impossible to make relatively thin casting.

Thermal history is critical for titanium castings. When heated above 800°C, a flaky oxide film forms. The ratio of the two forms of Ti (α-Ti which is h.c.p. and β-Ti which is b.c.c.) depends critically on thermal history (that is, cooling rate). Mechanical properties are very dependent on ratio of the two forms since β-Ti stronger but less ductile than α-Ti.

47.4.2 Titanium alloys

Examples include: Ti/Pd (70/30); Ti/Cu (80/20); Ti/V (85/15) and Ti/Al/V (90/6/4). These are mostly experimental materials; alloying elements can lower melting temperature and stabilize either the α- or β-form. Ti/A1/V is now available commercially. Because of casting difficulties, cast alloys with Ti can be radiographed to detect voids.

Table 47.1. General comparative properties of casting alloys

Material	Modulus of elasticity (GPa)	Pro-portional limit (MPa)	Ultimate tensile strength (MPa)	Elongat-ion (%)	Hard-ness	Melting range (°C)	Density (g/cm^3)
Au Type IV as cast	95	360	480	15	130-150 (BHN)	900	15
Au Type IV hardened	100	585	790	10	210-230 (BHN)	900	15
Co-Cr as cast	250	515	690	4	370 (BHN)	1300	8
Typical Ti alloy	115	560	700-985	18	210 (Vickers)	1600	5

47.5 WROUGHT WIRES

Wrought wires may be used in conjunction with castings. These may be made of Pt/Au/Pd or stainless steel, and soldered onto the framework with silver solder.

FURTHER READING

McGivney G P, Castleberry D J (1995). *McCracken's Removable Partial Prosthodonlics*, 9th edition. St Louis: Mosby. pp 248-257.

Blackman R, Barghi N, Tran C (1991). Dimensional changes in casting titanium removable partial denture frameworks. *Journal of Prosthetic Dentistry* **65**: 309-315.

Kononen M, Rintanen J, Waltimo A, Kempainen P (1995). Titanium framework removable partial denture used for patient allergic to other metals: a clinical report and literature review. *Journal of Prosthetic Dentistry* **73**: 4-7.

Vallittu P K, Kokkonen M (1995). Deflection fatigue of cobalt-chromium, titanium and gold alloy cast denture clasp. *Journal of Prosthetic Dentistry* **74**: 412-419.

Bridgeman J T, Marker V A, Hummel S K, Benson B W, Pace L L (1997). Comparison of titanium and cobalt-chromium removable partial denture clasps. *Journal of Prosthetic Dentistry* **78**: 187-193.

Chapter 48

Denture Teeth

Summary: Polymeric, ceramic and composite denture teeth are discussed and compared.

48.1 REQUIREMENTS

A number of considerations must be taken into account in the selection of denture teeth. These include size, form, color and material. In this chapter, a number of alternative materials are considered. In terms of desirable properties:

1. Interfacial properties. There should be durable bonding between denture base and teeth.
2. Chemical properties. Denture teeth should be resistant to oral fluids, and also should not be crazed by exposure to methyl methacrylate monomer either during the denture fabrication or on subsequent repair.
3. Mechanical properties. Teeth should be impact resistant to withstand forces during biting. They should also be abrasion resistant, with little wear. It must also be added that teeth should not be so hard that they cause wear of opposing natural dentition.
4. Other physical properties. Teeth should ideally have a similar coefficient of thermal expansion to the denture base, to reduce stresses at the bonded denture base/denture tooth interface during temperature changes in the mouth.
5. Esthetic properties. Color and translucency are of obvious importance. Surface texture is also important for anterior teeth since smooth surfaces with a high reflectance would have a lifeless appearance. It should be easy to characterize tooth surfaces using stains where necessary.

6. Practicability. Teeth should be easy to adjust by grinding and should be easy to repolish. Teeth should be able to absorb forces, so transmitting less force to the mucosa. They should make little impact sound on contact.

48.2 ACRYLIC TEETH

These may be manufactured by dough molding using permanent metal molds, but otherwise similar to the method of processing heat cured acrylic denture base materials. Alternatively injection molding or heat compression methods may be used. Some teeth contain an interpenetrating network of polymers (IPN).

A number of points of practical importance should be noted. The teeth will bond chemically with the acrylic denture base, providing that the tooth surface to be bonded is clean and free of wax. The presence of monomer, either on fabrication or repair of the denture, can cause crazing. For this reason, most acrylic teeth are cross-linked, which makes them more resistant to solvent action. The abrasion resistance of acrylic teeth is not ideal, and wear of teeth in service frequently occurs.

The properties of acrylic and porcelain teeth are compared in Table 48.1.

48.3 PORCELAIN TEETH

Porcelain can also be used for the construction of teeth; its composition and properties are discussed in Chapter 34.

Bonding to the denture base is usually achieved by means of pins or undercut holes. Recently, attempts have been made to bond porcelain teeth to acrylic by a combination of micromechanical retention and chemical bonding. The former is achieved by treating the ceramic with an etchant such as a hydrofluoric acid gel. Chemical bonding is attained by the use of a silane coupling agent.

Comparison with acrylic teeth is given in Table 48.1.

48.4 COMPOSITE TEETH

Polymer/ceramic composite teeth have been introduced, containing microfine filler particles of silica. They are claimed to be better than acrylic teeth in terms of wear resistance and superior to porcelain teeth in their ability to bond to denture base materials.

Table 48.1. Comparison of acrylic and porcelain teeth

Property	Acrylic teeth	Porcelain teeth
Interfacial properties	Chemical bonding if proper manipulation carried out	Mechanical bonding by pins or undercut holes. A combination of HF etching and silane treatment has been tested
Chemical properties	Reasonably resistant to chemical attack	Very resistant to chemical attack
Mechanical properties - bulk properties	Less brittle than porcelain	Brittle, chipping may occur
Mechanical properties - surface properties	Comparatively poor abrasion resistance	Excellent abrasion resistance
Effect on opposing dentition	None	May abrade tooth enamel
Coefficient of thermal expansion	Similar to acrylic denture base	Much less than acrylic denture base
Esthetic properties	Can be excellent. Teeth can be characterized by staining	Can be excellent
Practicability	Can be ground and then easily repolished	More difficult to grind and polish
In service	Considered to transmit less force to the mucosa; no clicking on contact with opposing teeth	Considered to transmit more force to the mucosa; clicking occurs on contact with the opposing teeth

FURTHER READING

Suzuki S, Sakoh M, Shiba A (1990). Impact resistance of highly crosslinked plastic denture teeth. *Journal of Biomedical Materials Research* **24**: 1661-1671.

Kawara M, Carter J M, Ogle R E, Johnson R R (1991). Bonding of plastic teeth to denture base resins. *Journal of Prosthetic Dentistry* **66**: 566-571.

Douglas W H, DeLong R, Pintado M R, Latta M A (1993). Wear rates of artificial denture teeth opposed by enamel dentition. *Journal of Clinical Dentistry* **4**: 43-47.

Lindquist T J, Ogle R E, Davis E L (1995). Twelve-month results of a clinical wear study of three artificial tooth materials. *Journal of Prosthetic Dentistry* **74**: 156-161.

Marchack B W, Yu Z, Zhao X Y, White S N (1995). Adhesion of denture tooth porcelain to heat-polymerized denture resin. *Journal of Prosthetic Dentistry* **74**: 242-249.

Hirano S, May K B, Wagner K C, Hacker C H (1998). *In vitro* wear of resin denture teeth. *Journal of Prosthetic Dentistry* **79**: 152-155.

Chapter 49

Denture Cleansers and Adhesives

Summary: The nature and properties of agents for cleansing dentures, and adhesives to assist in denture retention, are discussed.

49.1 DENTURE CLEANSERS

49.1.1 Deposits on dentures

If soft food debris clings to a denture, it can easily be removed by light brushing or rubbing, followed by rinsing. The hard deposits of calculus that can form on dentures are much more difficult to remove. The composition of these calcareous deposits varies from person to person, but essentially they consist of:

- An inorganic portion, shown to contain calcium phosphate, calcium carbonate and lesser quantities of other phosphates;
- An organic portion which bonds the deposit to the denture and is between 15 and 30% of the total deposit – this consists of mucoproteins.

49.1.2 Requirements

Ideally a material should have the following characteristics:

1. Non-toxic, easy to remove and leaving no traces of irritant material.
2. The ability to attack or dissolve both the organic and inorganic portions of denture deposits.
3. Harmless to all materials used in the construction of dentures, including denture base polymers and alloys, acrylic and porcelain teeth and resilient lining materials.
4. Not harmful to clothing, etc., if accidentally splashed or spilled.

5. Stable on storage.
6. Preferably bactericidal and fungicidal.

49.1.3 Classification and properties

The available types of material, their chief active constituents, and their main characteristics, are summarized in Table 49.1.

Table 49.1. Types of denture cleanser

Cleanser	Chief constituent	Properties
Oxygenating cleansers	Alkaline percarbonate or peroxide	Does not easily remove heavy deposits Harmful to soft lining materials
Hypochlorite solutions	Dilute sodium hypochlorite	May cause bleaching of denture material Can corrode chromium-containing alloys May leave an odor on the dentures
Dilute mineral acids	Hydrochloric acid	Corrosion of some alloys, though a corrosion inhibitor may be present
Denture cleansing powders	Abrasive agents	Abrasion of polymeric denture base and tooth materials
Denture cleansing pastes	Abrasive agents and/or acids	Abrasion of polymeric materials Can be difficult to remove paste completely from denture
Enzyme-containing materials	A protease	Ability to remove dental plaque

49.2 DENTURE ADHESIVES

49.2.1 Application

Adhesives are bought in large quantities by denture wearers, in attempts to improve the retention and function of their dentures. Denture adhesives may also be used in the following cases:

- As an aid in retention during the construction phase of a denture;
- As an aid to the retention of dentures and special appliances such as obturators, where there are physical limitations to the degree of retention that can otherwise be achieved;
- As a vehicle to aid application of drugs to the oral mucosa.

49.2.2 Constituents and mechanism of action

It is known that denture retention is enhanced by the presence of a high viscosity fluid between the denture and its supporting tissues. Denture adhesives contain polymeric constituents that dissolve to give a high viscosity solution at low concentration. In the available products, the active constituent(s) may be:

- Karaya gum (sterculia);
- Sodium carboxy methyl cellulose;
- Sodium carboxy methyl cellulose and poly(ethylene oxide);
- Sodium carboxy methyl cellulose and pectin and gelatin.

FURTHER READING

Keng S B, Lim M (1996). Denture plaque distribution and the effectiveness of a perborate-containing denture cleanser. *Quintessence International* **27**: 341-345.

McCabe J F, Murray I D, Kelly P J (1995). The efficacy of denture cleansers. *European Journal of Prosthodontics & Restorative Dentistry* **3**: 203-207.

Odman P A (1992). The effectiveness of an enzyme-containing denture cleanser. *Quintessence International* **23**: 187-190.

Dills S S, Olshan A M, Goldner S, Brogdon C (1988). Comparison of the antimicrobial capability of an abrasive paste and chemical-soak denture cleancrs. *Journal of Prosthetic Dentistry* **60**: 467-470.

Collys K D, Roma de Sousa A C, Smeyers-Verbeke J (1997). Soluble denture adhesives: pH and sodium content. *European Journal of Prosthodontics & Restorative Dentistry* **5**: 63-67

DeVengencie J, Ng M C, Ford P, Iacopino A M (1997). In vitro evaluation of denture adhesives: possible efficacy of complex carbohydrates. *International Journal of Prosthodontics* **10**:61-72.

Chapter 50

Implant Materials

Summary: This chapter classifies implants, and deals with choice of materials, including alloys and ceramics. Guided tissue regeneration is briefly discussed.

50.1 INTRODUCTION

The increasing use of dental implants to replace missing teeth has resulted in a wide range of implant types and materials. In the past, a variety of materials has been used to replace the roots of natural teeth, among these being, platinum, steel, cobalt alloys, titanium, carbon, porcelain and acrylic resin.

There are three types of dental implant:

1. The *subperiosteal* implant, which is essentially a framework resting beneath the periosteum on the bony ridge of the mandible. This carries the supports for a prosthesis which penetrate through the mucosa. Long term success rates are modest, with around 50% of implants still in position and functional at 15 years.
2. The *transosteal* implant, which penetrates from the upper surface of the mandible to the lower: there are few reports of success rates for this type.
3. The *endosseous* implant, which is anchored to the bone by a process termed osseointegration and which is partially submerged within the bone.

As success rates of endosseous implants are high, over 90% showing satisfactory function at ten years for some types, their use has become popular at the expense of the other two types. They have fewer clinical limitations than other types and may be obtained in a wide variety of sizes and designs. Success is dependent on intimate bone growth around the newly placed implant (*osseointegration*). This is an intimate interface between bone and implant.

Osseointegration requires a period of several months' stabilization, during which time the implant should be protected from the stresses of occlusion. In many types, the implant remains completely submerged during this time and is re-exposed at a later date. Some implants incorporate polymeric inserts which act as 'shock absorbers' (in the same manner as the periodontal membrane is considered to do for natural teeth), although these require replacement at regular intervals. Once osseointegration has occurred the implant transmits forces to the underlying bone and thereby supports a fixed or removable prosthesis. It is therefore apparent that the intimate contact between the implant and bone necessitates unique properties in terms of biocompatibility since the implant extends from the mouth through the epithelium into the underlying bone. Distribution of mechanical forces is also an important consideration. This is predominantly controlled by the shape and form of the implant but the microscopic distribution of forces is controlled by the properties of the material. There are a number of materials that appear to fulfil these criteria. However, correct surgical methods that minimize mechanical, chemical and thermal trauma to the tissues are also of fundamental importance.

Metals are the most commonly used implant materials in view of their suitable physical properties. Stainless steel and cobalt-chromium have previously been used because of their good corrosion resistance and acceptable biocompatibility, but these have largely been superseded by pure titanium or titanium alloys because of the excellent biocompatibility of titanium.

50.2 SURGICAL STAINLESS STEEL

This alloy is an iron-carbon (0.05% carbon) alloy with about 18% chromium added to impart corrosion resistance and 7-8% nickel to stabilize the austenitic structure (Section 13.7). It has been used for many years for dental and orthopedic implants. Its use is obviously contraindicated in patients who are allergic to nickel. It is used in a wrought and heat-treated condition that produces a high strength and highly ductile material that is resistant to fracture. The concept of surface passivation by a surface layer of oxide was first noted with stainless steel (Section 14.2.7). As this layer minimizes corrosion resistance it is important that it is not damaged. Stainless steel alloys may function for long periods of time without any apparent breakdown, but it has also been considered that the toxicity threshold for nickel may be reached, and that a sequestration reaction is the consequence. The low cost and good mechanical propertics are significant advantages.

50.3 TITANIUM AND ITS ALLOYS

Pure titanium is one of the materials of choice for implants in view of its good biocompatibility. It is highly reactive. In air and aqueous electrolytes is spontaneously oxidizes (passivates), forming a dense oxide film on its surface. This oxide layer of thickness about 1 nm thickness minimizes the potential for corrosion. Titanium is less dense than stainless steel and has a high strength to weight ratio. Its modulus of elasticity is approximately half that of cobalt chromium or stainless steel and five times greater than compact bone, which indicates that good design of the implant is essential in ensuring the correct distribution of mechanical forces. The biocompatibility and corrosion resistance of titanium are good, although titanium ions are released into bone and thereby into the circulation at a low level. There have been no reported adverse effects of this release and titanium remains the material of choice from the viewpoint of osseointegration and biocompatibility.

The limited mechanical strength of titanium has led to the development of titanium alloys, the most commonly used for implant use being 90% titanium, 6% aluminum and 4% vanadium by weight (Ti-6Al-4V – see Section 13.9). This alloy has a slightly higher modulus of elasticity than titanium, being 5.6 times that of compact bone, and, as with pure titanium, the surface oxidizes (passivates) readily. The potential for biodegradation of the various constituents of the alloy has been considered low and there have been few identifiable adverse sequelae to the use of this alloy in dental and orthopedic implants.

50.4 COBALT-CHROMIUM-MOLYBDENUM ALLOY

These surgical alloys of cobalt are not the same as those used for partial denture frameworks (Sections 13.8.1 and 47.3), although they are often used in the as-cast or cast-and-annealed conditions. Their composition is approximately 63% cobalt, 30% chromium and 5% molybdenum. Traces of carbon, manganese and nickel may also be present. These alloys have a principal use as subperiosteal frames. Chromium provides corrosion resistance by forming an oxide surface. Molybdenum and carbon contribute to the mechanical properties. These alloys have high resistance to corrosion, have a high modulus of elasticity and are the least ductile of the alloys used for dental implants. These alloys, and stainless steel, are lower in cost than titanium alloys and have provided good long-term success in many applications in dentistry and surgery. However, the greater biocompatibility and corrosion resistance of titanium have increased its use in dental implants.

50.5 OTHER METALS

Implant devices have also been constructed in reactive metals such as zirconium, tungsten and hafnium but their long-term success has still to be assessed. Gold has also been used as an implant material, but its low strength limits its applications. Most recently, implants have been constructed in a titanium substructure which has been coated with a thin layer (20 μm –100 μm) of calcium phosphate ceramic (see below) using the process known as flame or plasma-spraying. This 'bioactive', rough, coating promotes bone growth around the implant, producing a bond between bone and implant. It has been considered that this coating reduces the time required for osseointegration. However, the long-term success is dependent upon the maintenance of the bond between the metal and the ceramic coating. Current data suggests that some breakdown of the bond may occur.

50.6 CERAMICS

Because of their excellent biocompatibility and inertness, ceramics would appear to be logical materials for use as implants. Two types have been used:

1. Non-reactive materials such as aluminum oxide (Al_2O_3). This ceramic is well tolerated by bone, but does not appear to promote bone formation. However, although osseointegration does not occur in the manner associated with titanium implants, bone grows closely around these materials, thereby retaining the implant.
2. Bioactive calcium phosphate ceramic materials such as hydroxyapatite (HA) or tricalcium phosphate (TCP) have been used as non-resorbable implant materials for augmenting resorbed alveolar ridges. When used in such situations, the HA or TCP acts as a framework into which new bony

growth occurs. The strength of the integrated material is a combination of the ceramic and the infiltrating tissue. These materials were considered to possess advantages such as excellent biocompatibility, with similar constituents to those of normal tissue (calcium, phosphorus, oxygen and hydrogen), minimal thermal and electrical conductivity, and, modulus of elasticity similar to bone. Disadvantages include low tensile and shear strengths, relatively low attachment strengths and variable solubilities.

Another bioactive material is a dense ceramic Bioglass, prepared from CaO, Na_2O, P_2O_5 and SiO_2. This is a resorbable material. When used as an implant material, surface dissolution of the material occurs with the release of sodium, calcium and phosphate ions. Hydrogen ions from tissue fluid replace the sodium ions in the Bioglass. A calcium-phosphorus layer is formed on the surface of the material stimulating osteoblast proliferation and production of collagen fibrils that become enmeshed in the calcium-phosphorus layer. This produces a bond that is so strong that cohesive failure occurs within the Bioglass rather than at the interface when tested. A limiting factor is the brittle nature of the Bioglass; if this property can be improved, the material may show great potential.

50.7 BONE GROWTH PROMOTERS

A number of local bone growth promoters have recently been developed. These were originally only available from human and bovine sources but these proteins, called bone morphogenetic proteins (BMPs) may now be synthesized. An early trial using a collagen sponge impregnated with a BMP has produced sufficient bone augmentation in the antrum of a patient to permit implant placement.

50.8 CARBON COMPOUNDS

Carbon compounds have been used extensively in cardiovascular devices and have shown excellent biocompatibility. An advantage is a modulus of elasticity similar to that of bone, but clinical applications have so far been few, except for use as a coating on metallic and ceramic materials.

50.9 GUIDED TISSUE REGENERATION

This technique uses the principle of placing a resorbable or non-resorbable membrane into the area of a bone defect in order to prevent the ingrowth of soft tissue and allow the regeneration of bony tissue within a haematoma. The most commonly used non-resorbable membrane is expanded PTFE (polytetrafluoroethylene). This is available in several sizes and configurations for the varying sizes of defects. The major advantage of a resorbable membrane is that it will be absorbed by its host after its placement without the need for a second surgical procedure. Examples of resorbable materials are collagen, copolymers of glycolide and lactide, polylactic acid and polyurethane. Success rates appear to be dependent more upon the size and morphology of the periodontal defect, the care taken during the surgical procedure and the maintenance care provided rather than the barrier materials used. This technique may be employed to provide bony regeneration in conjunction with implants.

FURTHER READING

Trejo P M, Weltman R, Caffesse R G (1995). Guided tissue regeneration. A status report for the American Journal of Dentistry. *American Journal of Dentistry* **8**: 313-319.

Steinemann S G (1998). Titanium - the material of choice? *Periodontology 2000* **17** :7-21.

Schenk R K, Buser D (1998). Osseointegration: a reality. *Periodontology 2000* **17**: 22-35.

XIII

LABORATORY MATERIALS

Chapter 51

Cast and Die Materials

Summary: The composition and properties of cast and die materials are discussed, with particular reference to gypsum products.

51.1 INTRODUCTION

A *cast* is a replica of the teeth and/or the associated supporting bony tissues of one jaw, which is prepared from an impression. A *die* is a model of a single tooth, again prepared from an impression. Cast and die materials should have the following properties:

1. Mechanical properties. High strength is important, to reduce the likelihood of accidental breakage, particularly of teeth from a cast. The material should be as hard as possible, so that the surface will not be damaged during carving of a wax pattern.
2. Reproduction of detail. The ability to reproduce fine detail and sharp margins is essential.
3. Dimensional accuracy and stability. There should be little dimensional change on setting, and the material should remain dimensionally stable on storage.
4. Compatibility with impression materials. There should be no interaction between surface of impression and cast or die.
5. Color. Good color contrast with other materials being used, for example, inlay wax or porcelain, is important.
6. Economic considerations. Cheapness and ease of use are also important.

Casts and dies for dental use are frequently prepared from plaster of Paris, or from hard plaster materials, known as dental stones. Both these materials have calcium sulfate hemihydrate, $(CaSO_4)_2,H_2O$ (sometimes written $CaSO_4$, $\frac{1}{2}H_2O$) as their main constituent, prepared by heating calcium sulfate dehydrate (gypsum). This material is discussed next (Section 51.2) followed by consideration of alternative die materials (Section 51.3).

51.2 CALCIUM SULFATE HEMIHYDRATE

51.2.1 Classification

The hydrates of calcium sulfate are listed in Figure 51.1.

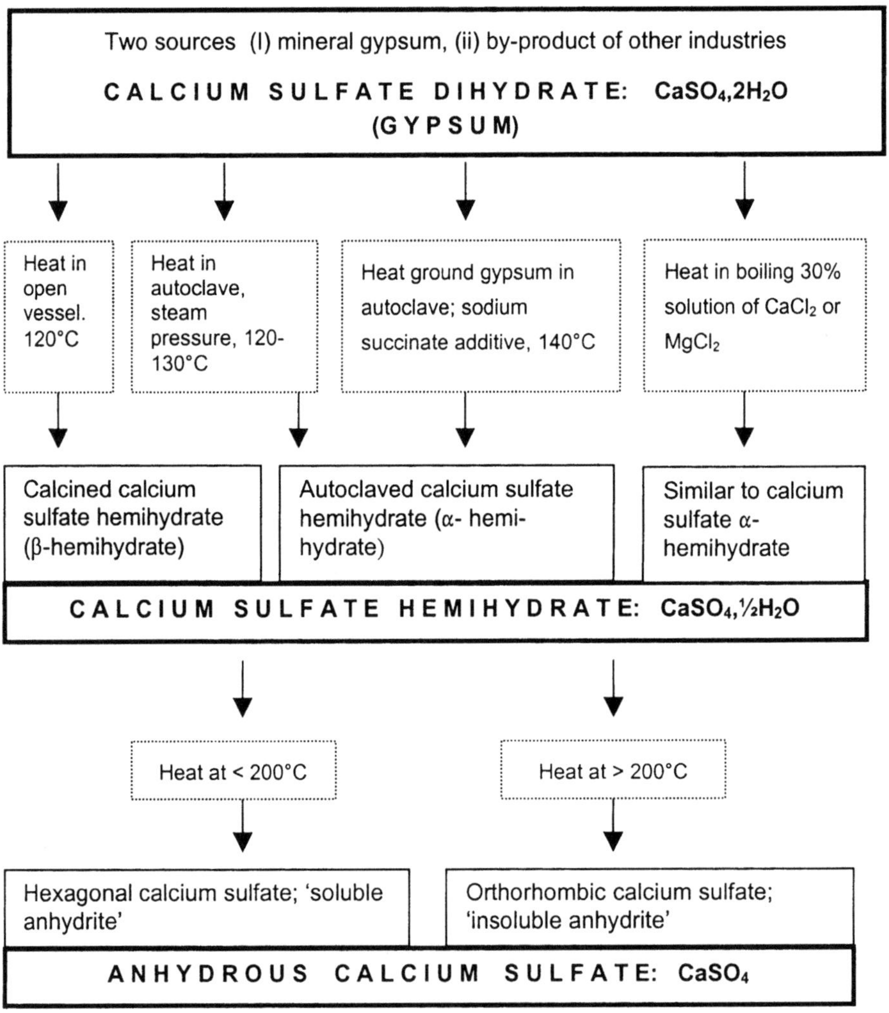

Figure 51.1. The hydrates of calcium sulfate.

In Figure 51.1 it can be seen that calcium sulfate hemihydrate is prepared from the dihydrate (gypsum) by a variety of heating methods:

$$CaSO_4{,}2H_2O \longrightarrow CaSO_4{,}{}^1/_2H_2O + {}^3/_2H_2O$$

Many dental materials contain calcium sulfate as their principal constituent, and these can be classified into a number of types:

- Type I. Plaster for recording impressions, including additives to control the setting expansion and time, as discussed in Chapter 31;
- Type II. Model plaster;
- Type III. Dental stone;
- Type IV. Dental stone, high strength;
- Type V. Dental stone, high strength, high expansion.

Types I and II are based on calcined (β) calcium sulfate hemihydrate. Types III - V stones contain the autoclaved material (α-hemihydrate), and are usually pigmented, to distinguish them from plaster which is white.

Another application of autoclaved calcium sulfate hemihydrate is their use as bonding agents in refractory mold materials for metal casting (Chapter 53).

51.2.2 The setting reaction of calcium sulfate hemihydrate

When hemihydrate is mixed with water, the dihydrate is formed, as follows:

$$CaSO_4,{}^1/_2H_2O + {}^3/_2H_2O \longrightarrow CaSO_4,2H_2O$$

This is the reverse of the reaction whereby hemihydrate is formed. From the above equation it can be calculated that 100 g of hemihydrate require about 18.6 ml water to give complete hydration. In practice, however, more water than this is used when mixing plaster or stone, to give a smooth workable mix.

On mixing the hemihydrate with water, some hemihydrate dissolves, giving Ca^{2+} and SO_4^{2-} ions. The solubility of hemihydrate in water at room temperature is about 0.8%. At this temperature, the solubility of the dihydrate is only about 0.2%. The dissolved hemihydrate forms the dihydrate in solution, which is then supersaturated. Crystal growth of the dihydrate from this solution then occurs.

Crystal growth occurs on nuclei of crystallization; in this case nuclei may be crystals of gypsum initially present as an impurity in the hemihydrate crystals. Diffusion, or movement, of the Ca^{2+} and SO_4^{2-} ions to these nuclei, also appears to be important. As the dihydrate crystallizes, so more hemihydrate dissolves and the process continues.

51.2.3 The setting process

Initially the mix of hemihydrate and water can be poured, provided the correct water/powder ratio is used. The material becomes rigid, but not hard ('initial set') – at this stage the material can be carved but not molded. The so-called 'final set' follows, when the material becomes hard and strong. However, at this stage the hydration reaction is not necessarily complete, nor has optimum strength and hardness been achieved. Heat is given out during setting, since the hydration of the hemihydrate is exothermic.

Dimensional changes also take place. A setting expansion can be observed. The linear expansion is in the range 0.3 to 0.4% for most plasters and 0.05 to 0.3% for dental stones. This expansion is caused by the outward thrust of the growing crystals of dihydrate. This expansion is, in fact, apparent. The expanded set material contains crystals of dihydrate and pores. The volume of crystals of the set material is less than the initial volume of the hemihydrate. The magnitude of this reduction in volume of the crystalline material can be calculated from the molecular weights and specific gravities of hemihydrate, water and dihydrate, and is approximately 7%.

If mixed plaster is placed under water at the initial set stage, a greater expansion on setting occurs. This is often termed *hygroscopic expansion* and is sometimes used to expand gypsum bonded investment materials (Section 53.4.3).

51.2.4 Differences between calcined and autoclaved hemihydrate

These two materials are chemically identical, but they differ in the following ways:

1. Manufacture. See Figure 51.1.
2. Particle size and shape. Calcined hemihydrate particles are larger, more irregular and porous. The particles of the autoclaved material are smaller, regular and non-porous (Figure 51.2).

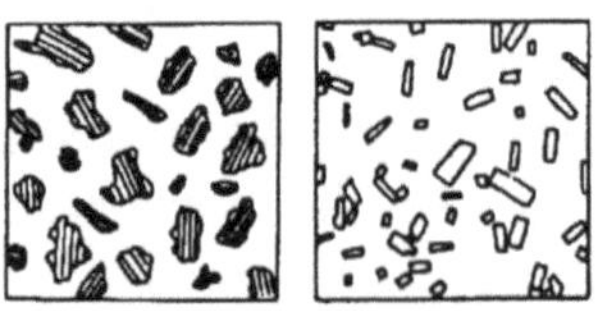

Figure 51.2. Particles of calcium sulfate hemihydrate; left:the calcined material; right: the autoclaved material. Approximate magnification x100.

3. Water/powder ratio. Theoretically this is 0.186. However, neither form of hemihydrate, when mixed with water to this ratio, will give a smooth workable mix. The ratios that are usually used in practice are:

- Types I and II: 50-60 ml water / 100 g plaster;
- Types III -V: 22 to 35 ml water /100 g stone.

The reason for the difference is that the porous particles of a calcined material soak up a considerable amount of water.

4. The set material. This consists of a network of interlocking dihydrate crystals; the spaces between these crystals are initially occupied by the excess water used in mixing the material (this water will contain calcium sulfate in solution). The greater the quantity of excess water, the more porous (or less dense) is the set material; thus the porosity of set plaster is greater than the porosity of set stone (Figure 51.3).

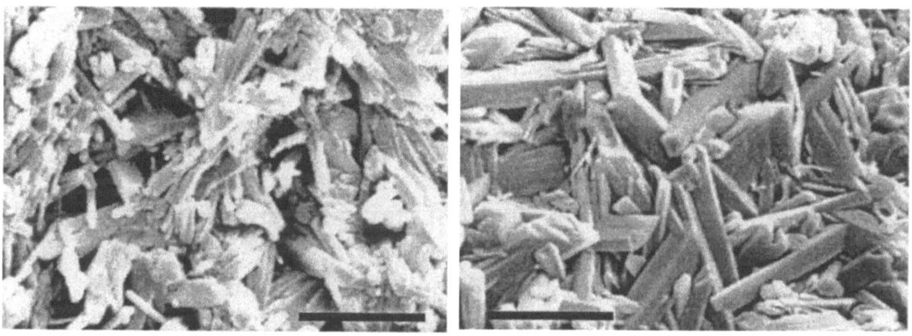

Figure 51.3 SEM showing structure of set gypsum; left: dental plaster (water/powder ratio = 0.55); right: type IV stone (water/powder ratio = 0.22). The horizontal bars represent 10 μm.

5. Mechanical properties of the set material. Strength and hardness depend on the density of the material; thus stone is harder and stronger than plaster.

6. Applications. Where strength and hardness are required, autoclaved hemihydrate, as in stone, is the material of choice. Examples are casts for construction of dentures, dies for crowns, bridge and inlay work, and binders for casting investments (Chapter 53). When mechanical properties are not of primary importance, plaster can be used, for example mounting casts and some orthodontic study casts.

51.2.5 The effects of additives

Nearly all acids and salts, when added to a mix of plaster or stone, affect the setting. The setting time may be increased or decreased. Accelerators include potassium sulfate, which accelerates setting by increasing the rate of solution of calcium sulfate hemihydrate. Gypsum accelerates by providing nuclei for crystal growth of further dihydrate. Potassium citrate and borax are examples of retarders. These either reduce the rate of dissolution of hemihydrate, or are adsorbed on to nuclei of crystallization, thus 'poisoning' these nuclei, so rendering them ineffective.

Additives may alter the setting expansion. Increased expansion is achieved by adding, for example, calcium acetate, which can give over 1% linear setting expansion. Decreased expansion is obtained by adding potassium sulfate, which can reduce the linear setting expansion down to 0.05%.

Additives usually reduce the strength of the material.

51.2.6 Manipulation

All gypsum products should be stored in closed containers, to prevent reaction with moisture from the atmosphere, which can cause formation of the dihydrate that can accelerate the setting. Contamination by traces of set gypsum and other impurities must be avoided.

Use of the correct water/powder ratio is essential. If stone is mixed with too much water, the set material may be as weak as plaster.

Incorporation of air into the material during mixing should be avoided. Vacuum mixing techniques are helpful in this regard. Mixing time of one minute is usually sufficient to give a smooth lump-free slurry.

Vibration is usually used in preparing a cast or die from an impression; this helps the slurry to flow well into the impression and helps to eliminate air bubbles. Over-vibration should be avoided as this may cause distortion of some impression materials.

A separating agent is applied to a stone die before preparation of a wax pattern on the die - this facilitates removal of the pattern from the die. Unfortunately these agents can soften the surface of the die.

51.2.7 Setting time

This is usually measured as the time taken for the setting material to become sufficiently rigid to withstand the penetration of a needle of known diameter under a known load. Two such pieces of apparatus are known as *Vicat* and *Gillmore* needles.

The setting time depends on the composition of the plaster or stone, as supplied by the manufacturer. For example, gypsum if present (possibly due to incomplete dehydration during the manufacturing process), will accelerate the setting. Hexagonal calcium sulfate, if present, will hydrate rapidly. Orthorhombic calcium sulfate, which can result from gross overheating of the gypsum during manufacture, reacts very slowly with water (sometimes known as *'dead-burnt' plaster*). Other impurities may be present, which either occurred in the gypsum starting material, or were introduced during the manufacturing process.

The setting times obviously also depends on the presence of added accelerators and/or retarders.

The physical form of the plaster or stone is also important. During manufacture grinding is usually carried out after the dehydration process. This accelerates the setting, since some of the ground crystals can act as nuclei for the crystal growth on setting. Grinding also increases the surface area of the hemihydrate exposed to water, thus increasing the rate of solution of the hemihydrate.

The temperature of the mix has very little effect on setting time up to 50°C. Table 51.1 gives results for one batch of dental stone. This is in contrast to most chemical reactions, which are accelerated considerably by an increase in temperature. This can be explained by assuming that the rate of reaction depends on the rate of random diffusion of Ca^{2+} and SO_4^{2-} ions to the growing dihydrate crystals. The rate of diffusion of ions in solution depends not only on the nature of the ions, but also on temperature and the concentration of ions. It can be shown that the rate of diffusion of Ca^{2+} and SO_4^{2-} ions at 50°C is approximately double the rate at 5°C. However the rate of diffusion of ions is directly proportional to their concentration. The solubility of hemihydrate is approximately 0.8% and 0.4% at 5°C and 50°C respectively. Thus at higher temperatures the rate of diffusion is reduced, owing to a decrease in concentration. The two factors above are opposite to each other and approximately equal in magnitude. Thus temperature has only a comparatively small effect on the rate of reaction within the range 5°C to 50°C. At higher temperatures, retardation of hydration occurs, and at 100°C there is no hydration - at approximately this temperature both hemihydrate and dihydrate have the same solubility.

Table 51.1. The effect of temperature on the setting time of dental stone

Temperature (°C)	Time for complete hydration of a dental stone (minutes)
5	65
25	75
30	60
35	50
40	45
45	40
50	55

Water/powder ratio has very little effect on the rate of hydration of the hemihydrate, although an increase in water content of a slurry gives a slower setting time as measured by the Vicat or Gillmore needle test. The reason is, that at a higher water/powder ratio, there are fewer growing dihydrate crystals per volume of mixed material. So in the more dilute slurries, more crystal growth has to occur before there is enough crystal contact to give sufficient rigidity to withstand the penetration of a setting time needle.

An increase in the mixing time can accelerate the set. Mixing can break up some of the formed dihydrate crystals, thus forming more nuclei of crystallization.

51.2.8 Strength

The strength of set gypsum depends on a number of factors. These include the material that is used - for example, autoclaved or calcined hemihydrate and the additives present. It also depends on the water/powder ratio (Table 51.2). For optimum properties, the plaster or stone should be left to hydrate for at least one hour (and preferably longer), and then dried to constant weight at 45 °C.

Table 51.2. The strength of plaster and stone

Material	Water/powder ratio	Condition	Compressive strength (MPa)
Plaster (Type II)	0.60	After 1 hour	10
Plaster (Type II)	0.60	Dried to constant weight	21
Stone (Type IV)	0.25	After 1 hour	30
Stone (Type IV)	0.25	Dried to constant weight	72

51.2.9 Assessment of cast and die materials based on calcium sulfate hemihydrate

How do these materials meet the requirements listed in Section 51.1?

1. Mechanical properties. These are not ideal – fracture of teeth from stone casts can occur with careless handling; also stone dies are not always sufficiently hard to resist abrasion during the carving of a wax pattern.
2. The ability to reproduce fine detail and sharp margins is excellent.
3. Dimensional accuracy and stability are good – the small linear setting expansion is not considered to be a significant source of error in most dental procedures.
4. Compatibility with impression materials. Some impression materials can cause a slight softening of the stone surface. Impression plaster has to be treated with a separating agent before casting up a cast in dental stone.
5. Color contrast. As noted above, dental stones usually contain pigments.

6. Dental stones are inexpensive and easy to use.

51.2.10 Recent developments

In attempts to improve abrasion resistance, some die stones contain a polymeric reinforcing agent.

51.3 ALTERNATIVE DIE MATERIALS

A wide range of alternative materials has been used for die production, some of which are materials designed for other dental applications. These include silicophosphate cements, dental amalgam, polymers and filled polymers (e.g. epoxy resins), and metal sprayed and electroplated dies.

FURTHER READING

Lewry A J, Williamson J (1994). Setting of gypsum plaster.
Part I. The hydration of calcium sulphate hemihydrate. *Journal of Materials Science* **29**: 5279-5284.
Part II. The development of microstructure and strength. *Journal of Materials Science* **29**: 5524-5528.
Part III. The effect of additives and impurities. *Journal of Materials Science* **29**: 6085-6090.

Chapter 52

Waxes and Baseplate Materials

Summary: Composition, properties and manipulation of many types of waxes for a number of dental applications are considered.

52.1 INTRODUCTION

Waxes were first used in dentistry in the early eighteenth century for the purpose of recording impressions of edentulous mouths. Although superseded by other impression materials, waxes are still employed in large quantities in various clinical and laboratory procedures. The construction of many dental appliances requires the use of waxes with specific and often markedly different physical properties. In order to obtain these requirements, dental waxes are usually blended from both natural and synthetic materials. Various resins and gums can be added to make waxes more adhesive.

52.2 CONSTITUENTS OF DENTAL WAXES

The basic constituents of dental waxes come from three main sources, that is, there are mineral, insect and vegetable waxes.

The structure and properties of the most important materials are classified in Table 52.1. Since the properties of these naturally occurring materials cannot be controlled, synthetic waxes (e.g. nitrogenous derivatives of fatty acids) or polymers of ethylene oxide may offer advantages.

52.3 PHYSICAL PROPERTIES OF WAXES

The most frequently quoted physical property of waxes is their melting point. While this may be of importance in industry it does not have the same significance in dentistry where blends of waxes are employed. The important physical properties of waxes used in dentistry, apart from ease of manipulation, are:

- Solid-solid transition temperature;
- Thermal expansion and contraction;
- Flow;
- Internal stress.

Table 52.1. Classification of naturally occurring waxes

Type	Example	Source	Structure and properties
Mineral	Paraffin wax	Obtained during the distillation of crude petroleum	Straight-chained hydrocarbon Polycrystalline Brittle at ambient temperature
Mineral	Microcrystall-ine wax or ceresin	As above	Branch-chained hydrocarbon Polycrystalline Less brittle than paraffin wax, due to their oil content.
Insect	Beeswax	Honeycombs	Less crystalline than paraffin wax When blended with parafin wax: - At room temperature makes it less brittle - At higher temperatures reduces the flow of the wax
Vegetable	Carnauba wax	South American palm trees	Hard lustrous and tough wax Blended with paraffin to harden it and raise its solid-solid transition temperature
Vegetable	Candelila wax	Plants	Similar to carnauba
Vegetable	Resins and gums	Trees	Used to add adhesive qualities to waxes

52.3.1 Solid-solid transition temperature

As the temperature of a wax is raised, a solid-solid transition occurs where the stable crystal lattice form (orthorhombic in most dental waxes) commences to change to a hexagonal form that is present below the melting point of the wax. It is during this progressive change from one lattice type to the other that waxes can be manipulated without flaking, tearing or becoming unduly stressed.

The existence of this solid-solid transition point and the temperature at which it occurs not only allows waxes to be manipulated satisfactorily, but also determines much of their physical behavior and suitability for various clinical and laboratory procedures. Waxes that should remain rigid in the mouth must have a solid-solid transition temperature above 37°C.

52.3.2 Thermal expansion and contraction

The coefficient of thermal expansion of waxes is higher than that of any other dental material. This is a potential source of error in dental procedures, since a pattern will shrink appreciably on cooling from its solidification temperature to room temperature. It can be shown that on cooling from 37°C to 20°C, a linear shrinkage of almost 0.6% can occur for a wax with a coefficient of thermal expansion of $350 \times 10^{-6}/°C$.

52.3.3 Flow

Waxes deform when subjected to a load for a period of time. This plastic deformation or percentage 'flow' depends on temperature and is found to be low when the temperature of the wax is below the solid-solid transition temperature, that is when the materials are in the stable crystal lattice form.

The flow property of waxes and wax mixtures increases as their temperature is raised above the transition temperature.

It is important in an inlay wax for use in the direct technique (Section 52.4.3) that there should be a large flow about 5°C above mouth temperature, so that good detail of the cavity will be obtained but negligible flow at 37°C, so that no distortion will occur on removal of the pattern from the cavity.

52.3.4 Internal stresses

Waxes have low thermal conductivity, so making it difficult to achieve uniform heating. If a wax is molded or adapted to shape without adequate heating to above the solid-solid transition temperature, considerable stresses will be set up in the material. If the wax is subsequently warmed, relief of the stresses will occur, resulting in distortion.

52.4 DENTAL APPLICATIONS OF WAXES

52.4.1 Modeling wax

This is used as a pattern material (Section 53.1), and for the registration of jaw relationships, in the construction of dentures. The desirable properties are that it should be easy to mold when softened, and not tear, flake or crack and it should be easy to carve. It should be capable of being melted and solidified a number of times without change of properties. No residue of wax should be left after applying boiling water and detergent to the mold formed about the wax.

The exact compositions of available modeling waxes are not usually revealed by the manufacturers, but suitable materials can be prepared using mixtures of such waxes as paraffin wax and beeswax, with a small quantity of a harder and tougher wax such as carnauba. A range of materials of different softening temperatures is available.

In the manipulation of the materials it is important that the wax is evenly heated throughout its whole bulk and adapted to shape before cooling, to minimize subsequent distortion due to relief of internal stresses.

Modeling waxes used for clinical procedures should show little or no dimensional change when they are heated to mouth temperature and subsequently cooled to room temperature.

52.4.2 Sheet casting wax

Sheet casting wax is supplied in sheets which have been rolled to a precise thickness. When such wax is being manipulated, care must be taken not to make it thinner. This can be avoided by heating the wax in hot water and using moist cotton-wool to adapt it to shape. It is important that both clasps and connectors of cast metallic dentures should be of the correct thickness.

Ready-formed polymeric components are available to simplify the waxing-up of a cast partial denture. Both casting waxes and polymeric components should burn out from the mold without leaving any residue.

52.4.3 Inlay wax

Inlay wax is used for the preparation of inlay patterns, either in the mouth, by the *direct technique*, or more usually these days on a model or die cast up from an impression – the *indirect technique*.

For use in the former application, it is important that the wax should have as low a thermal contraction as possible, though inevitably this must be high. It should have the correct flow properties and be colored (usually blue or green) to contrast with the oral tissues.

In addition, all inlay waxes should be easy to carve without chipping or flaking and burn out of the mold without leaving any residue.

The constituents of inlay waxes are similar to modeling waxes. The proportion of harder waxes is increased, however, to produce a blend capable of meeting the more stringent requirements of an inlay wax.

52.4.4 Carding and boxing-in-wax

This is a wax with a high flow value at room temperature and is easily moldable without the need for heating. It is used by manufacturers to attach artificial teeth to the mounts on which they are supplied, and is also used in the dental laboratory to 'box in' impressions prior to casting up.

52.4.5 Sticky wax

This is an adhesive brittle wax, usually made of beeswax and some naturally occurring resins. It should show no flow at room temperature. It is used in the dental laboratory for a variety of applications where temporary joining of articles is required, for example, joining together metal parts prior to soldering and joining fragments of a broken denture prior to the repair procedure. It should be easily removed by boiling water and should show minimal shrinkage on cooling to prevent movement of the parts to be joined.

52.4.6 Impression waxes

Impression, corrective and disclosing waxes are all characterized by their high degree of flow at mouth temperature.

52.5 THERMOPLASTIC BASEPLATE MATERIALS

These may be made of:
- Wax, similar to modelling wax;
- Shellac, or shellac with aluminum;
- A polymer such as polystyrene.

Baseplate materials should be readily adaptable to the required shape, rigid with little flow at mouth temperature and should not distort on standing, or in use.

FURTHER READING

Ito M, Yamagishi T, Oshida Y, Munoz C A (1996). Effect of selected physical properties of waxes on investments and casting shrinkage. *Journal of Prosthetic Dentistry* **75**:211-216.

Diwan R, Talic Y, Omar N, Sadig W (1997). Pattern waxes and inaccuracies in fixed and removable partial denture castings. *Journal of Prosthetic Dentistry*. **77**: 553-555.

Kotsiomiti E, McCabe J F (1997). Experimental wax mixtures for dental use. *Journal of Oral Rehabilitation* **24**: 517-521.

Chapter 53

Casting Investment Materials

Summary: Three types of refractory investment materials, used to form molds in the fabrication of cast metal restorations and prostheses, are discussed.

53.1 INTRODUCTION

When a restoration or appliance is being made by a 'lost wax' process, the wax pattern is embedded in an investment material. The wax is then removed from this mold, and the space that it occupied is filled by the material of which the restoration or appliance is to be made. For example, a wax pattern of a denture, in which the teeth have been set up is embedded in a two-part mold, made of plaster of Paris or dental stone (or a mixture of the two) contained in a two-part metal container (a *flask*). The wax is removed by means of boiling water and detergent, leaving the teeth embedded in the set gypsum. The space formerly occupied by the wax is subsequently filled with the polymeric denture base material (Chapter 45).

The wax pattern of an inlay or other cast restoration is embedded in a heat-resistant investment material, which is capable of setting to a hard mass. The wax is removed from such a mold usually by burning out, before casting the molten alloy. This chapter is primarily concerned with the latter materials, since details of plaster and stone are dealt with in Chapter 51.

53.2 REQUIREMENTS FOR INVESTMENT MATERIALS

All investment materials contain two principal constituents. There must be a refractory substance that will not decompose or disintegrate on heating. There is also a binder that sets and binds together the particles of the refractory substance to form the mold. The powder should be of a fine particle size to ensure a smooth surface on the casting. The mixed unset material should have a smooth consistency. The material should have a suitable setting time. The mold must expand to compensate for the shrinkage on cooling of the alloy. The set material should be permeable to allow air to escape as the molten alloy enters the mold. The strength of the material should be sufficient to withstand the force of the molten alloy entering the mold.

53.3 CLASSIFICATION OF INVESTMENT MATERIALS

Three types of investment materials are available. They all contain silica (SiO_2) as the refractory constituent. The chief difference between them is the type of binder used, as follows:

- Gypsum-bonded investments are widely used for gold alloys, but are unsuitable for alloys which melt at temperatures approaching 1200°C;
- Phosphate-bonded materials are used for casting cobalt-chromium alloys, since they can withstand higher temperatures;
- Silica-bonded investments are an alternative to the phosphate-bonded materials for high temperature casting.

53.4 GYPSUM-BONDED INVESTMENTS

53.4.1 Constituents

Silica is present in one of its allotropic forms (for example, cristobalite or quartz) to act as a refractory and to provide mold expansion by thermal expansion and inversion (Section 15.7).

Autoclaved calcium sulfate hemihydrate is present. It reacts with water and the resultant network of gypsum crystals binds the silica together. It also imparts strength to the mold. It can contribute to the mold expansion by the setting expansion that occurs.

Minor components include a reducing agent such as powdered charcoal, to reduce any oxide formed on the metal and a modifying chemical such as boric acid or sodium chloride, to inhibit shrinkage on heating

53.4.2 Manipulation

The mixing of an investment material is similar to that of dental stone (Chapter 51). Use of the correct water/powder ratio is important to ensure that the correct strength, setting time and expansion are obtained. Before investing the wax pattern, it is washed with a non-foam detergent to remove any oil or grease, and to facilitate the wetting of the pattern by the investment mix.

The casting ring is usually lined with a wet cellulose ('asbestos substitute') strip. This facilitates mold expansion (as outlined in the next section), since it can be compressed as expansion occurs, whereas a rigid ring on its own cannot do this. It contributes to the hygroscopic expansion.

Investing the pattern may be carried out under vacuum, to prevent trapping air on the surface of the pattern. Another technique is to paint investment material on to the pattern with a brush before carefully inserting it into the filled casting ring.

The mold is heated through 150 to 200°C; this dries out the excess water and burns off the wax. The mold is then slowly heated to above the temperature of inversion – usually to 700°C. It is held at this temperature for 30 minutes to ensure that the wax is completely burnt out.

53.4.3 Dimensional changes of the mold

Setting expansion is caused by the crystal growth of gypsum. In one technique the investment is immersed in water after setting has begun. A greatly increased setting expansion occurs (the *hygroscopic expansion*) so less thermal expansion is required. Increased hygroscopic expansion is obtained in the following cases:

- When a lower water/powder ratio is used;
- For an investment material of greater silica content;
- If water of higher temperature is used;
- For longer immersion in water.

Thermal expansion is also important. The thermal expansion of silica is discussed in Section 15.7.4. Investment materials containing cristobalite and quartz show rapid expansions between 200-300°C and 500-600°C respectively, due to displacive transformation of the silica (Figure 53.1). The amount of thermal expansion therefore depends on:

- Temperature;
- Quantity of silica in the material;
- Allotropic form of silica used; for example, the thermal expansion of cristobalite is greater than that of quartz at most temperatures (Figure 53.1);

– Water/powder ratio - thicker mixes have greater thermal expansion.

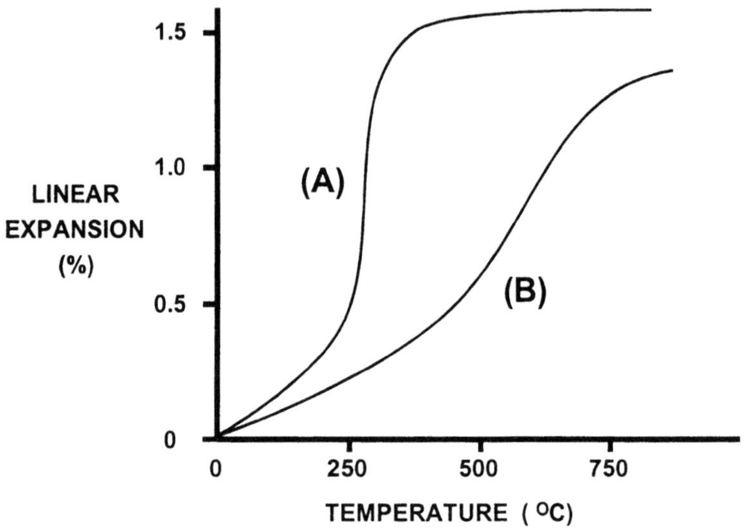

Figure 53.1. Thermal expansion of investments: (A) - containing cristobalite; (B) - containing quartz.

Shrinkage on heating must also be taken into account. This occurs due to the dehydration of the set gypsum in two stages:

$$CaSO_4,2H_2O \longrightarrow CaSO_4{}^1/_2H_2O + {}^3/_2H_2O$$

$$CaSO_4,{}^1/_2H_2O \longrightarrow CaSO_4 + {}^1/_2H_2O$$

The investment shrinkage is eliminated or reduced by the presence of small quantities of additives such as sodium chloride or boric acid.

53.4.4 Other properties

The total expansion of the mold is generally sufficient to compensate for the shrinkage on cooling of gold alloys (about 1.5% by volume). The investments containing finer particles of silica and calcium sulfate hemihydrate give smoother surfaces on the finished casting. Gypsum bonded investments are easy to manipulate giving a smooth consistency mix. The setting time of these materials can be easily controlled, as for stone and dental plaster. The set investment is porous and permeable to air, as is set gypsum - this helps to prevent back-pressure porosity in castings (Table 54.3). The strength of these materials, when set, if mixed at the correct water/powder ratio, is sufficient to withstand the forces of the molten alloy as it enters the mold. The autoclaved hemihydrate is used in preference to the calcined material for this reason (Section 51.2.9).

53.4.5 Limitations

Above around 1200°C a reaction can occur between calcium sulfate and silica:

$$CaSO_4 + SiO_2 \longrightarrow CaSiO_3 + SO_3$$

The sulfur trioxide gas that is evolved can causes porosity in the casting and may contribute to the corrosion of the casting. For this reason gypsum bonded investments are not used for the higher fusing dental alloys, such as cobalt-chromium. In this case phosphate- or silica-bonded materials are chosen.

53.5 PHOSPHATE-BONDED INVESTMENTS

53.5.1 Composition and setting

Magnesium oxide can react with a phosphate such as an ammonium phosphate in an aqueous system as follows:

$$MgO + NH_4H_2PO_4 \longrightarrow MgNH_4PO_4 + H_2O$$

The crystals of the magnesium ammonium phosphate bind together the particles of the silica refractory.

53.5.2 Manipulation

These materials are mixed with water, similar to gypsum-bonded investments. However, some differences in manipulation should be noted. Because of the strength of the set material, metal casting rings are not needed. In their place, plastic rings can be used; they are removed after the material has set, but before the investment is heated. The investment is heated to 1000°C to 1100°C.

53.5.3 Properties

The setting reaction is accompanied by an expansion, analogous to the crystal growth of gypsum. Also, thermal expansion occurs on heating.

A set phosphate-bonded material shows a certain degree of porosity and permeability to air, similar to the gypsum containing investments.

The set material increases in strength during heating, possibly due to chemical interaction between silica and the binder, giving complex silicophosphates.

53.6 SILICA-BONDED INVESTMENTS

53.6.1 Setting reactions

Stage 1 of the setting is a hydrolysis reaction. Ethyl silicate can be hydrolyzed to silicic acid, with liberation of ethyl alcohol:

$$Si(OC_2H_5)_4 + 4H_2O \longrightarrow Si(OH)_4 + 4C_2H_5OH$$

In practice, a polymerized form of ethyl silicate is used, yielding a sol of poly(silicic acid).

Stage 2 is a gelation process. The sol is mixed with cristobalite or quartz, then gel formation is made to occur under alkaline conditions by adding magnesium oxide. There is a slight shrinkage at this stage.

Stage 3 involves drying of the gel. On heating, considerable shrinkage occurs and there is a loss of alcohol and water, leaving a mold made of silica particles tightly packed together.

As an alternative to the above, simultaneous hydrolysis and gel formation can occur, when an amine such as piperidine is incorporated.

53.6.2 Properties

In terms of dimensional changes, there is a large amount of thermal expansion, due to the very large percentage of silica in the final material. This expansion is usually sufficient to compensate for both the setting shrinkage of the investment material and the casting shrinkage of the alloy.

The particles of the set material are packed so closely together that the porosity is negligible. Air spaces or vents must be left in the investment to permit escape of air from the mold.

FURTHER READING

Mori T (1993). Study of gypsum-bonded casting investments. Part 1. *Australian Dental Journal* **38**: 220-224.

McAloon J, Mori T (1993). Study of gypsum bonded casting investments. Part 2. *Australian Dental Journal* **38**: 306-308.

Luk H W-K, Darvell B W (1991). Strength of phosphate-bonded investments at high temperature. *Dental Materials* **7**: 99-102.

Chapter 54

Laboratory Procedures

Summary: An account of alloy casting, soldering, welding and abrasion and polishing.

54.1 CASTING

54.1.1 General method

This can be illustrated by considering the procedure used in the casting of an inlay in a gold alloy. The wax pattern has a sprue pin attached to it. The pattern is then invested. After setting of the investment material this pin is removed to provide a channel for the molten alloy to enter the mold. Attached to the sprue pin and the casting ring is a crucible former (or sprue base), which can be made of rubber or other polymers, or wax, or copper (Figure 54.1).

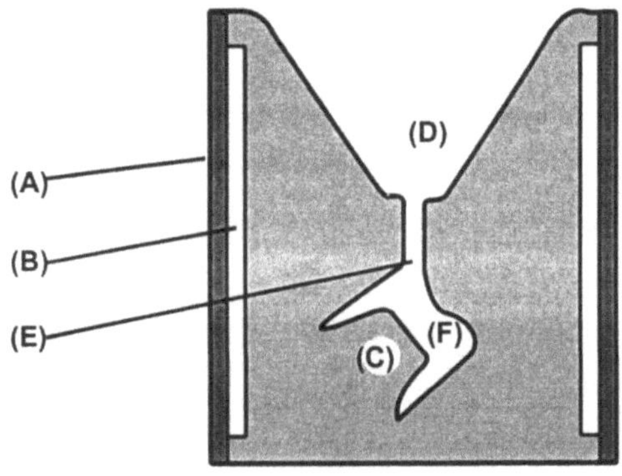

Figure 54.1. Cross section through an inlay casting mold, after removal of curcible former, sprue and wax: (A) - casting ring; (B) - ring lining; (C)- investment material; (D) - crucible former; (E) - sprue; (F) - inlay mold.

It is important that the correct diameter of sprue is used - this should be related to the size of the casting. A small inlay can have a sprue of 1.3 mm diameter; for most inlays it is 2.0 mm, and for very large crowns 2.6 mm. In some cases a reservoir may be needed. This is a piece of wax attached to the sprue about 1 mm away from the pattern. It can help to avoid porosity due to shrinkage. If the space occupied by the wax of the reservoir is of greater cross-section than the casting, the alloy that fills it will solidify later than in the main casting, and provide a reservoir of molten alloy to fill the space caused by shrinkage.

After removal of the sprue pin and the crucible former, the investment is heated in a furnace to burn out the wax and expand the mold. The alloy is melted by air/gas torches. The molten alloy is usually forced into the mold by a centrifugal method. As an alternative, air or steam pressure can be used.

Castings of larger dimensions than inlays – for example, the metal frameworks of partial dentures – usually necessitate the use of multiple sprues to ensure that the mold will be filled with the molten alloy before solidification of any part commences. When the casting is to be made in cobalt-chromium alloy, melting may be by an oxy-acetylene torch, or preferably by an electrical method, known as induction heating.

54.1.2 Faults in casting

Tables 54.1 to 54.5 give an analysis of the causes of casting faults, together with suggested methods of avoiding the problems. A casting may be dimensionally inaccurate (Table 54.1); have a rough surface (Table 54.2), be porous (Table 54.3), be contaminated (Table 54.4), and an incomplete casting may be obtained (Table 54.5).

Table 54.1. Causes of dimensional errors in castings

Problem	Cause	Method of prevention
Too large	Too much mold expansion	Use correct type of investment material at correct water/powder ratio and heat it to the correct temperature
Too small	Too little mold expansion	As above
Distortion	Distortion of wax pattern	Use correct handling techniques for wax

Table 54.2. Causes of rough surfaces and fins on castings

Problem	Cause	Method of prevention
Rough surface	Breakdown of investment material	Avoid having mold and alloy too hot
Rough surface	Air bubbles on the wax pattern	Use wetting agent on wax pattern and vacuum invest
Rough surface	Weak surface on investment	Avoid dilution of investment material by: - too high water/powder ratio - by use of too much wetting agent
Fins on casting	Investment material cracked	Avoid very rapid heating of investment

Table 54.3. Causes of porosity in castings

Problem	Cause	Method of prevention
Irregular voids	Shrinkage as alloy cools	Sprues of correct thickness should be used and they should be placed at the bulkiest section of the wax pattern
Irregular voids	Inclusion of particles of investment material	Heat mold upside down to permit particles to fall out of the mold
Spherical voids	Occluded gases in the molten alloy	Do not overheat the alloy
Rounded margins and regular large voids	Back pressure effect	Use adequate casting force; use investment of adequate permeability; avoid leaving reside of wax in mold; place pattern no more than 6-8 mm from end of casting ring
Porosity	Turbulent flow of molten metal	Place sprues correctly

Table 54.4. Causes of contamination of castings

Problem	Cause
Oxidation	Overheating of alloy; use of oxidizing zone of flame; failure to use flux
Sulfur contamination	Breakdown of investment owing to overheating

Table 54.5. Causes of incomplete castings

Insufficient alloy
Alloy insufficiently heated, so that premature solidification occurs
The mold is not hot enough, causing premature solidification
Blocked sprues, for example, by particles of investment material
Not enough centrifugal force in casting
Back pressure from gases unable to escape from the mold.

54.2 SOLDERING AND WELDING

54.2.1 Definitions

Soldering is the joining of metals by the fusion of an intermediary alloy which has a lower melting point. *Brazing*, a term used industrially, is a soldering operation at temperatures above about 500°C. In dentistry such a distinction is not usually made. *Welding* is a process in which the parts themselves are joined together, by the application of heat and/or pressure.

54.2.2 Soldering

There are a number of important requirements for dental solders. The fusion temperature must be at least 50°C to 100°C lower than the melting temperature of the alloys to be joined. The solder should ideally be as strong as the alloys being soldered. The molten material should flow freely and wet the components well. Good tarnish and corrosion resistance are essential. The color of the solder should be similar to that of the metals being joined.

Gold solders contain gold, silver and copper, with lesser quantities of zinc and tin. Gold contributes to the corrosion resistance. Zinc and tin help to lower the melting range by the formation of eutectic alloys. Their fusion range limits are typically 750°C to 900°C. They are suitable for most dental gold alloys.

Silver solders are essentially silver-copper alloys; zinc and cadmium may also be present to lower the fusion temperature. Fusion range limits are usually 600°C to 750°C. They are used for base metal alloys, and particularly useful for stainless steel; their lower fusion temperature reduces the likelihood of weld decay in the steel.

Fluxes are used in conjunction with soldering. A flux can protect the alloy surfaces from oxidation during soldering and dissolve metallic oxides as they are formed. Fluxes may be either borax or fluorides such as potassium fluoride. The latter flux is used particularly for the chromium-containing alloys, as it can dissolve the passivating oxide film. However, it should be noted that some fluoride-containing fluxes produce toxic fluorides when heated; the inhalation of such fumes should be avoided.

In soldering it is essential that the metallic parts to be joined are thoroughly clean. A solder of the correct fusion temperature should be selected. The reducing zone of the flame is used. The flame should be removed from the solder as soon as it flows. Immediately after soldering the work is quenched in water.

Investment soldering is used when very accurate alignment of the parts to be joined is required. The principles outlined in the previous section also apply here. The alignment is achieved by securing the parts together with sticky wax. After embedding in a refractory investment material, the wax is removed using boiling water and detergent, before soldering is carried out.

Soldering failures can usually be attributed to failure to clean the parts, improper fluxing, poor flow of solder if not sufficiently heated, or to overheating of solder - a pitted joint of low strength may result.

54.2.3 Welding

One example of welding (gold foil) is referred to in an earlier chapter (Section 13.5.1). Most other metals require higher temperatures to give successful welded joints. The most common method of achieving such hot-welding in dentistry is by the application of *resistance welding* or *spot welding*. In this procedure the pieces to be joined are pressed firmly together between two electrodes, usually made of copper. Grooved electrodes are available to give good contact with orthodontic wires. An electric current is passed through the electrodes and the pieces of metal. If the parts to be joined are relatively poor conductors of electricity they will heat up more than the electrodes when the current is passed. If sufficient heat is generated in the portion of metal in contact with the electrodes, and if enough pressure is applied, a welded joint is formed. Either the magnitude of the current, or the time for which it is passed, may be varied to give the desired optimum conditions. A current of 250 to 750 amperes is usually used, for a time of between 1/25th and 1/50th of a second. Too low a current, or too short a time, results in a weak joint; conversely, too much heating may thin the metal unduly.

This technique is not used for gold alloys that are good conductors of electricity. Also, it cannot be used for butt joints. Spot-welding is very successful for the formation of overlapping joints of stainless steel or other chromium-containing alloys.

54.3 ABRASION AND POLISHING

54.3.1 Introduction

It is important that all dental restorations and appliances should have a smooth surface. Food debris will be deposited on rough surfaces, from which it will be difficult to remove. Apart from poor oral hygiene, deposits can be a factor in causing corrosion of metallic materials. Also, patients do not normally tolerate rough surfaces in the mouth.

A rough surface is made smooth by a process known as *abrasion* in which hard sharp particles of abrasive are moved over the surface. Each particle of abrasive acts as a fine tool, cutting a groove in the surface of the article under treatment. The surface is thereby smoothed, but a series of scratches will be left, the dimensions of which will be dependent on the particle size of the abrasive. In any finishing process it is usual for a series of abrasives of increasing fineness to be used. The article should be washed thoroughly when changing from one abrasive to another. The work is moved continuously so that the scratches are produced in all directions.

The abrasive particles must be harder than the surface being abraded. These particles may be bonded together, as in a grinding wheel, disc or strip, or they may be carried across the surface by a brush or buff.

Unlike abrasion, polishing does not cut grooves in a material, but rather reduces irregularities. With some materials, particularly thermoplastic polymers, the surface flows to fill in any scratches, as it becomes heated.

54.3.2 Abrasion

A number of factors influencing the efficiency of abrasives. These include:

- The hardness of the abrasive particles; for example, diamond is the hardest material, whereas pumice, garnet, etc., are relatively mild abrasives;
- The shape of the abrasive particles; those with sharp edges will obviously be more efficient than those with obtuse angles;
- The particle size of the abrasive; larger particles will be able to cut deeper grooves;
- The mechanical properties of the abrasive; if the material breaks it should form a new cutting edge, thus brittleness can be an advantage;
- The rate of movement of the abrasive particles; slower abrasion produces deeper scratches;
- The pressure applied to the abrasive; too great a pressure may fracture an abrasive cutting instrument and increase the heat of friction that is evolved;
- The properties of the material that is being abraded - a brittle material can be abraded rapidly, whereas a malleable and ductile material (for example, pure gold) will flow instead of being removed by the abrasive.

The amount of heat generated during abrasion depends on the factors enumerated in the previous section. Cooling is often required, for example, in the cutting of tooth structure at high speeds, a water spray is required, and in abrading polymers, excessive heat should be avoided as it can cause stress relief and warpage.

There are a number of important abrasives that find application in dentistry:

- Diamond is the hardest known abrasive; its particles can be embedded in a ceramic or metallic binder, as in dental burs;
- Tungsten carbide is used mainly for the construction of burs and abrasive wheels;
- Silicon carbide may be supplied as a powder, or bonded with rubber to form the stones and wheels used in the dental laboratory;
- Alumina is used similarly to silicon carbide;
- Emery is a mixture of alumina and iron which is supplied as an abrasive coating on cloth or paper;
- Sand (silica) - this is used in sandpaper, in abrasive paper discs and in sandblasting procedures, particularly for cobalt-chromium alloys;
- Garnet is a milder abrasive, containing magnesium aluminum silicate, and used as a coating for paper discs;
- Cuttle-fish bone has similar used to garnet;
- Pumice is prepared by crushing pumice-stone, a porous volcanic rock; it is used as a suspension in water, particularly in the finishing of acrylic resins;
- Tripoli is a ground porous rock, which is mixed with a wax to form a 'brick' of material.

54.3.3 Polishing

The following are some of the main polishing agents used in dentistry:

- Whiting (or precipitated chalk) is used as a suspension in water for polishing plastics, such as acrylic;
- Zinc oxide in alcohol can be used for polishing amalgam restorations;
- Iron(III) oxide (rouge) is supplied in a soap base for polishing gold alloys; it is contra-indicated for polishing all chromium-containing alloys, as it can contaminate the surface and lead to corrosion;
- Chromium oxide is also used in a soap base, and is supplied for polishing stainless steel and cobalt-chromium alloys.

Electrolytic polishing is the reverse procedure to electroplating. The alloy to be polished is made the anode of an electrolytic cell. As the current is passed, some of the anode is dissolved leaving a bright surface. This is an excellent method for polishing the fitting surface of a cobalt-chromium alloy denture; so little material is removed that the fit of the denture is virtually unaltered.

54.3.4 Burnishing

Burnishing is a technique used to adapt the margins of a gold inlay. The instrument for this procedure can be made either of stainless steel or a chromium plated alloy. The instrument should not contain copper, which can become incorporated into the surface of the gold.

The ability of an alloy to be burnished may depend on high percentage elongation, low proportional limit and proof stress and a slow rate of work hardening.

APPENDICES

Appendix I

Units and Conversion Factors

In this book the SI system (Système International d'Unités) is used. Six basic units are listed in Table I.1.

Table I.1. Basic SI units

Physical quantity	Name of SI unit	Unit symbol
Length	metre	m
Mass	kilogram	kg
Time	second	s
Electric current	ampere	A
Temperature	kelvin	K
Luminous intensity	candela	Cd

Some derived units are given in Table I.2.

Table I.2. Derived SI units

Physical quantity	Name of SI unit	Unit symbol
Area	square metre	m^2
Volume	cubic metre	m^3
Force	newton	$N=kg.m/s^2$
Pressure, stress	newton per square metre	$N/m^2 = Pa$
Work, energy, quantity of heat	joule	J = Nm
Power	watt	W = J/s
Thermal conductivity	watt per metre degree Kelvin	W/mK

Prefixes can be used to form decimal multiples and sub-multiples of SI units, as listed in Table I.3

Table I.3. Prefixes for SI units

Factor by which the unit is multiplied	Prefix	Symbol
10^{12}	tera	T
10^{9}	giga	G
10^{6}	mega	M
10^{3}	kilo	k
10^{-3}	milli	m
10^{-6}	micro	μ
10^{-9}	nano	n
10^{-12}	pico	p
10^{-15}	femto	f
10^{-18}	atto	a

Table I.4 gives a useful list of conversion factors

Table I.4. Conversion factors

Unit	SI equivalent
Angstrom (Å)	10^{-10} m
*calorie (cal)	4.186 J
dyne	10^{-5} N
foot (ft)	0.3048 m
gram/cubic centimetre (g/cm^3)	1000 kg/m^3
inch (in)	24.4 mm
*kilogram-force/square centimetre (kgf/cm^2)	98.1 kPa
*kilogram-force (kgf)	9.81 N
*ounce (oz)	0.02835 kg
*ounce, fluid (fl oz)	28.41 cm^3
*pound (lb)	0.454 kg
*poundal (pdl)	0.1383 N
*pound-force (lbf)	4.448 N
*pound-force/square inch (lbf/in^2, psi)	6.895 kPa
square inch (in^2)	645.16 mm^2

*approximate values

Appendix II

Some Current Resin Composite Materials

Resin composite materials have been classified in Table 27.1. The purpose of this Appendix is to list the names of some representative materials that are currently available, and not to imply endorsement of any particular product.

Table II.1. Selected resin composite materials

Type	Material	Company
Microfilled	*Durafill*	Heraeus Kulzer
	Epic	Parkell
	Heliomolar	Ivoclar
	Perfection	Den-Mat
	Silux Plus	3M
Hybrid filled	*Aelitefil*	Bisco Dental
	Amelogen	Ultradent
	Ariston pHc	Vivadent
	Bisfil-P	Bisco Dental
	Brilliant New Formula	Coltene
	Concise	3M
	Glacier	Southern Dental
	HRV Herculite	Kerr
	Marathon	Den-Mat
	P50	3M
	Pertac II	Espe
	Pertac Hybrid	Espe
	Prisma APH	Dentsply/Caulk
	Prisma Spectrum	Dentsply/Caulk
	Prodigy	Kerr
	Tetric	Ivoclar
Continuum filled	*Restorative Z100*	3M
Flowable	*Aeliteflo*	Bisco Dental
	Compo-T VLC flowable with fluoride	Motloid
	Curay Match	Scientific Pharma
	Flow-it	Jeneric/Pentron
	Free-Flow	Health-Dent
	Revolution	Kerr

Type	Material	Company
	Wave	Southern Dental
Packable	*Alert* (with fibers)	Jeneric/Pentron
	Solitaire (porous filler particles)	Heraeus Kulzer
	Surefil (irregular filler particles)	Dentsply/Caulk

Appendix III

Dentin Bonding Systems

The objects of this Appendix are to list the major components of some current dentin bonding systems and to give chemical formulae of selected main constituents, where these have not already been presented in the text. Listing a product does not imply endorsement. Rapid changes are occurring in dentin bonding systems, and formulations of products may be changed.

ABC Enhanced (Chameleon)

*Conditioner: Nitric acid or phosphoric acid
*Primer: NTG-GMA (Figure III.1 below), pyromellitic acid glycerol dimethacrylate, acetone
*Bonding agent: Bis-GMA (Figure 11.13), hexanediol dimethacrylate, dimethylaminoethyl methacrylate

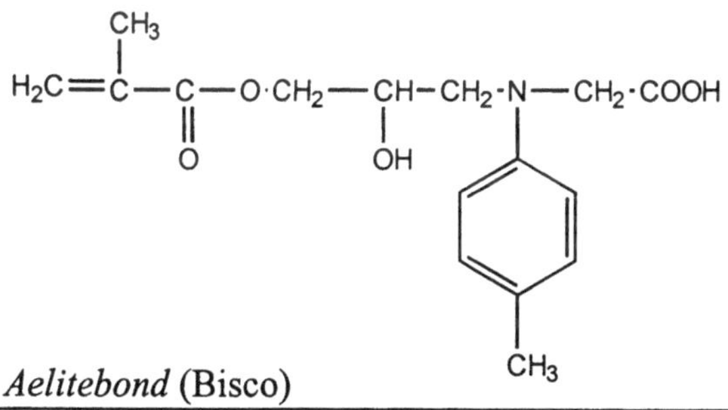

Figure III.1. N-tolylglycine glycidyl methacrylate (NTG-GMA).

Aelitebond (Bisco)

*Conditioner: Phosphoric acid
*Primer: Diarylsulfone dimethacrylate, hydroxyalkyl methacrylate, ethanol
*Bonding agent: Bis-GMA (Figure 11.13), urethane dimethacrylate (Figure 11.14), hydroxyalkyl methacrylate

All Bond 2 (Bisco)

*Conditioner: Phosphoric acid
*Primer: NTG-GMA (Figure III.1), BPDM (Figure 28.2)
*Bonding agent: Bis-GMA (Figure 11.13), HEMA (Figure 11.5), urethane dimethacrylate (Figure 11.14)

Amalgambond Plus (Parkell)

*Conditioner: Citric acid, ferric chloride
*Primer: HEMA (Figure 11.5), water
*Bonding agent: 4-META (Figure 28.3), methyl methacrylate, tri-n-butyl borane

Clearfil Liner Bond (J Morita)

*Conditioner: Citric acid, calcium chloride
*Primer: 5-NMSA (Figure III.2)
*Bonding agent: 10-MDP (Figure III.3)

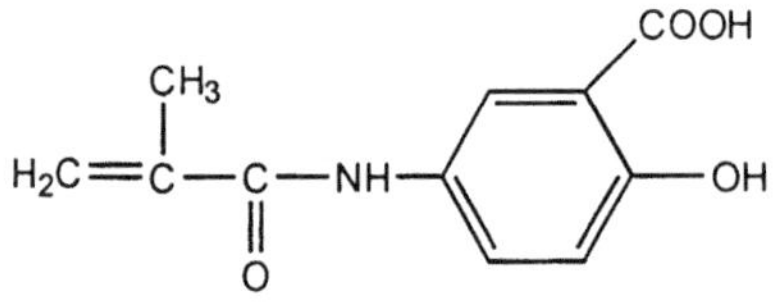

Figure III.2. N-methacryloyl-5-aminosalicylic acid (5-NMSA).

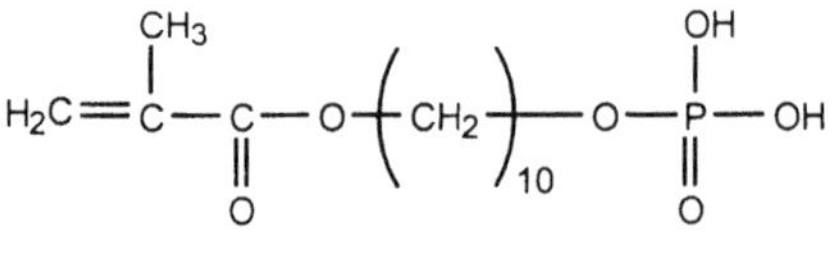

Figure III.3. 10-methacryloyloxy decyl dihydrogenphosphate.

Gluma 2000 (Bayer Dental)

*Conditioner: oxalic acid, aluminum nitrate, glycine
*Bonding agent: N-methacryloyloxyethyl-N-methyl formamide, Bis-GMA (Figure 11.13), acetic acid

One Step (Bisco)

*Conditioner: Phosphoric acid
*Primer: Bis-GMA (Figure 11.13), BPDM (Figure 28.2), HEMA (Figure 11.5), acetone

OptiBond, OptiBond FL (Kerr)

*Conditioner: Phosphoric acid
*Primer: HEMA (Figure 11.5), glycerophosphoric acid dimethacrylate (GPDM), 2-methacryloxy ethyl phthalate (MMEP), ethanol, water
*Bonding agent: Bis-GMA (Figure 11.13), HEMA (Figure 11.5), GPDM, barium aluminoborosilicate glass

Optibond Solo (Kerr)

A one-step bonding agent, claiming fluoride release, intended for bonding composite and amalgam restorations.

Prime and Bond 2.1 (Dentsply)

*Conditioner: Phosphoric acid
*Primer: PENTA (Figure 27.11), dimethacrylates, acetone

Scotchbond Multi-Purpose Plus (3M)

*Conditioner: Phosphoric acid
*Primer: HEMA (Figure 11.5), polyalkenoic acid co-polymer (Figure 26.4), water
*Bonding agent: Bis-GMA (Figure 11.13), HEMA (Figure 11.5)

Single Bond or *Scotchbond 1* (3M)

*Conditioner: Phosphoric acid
*Primer: HEMA (Figure 11.5), polyalkenoic acid co-polymer (Figure 26.4), Bis-GMA (Figure 11.13)

Tenure Quik (Den-Mat)

*Conditioner: Phosphoric acid
*Primer: sodium salt of NTG-GMA (Figure III.1)

Appendix IV

Dental Ceramics

The purpose of this Appendix is to classify some representative ceramic materials that are currently available, and not to imply endorsement of any particular product.

Table IV.1. A selection of current dental ceramics

Type	Material	Manufacturer
Powder-slurry ceramics	Duceram LFC	Degussa
	Optec HSP	Jeneric/Pentron
Castable ceramics	Dicor	Caulk/Dentsply
Machinable ceramics	Celay	Vident
	Cerec Vitablocs	Vident
	Dicor MGC	Caulk/Dentsply
Pressable ceramics	IPS Empress	Ivoclar
	Optec Pressable Ceramic	Jeneric/Pentron
Infiltrated ceramic	In-Ceram	Vident

Appendix V

Environmental Concerns

1. Mercury from dental amalgam. There are environmental concerns in relation to mercury from dental amalgam. Correct disposal of scrap amalgam has been stressed in Table 24.2. There may be a potential problem in relation to mercury vapor discharged from crematoria.

2. Bis-GMA resin. At one time there was reported concern about the estrogenic potential of Bis-GMA (Figure 11.13) which is widely used in pit and fissure sealants, resin composite restorative materials and dentin bonding systems. However, recent research has shown that this is not a problem.

3. Latex gloves. The use of latex gloves constitutes the production of a latex 'mountain' which is only minimally biodegradable. Enviromentally friendly alternatives to latex gloves are being gradually introduced but are not readily available at low cost.

4. Vinyl polysiloxane impression materials have been introduced into crown and bridge work, initially because of their superior dimensional stability, but their use has increased since disinfection of impressions was recommended as essential prior to delivery to the dental laboratory. Vinyl polysiloxanes are not readily biodegradable. The environmentally friendly alternative to impressioning, that is, computer-aided design and manufacture (CAD-CAM) is already available - at a cost- in the dental surgery. Hydrocolloid impression materials offer another environmentally friendly alternative.

5. Disposable plastics. Infection control has resulted in the increasing use of disposable, one-patient items to replace those that are difficult or costly to autoclave. However, this has resulted in increasing amounts of clinical waste from the dental surgery; this is disposed of by incineration. However, the plastics that are used in disposable items and devices may produce toxic fumes when incinerated.

6. Recycling. Dental offices may also generate substantial amounts of paper, as paper towels and wrappings for instruments, as well as office paper. Consideration should be given to its recycling.

7. Chemicals used in the developing of radiographs also present as an environmental issue. It is unacceptable to dispose of these through the sewerage system. The environmentally friendly answer is digital radiography.
8. Similarly, chemicals are used to disinfect work surfaces. Most of these are volatile and therefore do not require disposal; however, these should not be disposed of through the sewerage system.

Index